ACUTE AND CHRONIC WOUNDS

NURSING MANAGEMENT

ACUTE AND CHRONIC WOUNDS

NURSING MANAGEMENT

Edited by

RUTH A. BRYANT, MS, RN, CETN

Former Director
ET Nursing Education Program
Abbott Northwestern Hospital
Minneapolis, Minnesota
Clinical Consultant
Oklahoma City, Oklahoma

*With 86 illustrations
and 32 figures in color*

Coordinated with assistance from the
International Association for Enterostomal Therapy

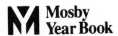

**Mosby
Year Book**

St. Louis Baltimore Boston Chicago London Philadelphia Sydney Toronto

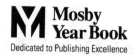

Mosby
Year Book
Dedicated to Publishing Excellence

Editor: Don Ladig, Terry Van Schaik
Developmental Editor: Jeanne Rowland
Project Manager: Mark Spann
Project Editor: Carl Masthay
Book and Cover Design: Gail Morey Hudson

Printed in the United States of America

Mosby–Year Book, Inc.
11830 Westline Industrial Drive, St. Louis, Missouri 63146

Library of Congress Cataloging-in-Publication Data

Acute and chronic wounds: nursing management / edited by Ruth A.
  Bryant; coordinated with assistance from the International
Association for Enterostomal Therapy.
     p.   cm.
   Includes index.
   ISBN 0-8016-0896-1
     1. Surgical wound infections—Nursing.   2. Skin—Ulcers—Nursing.
3. Wound healing.   I. Bryant, Ruth A.   II. International
Association for Enterostomal Therapy.
     [DNLM: 1. Wound Healing.   2. Wounds and Injuries—nursing.]
RD98.3.A38   1992
617. 1'06--dc20
DLC
for Library of Congress   91-37523
                                                                      CIP

92   93   94   95   96   CL/MY   9   8   7   6   5   4   3   2   1

Editorial Board

Contributors

BARBARA J. BRADEN, PhD, RN

Professor, Gerontological Nursing
Creighton University School of Nursing
Omaha, Nebraska

Chapter 5

RUTH A. BRYANT, MS, RN, CETN

Former Director, ET Nursing Education Program
Abbott Northwestern Hospital
Minneapolis, Minnesota

Chapters 1, 5, and 8

DENNIS L. CONFER, MD

Associate Professor of Medicine
Director, Bone Marrow Transplant Program
University of Oklahoma Health Science Center
Oklahoma City, Oklahoma

Chapter 10

DIANE M. COOPER, PhD, RN

Associate Professor, School of Nursing
Adult Health Division
Assistant Professor, Director of Plastic Surgery
Department of Surgery
University of Texas Medical Branch Galveston
University of Texas
Galveston, Texas

Chapters 3 and 4

DOROTHY B. DOUGHTY, MN, RN, CETN

Director, ET Nursing Education Program
Emory University
Atlanta, Georgia

Chapter 2

RITA A. FRANTZ, PhD, RN, FAAN

Associate Professor, College of Nursing
The University of Iowa
Iowa City, Iowa

Chapter 10

G. ALLEN HOLLOWAY, Jr., MD

Director, Vascular Laboratory, Department of Surgery
Maricopa Medical Center
Phoenix, Arizona

Chapter 6

ALISON JUNEN, BSN, RN

Charge Nurse, Hyperbaric Medicine Unit
Humana Hospital
Huntsville, Alabama

Chapter 10

NANCY NUWER KONSTANTINIDES, MS, RN, CNSN, CANP

Metabolic Nurse Specialist
University of Minnesota Hospitals and Clinics
Minneapolis, Minnesota

Chapter 9

ELAINE McCLURE, BSN, MA, RN

Formerly at Jewish Hospital of St. Louis at Washington University Medical Center
St. Louis, Missouri

Chapter 7

SUSAN MITCHELL, MSN, RN

Emergency Department Supervisor
Humana Hospital
Huntsville, Alabama

Chapter 10

DONALD J. MORRIS, MD

Chief, Section of Plastic Surgery
Carney Hospital
Dorchester, Massachusetts

Chapter 5

PAUL M. NEMIROFF, PhD, MD

Clinical Associate Professor of Surgery, Vanderbilt University
Medical Director, Hyperbaric Medicine Unit
Humana Hospital
Huntsville, Alabama
Consultant to Surgeon General USAF (Hyperbaric Medicine)
Member, National Hyperbaric Oxygen Committee

Chapter 10

JULANNE PALMER, ADN, RN

Staff Nurse, Hyperbaric Medicine Unit
Humana Hospital
Huntsville, Alabama

Chapter 10

BARBARA PIEPER, PhD, RN, CETN

Associate Professor, College of Nursing
Wayne State University
Clinical Nurse Specialist, ET Nursing
Detroit Receiving Hospital
Detroit, Michigan

Chapter 5

PAUL ROUSSEAU, MD

Chief, Geriatrics, Veteran's Administration Medical Center
Phoenix, Arizona
Adjunct Professor, Adult Development and Aging
Arizona State University
Tempe, Arizona

Chapter 6

MARY L. SHANNON, EdD, RN

Professor and Chairwoman, Adult Health Department
University of Texas School of Nursing at Galveston
Galveston, Texas

Chapter 5

KATHI THIMSEN-WHITAKER, RN, CETN

Private practice, Formerly Director, ET Nursing Services
Jewish Hospital of St. Louis at Washington University Medical Center
St. Louis, Missouri

Chapter 7

ANNETTE B. WYSOCKI, PhD, RN C

Director, Nursing Research, Research Assistant Professor
New York University Medical Center;
Adjunct Assistant Professor, New York University
New York, New York

Chapter 1

MICKEY YOUNG, BSN, RN, CETN

ET Nurse Practitioner, DePaul Health Center
St. Louis, Missouri

Chapter 7

MARY ZINK, BSN, RN, CETN

Faculty, ET Nursing Education Program
Abbott Northwestern Hospital
Minneapolis, Minnesota

Chapter 6

Preface

A major component of nursing care is the maintenance of skin integrity and the management of wounds, both acute and chronic. Maintenance of skin integrity and management of wounds transcends all nursing specialties, patient populations, and care settings. Whether the problem is perianal irritation on an infant, an open abdominal wound on a new postoperative patient, or a reddened pressure point on a hospice patient, nurses make assessments and plan interventions related to skin integrity and wound management on a daily basis.

Concern and interest in skin integrity and wound management has increased as our population ages and as the frequency of chronic diseases increases. The prevalence of chronic ulcerated skin lesions is estimated to be 120 per 100,000 persons 45 to 64 years of age, 150 per 100,000 persons 65 to 74, but over 800 per 100,000 persons 75 years and older.* These chronic lesions include ulcers caused by pressure, venous hypertension, arterial insufficiency, and diabetic neuropathy. Although these numbers are quite staggering, they fail to capture the venous ulcers that are not reported to the physician, the stage one pressure ulcers that are overlooked, or the acute wounds such as surgical wound dehiscence, intravenous extravasation, or chemical denudation around a percutaneous gastrostomy tube site.

At some point in our basic nursing education, we were taught how to "tend" wounds. We learned how to irrigate wounds and how to pack wounds; we learned how to use sterile techniques and how to redress incisions. We were left with the impression that wound repair was a process that just transpired with very little intervention on the part of health care professionals. We provided technical care with little true understanding of wound repair or the effect of our modest interventions at the cellular wound level. This approach is no longer appropriate.

The physiology of wound healing and implications for wound management have been the focus of considerable research in the past two decades. Research has shown clearly that effective wound management requires correction of etiologic factors, control of infection,

[1]Allman RM: Epidemiology of pressure sores in different populations, Decubitus 2(2):30+, 1989.

enhancement of medical and nutritional state, and topical therapy that provides a microenvironment for healing.

Nurses are now challenged to provide wound management that is based on physiologic principles and research findings. To do so, we as nurses need both the art and science of wound management. We need knowledge regarding maintenance of skin integrity and skills in wound assessment and wound management. Because effective wound management requires a multidisciplinary approach, nurses must also practice collaboratively, consulting with specialists such as dieticians, physical therapists, surgeons, and orthotists.

Written by enterostomal therapy (ET) nurses and other wound care experts, this book provides a comprehensive resource for health care providers challenged with the care of acute surgical wounds and all types of chronic wounds. Each chapter opens with a list of learning objectives and closes with review questions that allow the reader to assess mastery of the material just presented. The structure of the skin, its functions, types of skin damage, physiology of wound healing, and general principles of wound management are presented in Chapters 1 and 2. These chapters provide the framework needed to understand and consequently minimize threats to the skin. Chapter 3 is a review of current wound assessment and evaluation techniques (tools and macroscopic indices). Gaps, inadequacies, opportunities for research, and the need for objective and regular wound observations are identified. The differences in the pathophysiology and management of acute versus chronic wounds with guidelines for optimizing the healing of acute surgical wounds are presented in Chapter 4. Chapters 5 and 6 address the pathophysiology, risk factors, preventive measures, assessment, and management (nursing, medical, and surgical) of pressure and lower extremity ulcers. The management of percutaneous tubes, draining wounds, and fistulas is presented in Chapters 7 and 8. The effects of malnutrition on the wound-healing process and nursing interventions to provide nutritional support are explained in Chapter 9. Evolving methods of wound management such as growth factors, hyperbaric oxygenation, and electrical stimulation are explored in Chapter 10. Appendices include a glossary, pressure ulcer risk assessment scales, and listings of support surfaces and wound dressings. With this background the nurse is better prepared to develop a comprehensive care plan for the patient with a wound or, better yet, to recognize a patient's risk for skin damage and develop a plan of care aimed at prevention.

This book strives to convey a comprehensive and current understanding of the biology, pathophysiology, and management of dermal wounds. In the process, however, numerous unanswered questions become glaringly apparent. What is the relevance of acute wound repair models to chronic wound repair? What are the indicators of a wound that is healing properly? What is the proper terminology for pressure-induced skin damage—pressure ulcer or pressure sore? Is tissue interface pressure the best measure of impending pressure damage? It behooves all health care professionals to develop a sincere respect for the wound and the wound repair process. We have much to learn about the process and the consequences of our actions.

Ruth A. Bryant

Acknowledgments

I would like to offer my sincere appreciation and gratitude to many people who were instrumental in helping me make this book a reality.

My husband, Dennis Confer, who tolerated my obsession for this project, accepted my frantic pace, and assisted me with content, computer literacy, and realism.

The editorial board, for their tireless work and rearranged calendars: Donna Brewer, Dorothy Doughty, Beverly Hampton, Michiko Ooka, Paula Erwin-Toth, and Joan Van Niel.

Dorothy Doughty, for her humor and brilliant ability to prioritize, synthesize, and empathize.

Jeanne Rowland, nursing developmental editor, for her persistence, direction, and patience.

My co-workers at Abbott Northwestern Hospital (Mary Zink, Dee Brown, Deb Thayer, and Andrea Blosberg), for supporting my efforts with their work and words.

The Abbott Northwestern ET Nursing Education Program graduates, for their affirmation that this was indeed a worthwhile and urgent project.

Nancy Borstad, my boss at Abbott Northwestern Hospital, for providing the environment in which I could grow and specialize.

The people at ConvaTec, for their generous financial support of the project.

My parents (Marilyn and Dodd) because in many respects, none of this would have been possible without their love, support, and encouragement.

Ruth A. Bryant

Contents

1   **Skin,** 1

Skin integrity, 2

Annette B. Wysocki

Skin layers, 2
Skin functions, 5
Factors altering skin characteristics, 8

Skin pathology, 10

Ruth A. Bryant

Types of skin damage, 10
Conclusion, 25

2   **Principles of Wound Healing
    and Wound Management,** 31

Dorothy B. Doughty

Physiology of wound healing, 32
Factors affecting wound healing, 42
Principles of wound management, 46
Summary, 61

3   **Wound Assessment and
    Evaluation of Healing,** 69

Diane M. Cooper

Wound evaluation, 70
Macroscopic indices of healing, 80

Documentation guidelines, 84
Recommendations for more accurate
    wound assessment, 84
Summary, 86

4   **Acute Surgical Wounds,** 91

Diane M. Cooper

Definition of the acute surgical wound,
    92
Factors affecting healing of the acute
    surgical wound, 93
The incision, 96
Wound measurement, 98
Summary, 100

5   **Pressure Ulcers,** 105

Ruth A. Bryant
Mary L. Shannon
Barbara Pieper
Barbara J. Braden
Donald J. Morris

Economic impact, 107
Scope of the problem, 107
Summary, 109
Terminology, 109
Etiology, 110
Pathophysiologic changes, 117
Prevention of pressure ulcers, 120

Management of pressure ulcers, 139
Surgical interventions for pressure
   ulcers, 141
Summary, 152

6 Lower Extremity Ulcers, 164

Mary Zink
Paul Rousseau
G. Allen Holloway, Jr.

Arterial ulcers, 165
Peripheral neuropathy, 192
Venous ulcers, 195
Summary, 204

**7 Management of Percutaneous
     Tubes,** 213

Mickey Young
Elaine McClure
Kathi Thimsen-Whitaker

Gastrostomy and jejunostomy tubes,
   215
Empyema (chest) tubes, 230
Percutaneous nephrostomy tubes, 234
Percutaneous biliary catheters, 240
Summary, 243

**8 Management of Drain Sites and
     Fistulas,** 248

Ruth A. Bryant

Incidence and etiology, 249
Terminology, 250
Manifestations, 251
Medical management, 252
Nursing management, 259
Summary, 281

**9 Principles of Nutritional
     Support,** 288

Nancy Nuwer Konstantinides

Definition and incidence of
   malnutrition, 289

Effects of malnutrition, 289
Causes of malnutrition, 289
Nutritional assessment, 290
Nutritional support, 294
Summary, 296
Case study, 297

**10 Evolving Wound Care
       Modalities,** 301

Molecular regulation, 302

Dennis L. Confer

Electrical stimulation, 308

Rita A. Franz

Hyperbaric oxygen, 311

Paul M. Nemiroff
Alison Junen
Susan Mitchell
Julanne Palmer

Evaluating clinical trials, 314

Dennis L. Confer

Glossary, 322

Appendixes

A Risk assessment scales, 325
   Gosnell scale, 326, 327
   Braden scale for predicting pressure
      sore risk, 328
   Norton scale, 329

B Topical wound care products, 330

C Support surfaces, 333

Chart with Fig. 5-2, 335-336

Color Plates, facing p. 288

1 Skin

ANNETTE B. WYSOCKI
RUTH A. BRYANT

OBJECTIVES

1. Explain the importance of normal skin integrity.
2. Identify the major layers of the skin.
3. Define the following terms: stratum corneum, stratum granulosum, stratum spinosum, stratum germinativum, rete ridges, keratinocytes, melanocytes, basement membrane zone.
4. Identify the five major functions of the skin.
5. Identify three ways in which the skin protects against pathogenic invasion.
6. Explain the relationship between skin pigmentation and protection against ultraviolet radiation.
7. Identify the two mechanisms by which the skin provides thermoregulation.
8. Describe at least two effects each of the following have on the skin: aging, ultraviolet radiation, topical preparations, medications.
9. State seven categories or types of skin damage.
10. Distinguish between the following lesions:
    macule   papule   plaque
    nodule   wheal   pustule
    vesicle   bulla
11. Differentiate between erosion and ulcer.
12. Describe four types of mechanical trauma by the extent of tissue damage associated with each.
13. Discuss at least three interventions to prevent each type of mechanical trauma.
14. For three common causes of chemical damage, describe three preventive interventions.
15. Describe the process of an allergic contact dermatitis.

1

16. Identify factors that predispose a patient to candidiasis.

17. Describe the types of lesions common to candidiasis, folliculitis, impetigo, and bullous impetigo.

18. Distinguish between herpes simplex and herpes zoster according to cause, onset, clinical presentation, and treatment.

19. Describe the process of tissue damage caused by radiation.

Skin integrity

ANNETTE B. WYSOCKI

The skin is the one organ of the body that is constantly exposed to a changing environment. Maintaining its integrity is a complex process and major assaults from surgical incisions, injuries, or burns can lead to life-threatening consequences (without appropriate treatment).

Human skin is divided into two major layers, the epidermis, or outermost layer, and the dermis, or innermost layer (Plate 1). These two layers are separated by a structure called the basement membrane. Underneath the dermis is a layer of loose connective tissue, the hypodermis. Major functions of the skin are protection, thermoregulation, sensation, metabolism, and communication.[15,21,47]

The skin of the average adult covers approximately 3000 square inches, or an area almost equivalent to two square meters. From birth to maturity the skin covering will undergo a sevenfold expansion. It weighs about 6 pounds and receives one third of the body's circulating blood volume. The skin forms a protective barrier from the external environment while maintaining a homeostatic internal environment. Epidermal appendages—nails, hair follicles, sweat or sebaceous glands—which are lined with epidermal cells, are also present in the skin. During the healing of partial-thickness wounds, these epidermal cells migrate to resurface the wound. This organ is capable of self-regeneration and can withstand limited mechanical and chemical assaults. The skin varies in thickness from 0.5 mm in the tympanic membrane to 6 mm in the soles of the feet and the palms of the hand. Variations are attributable to differences in the thickness of the skin layers covering underlying organs, bones, muscle, and cartilage.

SKIN LAYERS

Epidermis

Epidermis, the outermost skin layer, is avascular and is derived from embryonic ectoderm. The epidermal layer is composed of stratified squamous epithelial cells or keratinocytes and is divided into five layers as shown histologically in Plate 1. These layers, beginning from the outermost to the innermost, are stratum corneum, stratum lucidum, stratum granulosum, stratum spinosum, and stratum germinativum or, simply, basal layer.

Stratum Corneum. The stratum corneum, or horny layer, the top layer, is composed of dead keratinized cells. These squames, or corneocytes, are the cells that are abraded by the daily mechanical and chemical trauma of handwashing, scratching, bathing, exercising, and changing of clothes. Stratum corneum is composed of layers of thin, stacked, pancake-appearing, anucleate cells. These cells are almost entirely filled with the protein keratin; hence they are called keratinocytes. These keratinocytes are initially formed in the basal layer and undergo the process of differentiation. The normal stratum corneum is composed of completely differentiated keratinocytes. Keratin, the tough fibrous insoluble protein found in these cells, is resistant to changes in temperature or pH and to chemical digestion by trypsin and pepsin. This same protein is found in hair and nails; in these structures keratin is referred to as "hard" keratin compared to the "soft" keratin of the skin.[15,37]

Stratum Lucidum. The stratum lucidum is the layer directly below the stratum corneum. This layer is found in areas where the epidermis is thicker, such as the palms of the hands or soles of the feet, where it is prominent but is absent from thinner skin, such as the eyelids. This layer can be one to five cells thick and is transparent, and cell boundaries are often hard to identify in histologic sections under the light microscope.[15]

Stratum Granulosum. The stratum granulosum, or granular layer, is beneath the stratum lucidum when present; otherwise it lies beneath the stratum corneum. This layer is one to five cells thick and is so named because of the granules present in the keratinocytes of this layer. The cells of this layer have not yet been compressed into a flattened layer and are diamond shaped. The structures contained in these cells are keratohyalin granules, which become intensely stained with the appropriate acid and basic dyes. The protein contained in these granules helps to organize the keratin filaments in the intracellular space.[21,44]

Stratum Spinosum. The stratum spinosum is the next layer below the stratum granulosum. This layer is often described as the prickly layer because cytoplasmic structures in these cells take on this morphology. Generally the cells of this layer are polyhedral in shape. A prominent feature of the prickle layer are desmosomes, a type of cell-cell junction.[21]

Stratum Germinativum. The stratum germinativum is the innermost epidermal layer. It is often referred to simply as the "basal layer" and can be seen in Plate 1. It is a single layer of mitotically active cells called basal keratinocytes, or basal cells. Once cells leave the basal layer they begin an upward migration, which can take 2 to 3 weeks. After leaving the basal layer the cells begin the process of differentiation. All layers of the epidermis consist of peaks and valleys. This arrangement is more dramatic in the basal layer. In fact, the epidermal protrusions of the basal layer that point downward into the dermis are called rete ridges, or rete pegs. Rete ridges are partly responsible for anchoring the epidermis, thus providing structural integrity. Also distributed in this layer are melanocytes, the cells responsible for skin pigmentation. These are dendritic cells arising from the neural crest that synthesize melanin. In normal skin the number of melanocytes present is nearly the same regardless of skin color. The primary difference between light- and dark-skinned individuals is the size and distribution of the melanosomes, the structures containing the melanin pigment, and the activity of the melanocytes. Carotene or carotenoids are responsible for imparting the yellow hue to the skin of some individuals.[15,32,37]

Basement Membrane Zone

The basement membrane zone (BMZ) is the area that separates the epidermis from the dermis. Texts also often refer to this as the dermoepidermal junction. Closer examination of the BMZ in the past decade has revealed it to be more complex than previously believed.

The BMZ is subdivided into two more or less distinct zones, the lamina lucida and the lamina densa. The lamina lucida is so named because it is an electron-translucent zone compared to the electron-dense zone of the lamina densa. The major proteins found in the BMZ are fibronectin, an adhesive glycoprotein, laminin, also a glycoprotein, type IV collagen, a non–fiber forming collagen, and heparan sulfate proteoglycan, a glycosaminoglycan that probably acts as a type of ground substance.[32]

Dermis

The dermis, or corium, is the thickest skin layer and compared to the cellular epidermal layer is sparsely populated by cells. The major proteins found in this layer are collagen and elastin. Fibroblasts are the cells distributed in this layer that synthesize and secrete these proteins. This layer is a matrix supporting the epidermis and can be divided into two areas, the papillary dermis and the reticular dermis, as seen in Plate 1.

Papillary Dermis. The papillary dermis lies immediately below the basement membrane and forms interdigitating structures with the rete ridges of the epidermis called dermal papillae. The dermal papillae contain capillary loops (shown in Plate 1), which supply the necessary oxygen and nutrients to the overlying epidermis via the BMZ. The collagen fibers contained in the papillary dermis are much smaller in diameter and form smaller wavy cable-like structures compared to the reticular dermis.

Reticular Dermis. The reticular dermis is the area below the papillary dermis and forms the base of the dermis. The collagen fibers in this layer are thicker in diameter and form larger cable-like structures. There is no clear separation of papillary and reticular dermis, rather the collagen fibers change in size gradually from papillary to reticular dermis. A complex of cutaneous blood vessels is also found in this part of the dermis.

Dermal Proteins

Collagen. Collagen is the major structural protein found in the dermis and is secreted by dermal fibroblasts as tropocollagen. After additional extracellular processing mature collagen fibers are formed. Normal human dermis is primarily composed of type I collagen, a fiber-forming collagen. Type I collagen represents about 85% of the collagen present, and type III collagen, also a fiber-forming collagen, represents the remaining 15%.[11] Collagen is the protein that gives the skin its tensile strength. Chemically processed collagen from bovine sources results in leather handbags, valued for their strength and long life. The primary constituents of collagen are proline, glycine, hydroxyproline and hydroxylysine.

Elastin. Elastin, another protein found in the dermis, provides the skin with its elastic recoil. This prevents the skin from being permanently reshaped. Elastin is a fiber-forming protein like collagen and has a high amount of proline and glycine but, unlike collagen, lacks large amounts of hydroxyproline. Elastin fibers form structures similar to a spring or coil that allow this protein to be stretched and, when released, to return to its inherent configuration.[21,32]

Hypodermis

Hypodermis, or superficial fascia, forms a subcutaneous layer below the dermis. This is an adipose layer containing a subdermal plexus of blood vessels giving rise to the cutaneous plexus in the dermis, which, in turn, gives rise to the papillary plexus and loops of the papillary dermis (Fig. 1-1). Hypodermis attaches the dermis to underlying structures.

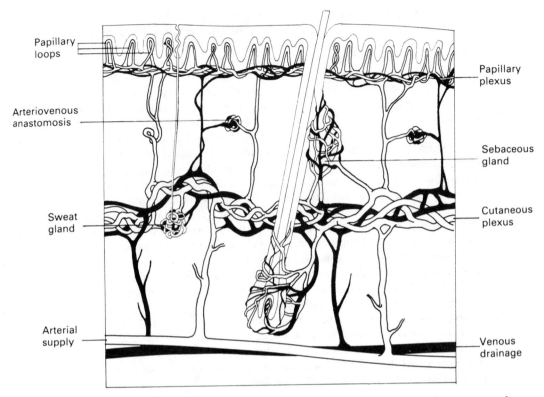

Fig. 1-1   Blood circulation in the skin with papillary loops, which supply oxygen and nutrients to the epidermis, and dermal cutaneous plexuses, which arise from the deeper blood supply located in the hypodermis. (From Wheater PR, Burkett HG, and Daniels VG: Functional histology: a text and colour atlas, ed 2, Edinburgh, 1987, Churchill Livingstone.)

SKIN FUNCTIONS

Protection

The skin provides protection against aqueous, chemical, and mechanical assaults, bacterial and viral pathogens, and ultraviolet radiation (UV). It also prevents excessive loss of fluids and electrolytes to maintain the homeostatic environment. The effectiveness of the skin in preventing excess fluid loss can be seen in burn patients; patients with burns involving 30% of their body can lose up to 4.1 liters of fluid compared to 710 ml for a normal adult.[31] Injury against mechanical assaults is mainly provided by the tough fibroelastic tissue of the dermis, collagen, and elastin. Collagen, the most abundant protein in mammals, represents 25% of total weight[40] and provides tensile strength, which makes the skin resistant to tearing forces. Elastin is distributed with collagen but in smaller amounts. Large concentrations of elastin are present in blood vessels, especially the aortic arch near the heart.

Protection Against Pathogens. Protection against aqueous, chemical, bacterial, and viral pathogens is provided by the stratum corneum, secretions from the sebaceous glands, and the skin immune system. The primary line of defense against all these agents is an intact stratum corneum.[27] As already mentioned, the insoluble protein keratin found in the horny layer provides good resistance. In addition the constant shedding of squames from the stratum corneum prevents the entrenchment of microorganisms.

Sebum, a lipid-rich oily substance secreted by the sebaceous glands onto the skin surface, usually via hair follicles and shafts, provides an acidic coating ranging from pH 4 to 6.8,[38] with a mean pH of 5.5.[27] This acidity and natural antibacterial substances found in sebum retards the growth of microorganisms. These glands are stimulated by sex hormones, androgens, and become very active during adolescence. Sebum, along with keratin, provides resistance to aqueous and chemical solutions. When sebaceous glands occur in association with hair follicles, they are called a pilosebaceous unit. Sebaceous glands are not found on palms or soles and occur in areas that lack hair such as the lips.

Resistance to pathogenic microorganisms is also provided by normal skin flora by bacterial interference.[41] Conceptually, there are two categories of skin flora: resident, the bacteria normally found on a person, and transient, bacteria that are not normally found on a person, and are usually shed by daily hygenic practices such as bathing and hand washing. Resident bacteria are found on exposed skin, moist areas such as the axilla, perineum, and toe webs, and covered skin. So-called bacterial microcolonies are found in hair follicles and at the edges of squames as halos in the upper loose surface layers. The following species of bacteria are found in human skin: *Staphylococcus, Micrococcus, Peptococcus, Corynebacterium, Brevibacterium, Proprionibacterium, Streptococcus, Neisseria,* and *Acinetobacter.* The yeast *Pityrosporum* and the mite *Demodex* are also found. Not all species are found on any one individual, but most carry at least five of these genera. Normal viral flora are not known to exist.[22]

Protection Against Ultraviolet (UV) Radiation. Protection against ultraviolet radiation is provided by skin pigmentation, which results from synthesis of the pigment melanin. Harmful effects are attributable to the long-wave form of UV radiation, or UV-A, which ranges spectrally from 320 to 400 nm;[7] the shorter the waves the more dangerous they become. Because of the increased synthesis, amount, and distribution of melanin in dark skin, these individuals are better protected against skin cancer. Melanin is distributed in all layers of the epidermis in dark skin in contrast to light skin where it is not found in large quantities in all layers.[38]

Skin Immune System. The skin immune system also provides protection against invading microorganisms and antigens. The cells of the skin that provide immune protection are the Langerhans cells, an antigen-presenting cell found in the epidermis, tissue macrophages, which ingest and digest bacteria and other substances, and mast cells, which contain histamine (released in inflammatory reactions). Both macrophages and mast cells are found in the dermis.[2,3,46]

Thermoregulation

Thermoregulation of the body is provided by the skin, which acts as a barrier between the outside and inside environment to maintain body temperature. The two primary thermoregulatory mechanisms are circulation and sweating. Blood vessels can either dilate to dissipate heat or constrict to shunt heat to underlying body organs. When dilated, these vessels have an increased blood flow and release heat by conduction, convection, radiation, and evaporation. Vasoconstriction is often accompanied by actions of the arrector pili muscle attached to hair follicles, which results in the hair standing vertically. In mammals that depend on hair for warmth this action fluffs up the fur to increase thermal capacity. The bulge around the hair shaft that is visible when this occurs is commonly referred to as "goose bumps." In humans shivering is more important for maintaining body temperature when the outside environment is cold than the vertical orientation of hair.[15,32]

Sweating occurs when there is an increase in the activity of the sweat glands. Sweat glands are of two types, eccrine and apocrine. Eccrine glands arise from epidermal invagination and are found abundantly on the palms of the hand and soles of the feet. These glands are largely under control of the nervous system responding to temperature differences and emotional stimulation. Muscular activity also influences their secretory activity. These glands, located in the dermis as a coil, secrete fluid consisting of sodium chloride, urea, sulfates, and phosphates.[37,38] Thermoregulatory control occurs as a result of cooling when fluid is evaporated from the skin surface, since such evaporation requires heat. The odor associated with sweat is largely a result of bacterial action.

Apocrine sweat glands are usually found in association with hair follicles but do not play a significant role in thermoregulation. These coiled tubular glands are present in the axilla and anogenital area; modifications of these glands are found in the ear and secrete ear wax, cerumen.[38]

Sensation

Nerve receptors located in the skin are sensitive to pain, touch, temperature, and pressure. When stimulated, these receptors transmit impulses to the cerebral cortex where it is interpreted. Combinations of these four basic types of sensations result in burning, tickling, and itching.[15] These sensations are propagated by unmyelinated free nerve endings, Merkel cells, Meissner corpuscles, Krause end bulbs, Ruffini terminals, and pacinian corpuscles. Identification of particular responses with specific nerve structures has not been successful. In part the reason is that some receptors seem to respond to a variety of stimuli. However, it is known that Meissner corpuscles are involved in touch reception; pacinian corpuscles (see Plate 1) respond to pressure, coarse touch, vibration and tension; and free nerve endings respond to touch, pain, and temperature.[44]

Metabolism

Synthesis of vitamin D occurs in the skin in the presence of sunlight. Ultraviolet radiation converts a sterol, 7-dehydrocholesterol, to cholecalciferol, vitamin D. This vitamin participates in calcium and phosphate metabolism and is important in the mineralization of bone. Because vitamin D is synthesized in the skin but then transmitted to other parts of the body, it is considered an active hormone when converted to calcitriol, 1,25-dihydroxy-cholecalciferol.[17,40]

Communication

In addition to its biologic, structural, functional, and physiologic functions, human skin also functions as an organ of communication and identification. The skin over our face is especially important for identification of a person and plays a role in internal and external assessments of beauty. Injury to the skin can result in not only functional and physiologic consequences, but also changes in body image. Scarring from trauma, surgery, or incisions can lead to changes in clothing choices, avoidance of public exposure, and a decrease in self-esteem. Research[33] indicates that with increased scarring from facial acne, the self-image is progressively reduced. Adolescents are especially sensitive to physical appearances.[5] As an organ of communication facial skin along with underlying muscles is capable of expressions such as smiling, frowning, and pouting. The sensation of touching can also convey feelings of comfort, concern, friendship, and love.

FACTORS ALTERING SKIN CHARACTERISTICS

Age

Age is an important factor in altering skin characteristics. More recently the scarless healing of fetal tissue has come under more intense investigation.[19,34] It has been found that wounds heal without scarring in fetal lambs up until 120 days of gestation. Collagen deposition in fetal wounds occurs more rapidly and in a normal dermal pattern.[19] In addition, an important difference between fetal and adult skin is the amount of hyaluronic acid, a glycosaminoglycan. In the laboratory setting, topical application of hyaluronic acid has been associated with a reduction in scar formation in postnatal wounds. This glycosaminoglycan is associated with collagen, and it has been proposed that a hyaluronic acid-collagen-protein complex plays a role in fetal scarless healing.[34]

At birth the skin and nails are thinner than those in an adult but will gradually increase in thickness with aging. The next period of change occurs in adolescence when hormonal stimulation results in increased activity of sebaceous glands and hair follicles. Sebaceous glands increase their secretory rate, and hair follicles, giving rise to secondary sexual characteristics, become activated.

From adolescence to adulthood there is a gradual change in skin characteristics. By the time the skin reaches mature adulthood several changes become apparent. The dermis decreases in thickness by about 20%, whereas the epidermis remains relatively unchanged. Epidermal turnover time is increased; this means that wound healing may take longer. For instance, in young adults epidermal turnover takes about 21 days, but by 35 years of age this turnover time is doubled. Barrier function is reduced, and such reduction may increase the risk of irritation. Sensory receptors are diminished in capacity, meaning that the skin is more likely to be burned or traumatized without perception. Vitamin D production is decreased and may be a factor in osteomalacia. There is a decrease in the number of Langerhans cells, which affects the immunocompetence of the skin and can lead to an increased risk of skin cancer and infection by invading microorganisms. The inflammatory response is decreased, and such a decrease may alter allergic reactions and healing. A decrease in the number of sweat glands, diminished vascularity, and a reduction in the subcutaneous fat present compromise the thermoregulatory capacity of the skin. Epidermodermal junction changes, such as the flattening of the prominent dermal papillae and of the rete ridges, alter junctional integrity. Consequently, the skin is more easily torn in response to mechanical trauma, especially shearing forces. Because the hypodermis also becomes thinner, mature individuals are more prone to pressure necrosis.[12] Age-related changes in active melanocytes results in gray hair commonly seen in mature adults.[35] Other overt changes are wrinkling and sagging, which occur as a result of loss of underlying tissue.

Sun

Excess exposure to ultraviolet radiation can have a range of harmful effects that accelerate aging of the skin. For this reason the condition associated with UV-damaged skin is referred to as photoaging. Dermatologically it is called dermatoheliosis. Obvious clinical signs of photodamaged skin are dryness, tough leathery skin, and wrinkling (as a result of collagen and elastin degeneration) and irregular pigmentation (from changes in melanin distribution).[35] Excessive exposure to UV radiation increases the risk of developing skin cancers such as basal or squamous cell carcinoma and malignant melanoma. Damage to the DNA of skin cells leads to transformation of cells and cancer.[7] Changes also occur in epidermal and dermal cells; epidermal cells become thickened, fibroblasts become more numerous, and dermal vessels become dilated and tortuous. Langerhans cells are reduced in number by about 50% thereby diminishing the immunocompetence of the skin.[18]

Immediate short-term exposure to UV radiation can lead to sunburn. This type of red sunburn is the result of a vasodilatory response that increases blood volume. Whether an individual will become sunburned depends on the extent of skin pigmentation. Naturally, those with the least pigmentation are more prone to sunburn and the harmful long-term effects of UV radiation. Severe short-term exposure of unprotected lightly pigmented skin can lead to blistering, a second-degree burn.

Hydration

Adequate skin hydration is normally provided by sebum secretion and an intact stratum corneum with its keratinized cells. Several factors can affect skin hydration; among these are relative humidity, removal of sebum, and age. Each of these factors increases water loss from the skin leading to dryness and scaling. Application of emollients to the skin replaces the barrier function of lost sebum or decreased evaporative water loss when the relative humidity is low. Retention of water in the epidermal layers after application of a lotion leads to swelling of the skin, which is perceived as smoothness and softness. Often various products are promoted with claims of superiority over others without adequate in vitro, in vivo, or clinical data. The superiority of oil baths over water baths was found to be only marginal.[39] Twenty minutes after both kinds of bath, skin hydration was increased when measured by water evaporation and electrical conductance and capacitance. A small but significantly greater amount of water was bound in the skin after the oil bath, whereas no change was seen in evaporation, conductance, or capacitance. Thus, increases in water-holding capacity of the skin after an oil bath may not be of importance. On the other hand, a difference was found in skin-surface lipids, which lasted at least 3 hours. This effect is comparable to application of a traditional moisturizing lotion. The authors of this study concluded that because daily use of bath oil is not practical, application of moisturizing lotions may be more advantageous and that the beneficial effects of bath oils is related to lipidization of the skin surface.[39]

Soaps

Washing or bathing with an alkaline soap reduces the thickness and number of cell layers in the stratum corneum.[45] Generally, soap emulsifies the lipid coating of the skin and removes it along with resident and transient bacteria. Excessive use of soap or detergents can interfere with the water-holding capacity of the skin and may impair bacterial resistance. Use of alkaline soaps increases skin pH, which may change bacterial resistance. The time for recovery to normal skin pH of 5.5 depends on the length of exposure. Ordinary washing requires 45 minutes to restore skin pH, whereas prolonged exposure can require 19 hours.[6] Other agents that can lead to delipidization or dehydration of skin are alcohol and acetone.

Nutrition

Normal healthy skin integrity can be maintained by an adequate dietary intake of protein, carbohydrate, fats, vitamins, and minerals. Under normal conditions increased nutrition is not beneficial. If the skin is damaged, increased dietary intake of some substances such as vitamin C for collagen formation may be beneficial. A healthy diet of protein breaks down to supply the necessary amino acids for protein synthesis. Fats are broken down into essential fatty acids, which can then be used by cells to form their lipid bilayer. Carbohydrates are digested to supply energy for cell metabolism. Vitamins C, D, and A; the B vitamins pyridoxine and riboflavin; the mineral elements iron, zinc, and copper; and many others are needed to maintain a normal healthy skin. Adequate dietary intake can be ensured by ingestion of amounts consistent with the recommended daily allowances (RDA).[26]

Medications

Various medications are known to affect the skin. One of the best studied are the corticosteroids, which are known to interfere with epidermal regeneration and collagen synthesis.[10,23] Photosensitive and phototoxic reactions are also known to occur from medications. Among the categories of medications that can affect the skin are antibacterials, antihypertensives, analgesics, tricyclic antidepressants, antihistamines, antineoplastic agents, antipsychotic drugs, diuretics, hypoglycemic agents, sunscreens, and oral contraceptives.[24] Skin flora can be changed by the use of antibacterials, orally administered steroids, and hormones. Analgesics, antihistamines, and nonsteroidal antiinflammatory agents can alter inflammatory reactions. Thus, whenever drugs are prescribed or skin reactions occur, medications should always be examined to check whether they are responsible.

Skin pathology

RUTH A. BRYANT

TYPES OF SKIN DAMAGE

Normal skin integrity can be jeopardized or compromised by several factors: mechanical, chemical, vascular, infectious, allergic, thermal, and miscellaneous assaults such as radiation and extravasation. Each type of injury creates a unique characteristic skin response such as erythema, macule, papule, vesicle, erosion, or ulcer. Figs. 1-2 and 1-3 define the terminology appropriate for these skin responses. Primary lesions such as pustules and bullae can evolve into secondary lesions like an erosion and, ultimately, an ulcer. The nurse who cares for wounds must be familiar with these terms to describe skin manifestations accurately.

Before a treatment plan for a chronic or acute wound is initiated, it is imperative that the underlying cause for the wound be determined. Clues to the cause can be found by assessment of the following parameters: location, characteristics, distribution, and the patient's subjective comments (Table 1-1). Once the cause of the wound is identified, realistic goals for the wound can be established and a comprehensive, multidisciplinary treatment plan devised. This section is a brief description of the pathophysiologic process of each type of skin damage and appropriate interventions.

MACULE

A circumscribed, flat discoloration, which may be brown, blue, red, or hypopigmented

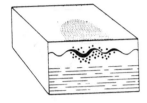

PLAQUE

A circumscribed, elevated, superficial, solid lesion more than 0.5 cm in diameter, often formed by the confluence of papules

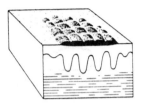

PUSTULE

A circumscribed collection of leukocytes and free fluid that varies in size

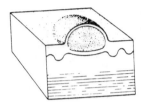

VESICLE

A circumscribed collection of free fluid up to 0.5 cm in diameter

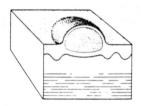

BULLA

A circumscribed collection of free fluid more than 0.5 cm in diameter

NODULE

A circumscribed, elevated, solid lesion more than 0.5 cm in diameter; a large nodule is referred to as a tumor

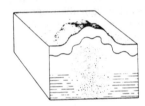

PAPULE

An elevated solid lesion up to 0.5 cm in diameter; color varies; papules may become confluent and form plaques

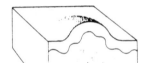

WHEAL

A firm edematous plaque resulting from infiltration of the dermis with fluid; wheals are transient and may last only a few hours

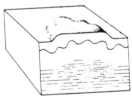
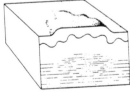

Fig. 1-2 Definition of primary skin lesions. (From Habif TP: Clinical dermatology: a color guide to diagnosis and therapy, ed 2, St. Louis, 1990, Mosby–Year Book, Inc.)

SCALES
Excess dead epidermal cells that are produced by abnormal keratinization and shedding.

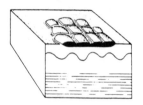

EROSIONS
A focal loss of epidermis; erosions do not penetrate below the dermoepidermal junction and therefore heal without scaring

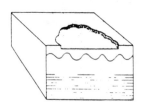

ULCERS
A focal loss of epidermis and dermis; ulcers heal with scarring

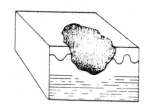

CRUSTS
A collection of dried serum and cellular debris; a scab

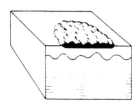

SCAR
An abnormal formation of connective tissue implying dermal damage; after injury or surgery scars are initially thick and pink but with time become white and atrophic

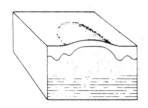

ATROPHY
A depression in the skin resulting from thinning of the epidermis or dermis

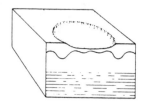

FISSURE
A linear loss of epidermis and dermis with sharply defined, nearly vertical walls

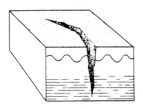

Fig. 1-3   Definition of secondary skin lesions. (from Habif TP: Clinical dermatology: a color guide to diagnosis and therapy, ed 2, St. Louis, 1990, Mosby–Year Book, Inc.)

Table 1-1 Common clues to the causes of wounds

Cause	Location	Characteristics
Pressure	Bony prominences in immobile patient	Deep lesion (stage IV)
Shear	Surfaces exposed to bed or chair surface in patient with reduced mobility or poor tissue turgor	Shallow or deep tissue damage common (stage II, III, IV) May present as hematoma
Friction	Surfaces exposed to bed or chair surface	Superficial (stage I or II)
Chemical (such as incontinence)	Areas exposed to urine, stool, or drainage	Superficial (stage I or II)
Moisture	Intertriginous areas	Superficial (stage I or II)
Venous hypertension	Medial malleolus	Hyperpigmentation or edema of surrounding tissue Crusting
Ischemia	Distal or in areas of trauma	Surrounding tissue cool and pale Diminished or absent pulses Delayed capillary refill Pain
Neuropathy	Areas of sensory loss exposed to trauma or pressure (such as feet and heels)	Common in patients with diabetes May be associated with abnormal gait

Mechanical Damage

Mechanical damage is created by those forces that are applied externally to the skin such as pressure, shear, friction, and epidermal stripping. Each may occur in isolation or in combination with other mechanical injuries.

Pressure. Pressure is the most familiar form of mechanical damage. When externally applied pressure exceeds capillary closing pressure, capillary occlusion occurs. With unrelieved pressure, tissue ischemia develops and metabolic wastes accumulate in the interstitial tissue. Anoxia and cellular death is the result.[1]

Pressure ulcers most commonly occur over a bony prominence such as the trochanter, sacrum, or calcaneus. The tissue damage associated with a pressure ulcer is greatest at the bone-tissue interface; therefore these wounds typically extend into subcutaneous tissue or deeper (that is, muscle, tendon, or bone). Necrotic tissue will be present initially. Braden and Bergstrom[9] describe a conceptual schema for studying the etiology of pressure-induced skin damage. According to this schema, intensity of pressure, duration of pressure, and tissue tolerance determine pressure-ulcer development. A detailed discussion of the pathophysiologic process of pressure-ulcer development, risk factors, and prevention can be found in Chapter 5.

It is widely believed that wounds caused by pressure can be prevented with current technology and resources. The first step in a prevention plan is to identify patients at risk for pressure-ulcer development. A risk assessment tool that is valid and reliable should be used to quantify the patients risk for developing a pressure ulcer. Factors known to increase risk include immobility, advanced age, malnutrition, impaired perception or sensation, moisture (such as incontinence), friction, and shear.

Box 1-1   MECHANICAL SKIN DAMAGE PREVENTION
Intervention (rationale)

PRESSURE

Implement pressure reduction if the patient is able to reposition or the wound is on only one surface. (Redistributes weight over larger surface area.)

Implement pressure relief is the patient unable to reposition or the wound is on more than one surface. (Limited intact body surfaces that can be used to absorb and redistribute weight.)

Establish turning schedule. (Compliance and continuity of care will be enhanced.)

Reposition patient between supine position and 30-degree lateral position. (30-degree lateral position does not exert pressure on any bony prominence.)

Keep pressure of heels by using positioning aids and pillows. (Heel interface pressures often exceed capillary closing pressure regardless of support surface.)

SHEAR

Limit elevating head of bed to no more than 30 degrees and for limited times. (Reduces pull of gravity and sliding of tissues.)

Position feet against a foot board. (Prevents sliding down in bed.)

Use knee gatch when head of bed elevated. (Prevents sliding down in bed.)

Use lift sheet to reposition patient. (Prevents dragging of patient's skin across bed.)

FRICTION

Apply transparent dressing or skin sealant to skin surface. (Provides a barrier to friction.)

Use sheepskin elbow or heel protectors. (Reduces exposure of skin to friction.)

Apply moisturizers to skin. (Adequately maintained epidermis more resistant to stressors.)

Reduce shear. (Friction always occurs in combination with shear.)

EPIDERMAL STRIPPING

Apply tape without tension. (Prevents blistering of skin under tape.)

Use porous tapes. (Allows moisture to evaporate.)

To remove tape, slowly peel tape away from anchored skin. (Decreases trauma to epidermis and dermoepidermal junction.)

Secure dressings with roll gauze, tubular stockinette, or self-adhering tape. (Avoids unnecessary tapes on skin.)

Use skin sealants or solid-wafer skin barriers under adhesives. (Provides protective layer over skin for adhering tapes.)

Secure dressings with Montgomery straps. (Prevents repeated tape applications.)

NOTE: When protective devices are used to protect the skin from mechanical trauma, the product should be removed at regular intervals to allow inspection and assessment of the area.

Several modalities are available to prevent pressure ulcers (see Box 1-1). Prevention involves maintenance of healthy skin, frequent repositioning, and the appropriate utilization of support surfaces.[4] Because of unique patient needs and the constraints on staff, frequent repositioning is difficult to consistently provide, therefore repositioning is often an adjunctive intervention to the use of a support surface and is seldom an isolated intervention. Chapter 5 describes in detail the process of pressure-ulcer prevention.

Shear. Shear force is created by the interaction of both gravity and friction (resistance) against the surface of the skin.[1] Friction is always present when shear force is present. The classic example of shear is when a patient is in a semi-Fowler's position; while the torso slides downward to the foot of the bed, the bed surface generates enough resistance that the

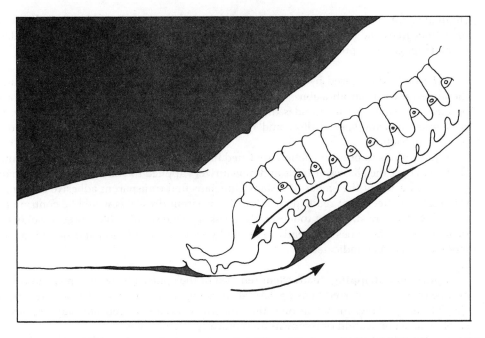

Fig. 1-4 Shearing force. (From Loeper JM, Flinn NA, Irrgang SJ, and Weightman MM: Therapeutic positioning and skin care, Minneapolis, 1986, Sister Kenny Institute.)

skin over the sacrum tends to remain in the same location (Fig. 1-4). Ultimately, the skin is held in place while the skeletal structures pull the body (by gravity) toward the foot of the bed. Consequently blood vessels in the area are stretched and angulated, and such changes may create small vessel thrombosis and tissue death.

Shear may cause shallow or deep ulcers and extends the tissue damage seen with pressure ulcers. This extension is manifested in the pressure ulcer by the presence of undermining (dissection or separation of tissue parallel to the skin surface).

Shear injury is predominately localized at the sacrum or coccyx and is most commonly a consequence of elevating the head of the bed or of improper transfer technique. Prevention requires an awareness of those situations in which the skin is exposed to shear force. For example, the patient with pulmonary distress will require the head of the bed to be elevated to facilitate adequate ventilation; however the patient is at great risk for shear injury. Likewise, the patient with a cerebrovascular accident may experience shear injury when being transferred from the bed to the wheelchair.

Strategies for prevention of shear are listed in Box 1-1. Because shear is an important contributing factor to pressure-ulcer development, strategies to prevent shear and pressure simultaneously are often warranted. It should be noted that although the use of sheepskin (preferably genuine sheepskin) is advocated to reduce shear, no research has been conducted to support this as an intervention.[4] Sheepskin, however, should not be confused with pressure-reduction measures. There are also available many support surfaces that have a slick fabric covering, which is believed to reduce shear. The primary intervention nurses should use is lift sheets to reduce shear when repositioning the patient; this method would eliminate drag on the sacral skin. Elevation of the head of bed should be limited to no more than 30 degrees and be limited to short periods of time. Finally, the knee gatch can be used to interrupt gravity's pull on the body toward the foot of the bed.

Friction. Skin injured by friction results from two surfaces rubbing together and has the appearance of an abrasion. This type of injury is frequently seen on elbows or heels because the patient easily abrades these surfaces against sheets when repositioning. Injury is characteristically very shallow and limited to the epidermis. Tissue necrosis does not occur with friction.

Interventions to prevent friction are listed in Box 1-1. These involve the use of protective sheepskin over the elbows or heels and moisturizers applied to vulnerable areas to maintain proper hydration of the epidermis. Many clinicians find transparent adhesive dressings and skin sealants effective at reducing friction. Transparent dressings would be contraindicated if the friction were sufficient to loosen the dressing. One should check braces, splints, prosthetic devices, and shoes frequently to assess for evidence of friction and should implement modifications when indicated.

Epidermal Stripping. Inadvertent removal of the epidermis by such mechanical means as tape removal is referred to as epidermal stripping. Typically, these lesions are irregularly shaped and shallow, involving only the epidermis. Frequent, repeated tape removal and careless tape application or removal can remove epidermal cells.

Epidermal stripping can be prevented by (1) recognition of fragile, vulnerable skin, (2) appropriate application and removal of tape, (3) use of solid-wafer skin barriers or skin sealants under adhesives, (4) use of porous tapes, and (5) avoidance of unnecessary tapes (see Box 1-1).[6]

Both immature and aging skin are particularly vulnerable to epidermal stripping. The premature infant's skin is vulnerable because the dermoepidermis junction is undeveloped and weak.[16] Because of reduced collagen and elastin present in the aging skin, removal of epidermal cells with tape removal can be a problem.[13] Likewise, patients receiving corticosteroid therapy will also experience reduced tissue collagen strength thereby increasing the risk for epidermal stripping. In general, it is best to avoid applying adhesives in an area receiving irradiation.

Appropriate tape application and removal techniques can also help prevent skin stripping. Proper tape application implies that the tape is applied without tension or "pinching" of the epidermis. Often tape is applied appropriately after a surgical procedure, but as edema develops at the surgical site over the ensuing 24 hours, the tape begins to pull on the underlying skin. Blisters then develop under the tape. To alleviate the tension that develops as the skin becomes normally edematous after surgical manipulation, it may be advisable to remove and reapply dressings 24 hours postoperatively.

Proper tape removal entails slowly peeling the tape away from the skin while stabilizing the skin. Solvents can be used to break the adhesive skin bond, though solvents have a drying effect on the skin. Plain tap water can often serve this purpose quite effectively.

Solid-wafer skin barriers can also be applied around a wound; wound dressings are then secured by anchoring of the tape to the solid-wafer skin barrier. One can easily apply the tape and reapply it to the barrier wafer without traumatizing the epidermis. Wafers can remain in place for several days.

Finally, skin sealants may be applied to the skin before the tape is applied to provide protection from epidermal stripping. Skin sealants should not be applied to denuded tissue, however, because the alcohol content can cause temporary discomfort. It is important to allow the skin sealant to dry completely before applying tape. Many central-line dressing kits, for example, are prepackaged with a skin sealant.

Unnecessary use of adhesives and tapes should be avoided, particularly on vulnerable, fragile skin. Nurses can become quite creative when securing dressings without applying tape to the skin. For example, tubular stockinette, roll gauze, or self-adhering tape can be used.

Chemical Factors

The presence of chemicals on the skin is a common source of skin damage and can result from fecal incontinence, harsh solutions such as povidone-iodine complex (Betadine), improper use of products (such as, skin sealants), and drainage around percutaneous tubes or drains. The presence of these solutions or secretions on the skin will destroy or erode the epidermis. Early manifestations start with erythema or an erythematous macular rash and can quickly progress to denudement if exposure continues. (See Plate 2.)

Chemical irritation or dermatitis is also referred to as an irritant contact dermatitis. Skin damage may be evident in only a few hours in the presence of a strong irritant (such as small bowel discharge). On the other hand, repeat exposures over several days may be necessary when the irritant is weak. Chemical dermatitis can be distinguished from an allergic reaction by its irregular borders and always requires the presence of drainage or chemicals. Subjectively chemical dermatitis is very uncomfortable for the patient because of the shallow (epidermal and dermal) nature of the lesions.

Chemical irritation can be prevented by (1) identification of patients at risk for chemical irritation, (2) prevention of drainage around catheters or drains from contacting the skin, (3) avoidance of the presence of harsh substances on the skin, and (4) appropriate use of skin-care products (soaps, barriers, adhesives, or solvents).

Moisture-barrier ointments, gentle skin cleansing, and creative uses of skin barriers are the cornerstone to the prevention of chemical irritation when patients are identified at risk.[42] For example, it should be anticipated that the patient with a low serum albumin level who is receiving antibiotics is at risk for developing diarrhea once enteral feedings are initiated. The nurse should initiate a care plan of gentle skin cleansing (no harsh soaps or rough cloths)[4] and ointments to prevent chemical irritation.[13] The infant with increased stooling frequency requires more frequent diaper changes, gentle cleansing, and appropriate use of ointments. Likewise, the adult may experience diarrhea for a wide variety of reasons (such as gastrointestinal bleeding or antibiotic therapy). Diligent and appropriate use of moisture-barrier ointments can help prevent denudation or ulceration.

When moisture-barrier ointments are overwhelmed by the frequency or volume of diarrhea, moisture-barrier pastes and rectal pouches may be indicated temporarily to protect the skin from diarrhea.[42] Rectal pouches are adhesive ostomy pouches specifically designed to fit the perianal contours and contain the incontinent stool. These products can be extremely cost effective by providing skin protection from chemicals and moisture buildup, reducing linen changes, freeing up nursing time for other types of care and activities, and preserving the patient's dignity. Step-by-step instructions to apply a rectal pouch are listed in Box 1-2.

Drainage around catheters and tubes should be managed in such a way that the drainage is either eliminated when possible or the skin is not directly exposed to the

---

Box 1-2   RECTAL POUCHING PROCEDURE

1. Assemble equipment: pouch, paste, clip, cloth, bag for waste, razor.
2. Prepare pouch:
    a. Remove paper backing from skin barrier and tape.
    b. Apply a thick bead of paste around the center opening; set aside.
3. Remove and apply pouch:
    a. Loosen tape and gently push skin away from adhesive.
    b. Discard pouch and save clip (if one is used).
    c. Remove any paste residue, using a dry tissue.
    d. Wash skin with soft cloth and warm water; be sure to remove any greasy residue, using a gentle soap and water. Rinse and dry thoroughly.
    e. Shave perianal hair, if present.
    f. To create a smooth adhesive surface, apply a bead of paste in the gluteal fold and between the anal opening and the scrotum or vagina.
    g. Before applying pouch, fold skin barrier surface of pouch vertically (lengthwise).
    h. Align pouch between scrotum or vagina and anal opening, and apply to skin.
    i. Slowly unfold pouch and adhesive to apply to skin in smooth fashion.
    j. Encourage seal by massaging the adhesive for 1 minute.
    k. Attach clip to open end of pouch or attach spout to straight drainage.
    l. Change pouch only if it leaks.
    m. Reposition patient carefully to avoid undue stress on pouch seal.

NOTE: Skin-barrier powders must be used to dry moist denudation, when present, before the pouch is applied.

---

drainage. For example, when leakage occurs around a gastrostomy tube, the first step is to ascertain proper placement and stabilization of the tube. If drainage persists once this is accomplished, appropriate use of skin barriers (particularly moisture-barrier ointments or solid-wafer skin barriers) are indicated. A solid-wafer skin barrier can be trimmed to fit around a tube site, remain in place for several days, and be changed only as it loosens at the tube site. Ointments should be reapplied periodically throughout the day to assure adequate skin protection. Gauze dressings are then applied over the skin barrier to absorb drainage and are changed when moist.

Solutions such as acetic acid and Betadine are at times used in wounds, though controversial. The constant prolonged presence of such substances against the skin can also jeopardize skin integrity and create chemical damage.

Damage can be prevented by (1) monitoring of appropriate dressing technique so that gauze dressings contact only the wound bed and are not contacting surrounding intact skin and (2) bracketing of the wound with skin barriers (ointments, solid wafers, or skin sealants).

Improper use of skin-care products such as skin cleansers, solvents, adhesives, and skin sealants can contribute to chemical irritation. Skin cleansers and solvents must be thoroughly rinsed from the skin to prevent buildup of harmful substances. Skin cleansers or soaps should be used sparingly to avoid disruption of the normal acid pH of the skin.[6,45] Adhesives, such as cements, and skin sealants must be allowed to dry adequately so that solvents evaporate before other products are applied.

Vascular Damage

Ulcerations, particularly on the legs or feet, also occur as a result of venous hypertension, arterial insufficiency, or neuropathy, or a combination of these factors. Although these types of lesions commonly develop incidentally to benign trauma (that is, by bumping against the leg of a chair), each ulcer has very distinct distinguishing features, pathologic processes, and treatment regimen.

Arterial. Arterial insufficiency, whether acute or subacute, can precipitate ulcerations of the skin when exposed to harmless trauma. Clinical arterial diseases that are characterized by peripheral ischemia and reduced skin blood flow include arteriosclerosis obliterans, thromboangitis obliterans, diabetes mellitus, Raynaud's disease, and sickle cell disease.[14,30] Arterial ulcers are frequently located on the feet, toes, and lower leg and are extremely painful. This pain is exacerbated when the patient is in a recumbent position with the leg resting on the bed but quickly resolves when the leg is allowed to dangle over the edge of the bed; arterial perfusion is thus enhanced by gravity.

Arterial ulcers are typically deep ulcers with a pale wound bed and distinct wound margins. Ischemic changes in the leg are also visible and include thin, hairless leg, thickened toenails, and dry epidermis.

When arterial perfusion is jeopardized, care should be taken to prevent the development of arterial ulcerations. Prevention focuses on avoidance of compression, avoidance of constricting garments (such as elastic ribbing on stocking), avoidance of mechanical, chemical, or thermal trauma and adequate remoisturizing of the epidermis. A complete review of causative factors, prevention, ulcer characteristics, diagnostic studies, and management is presented in Chapter 6.

Venous. Venous hypertension, which develops as a result of incompetent perforator veins, also contributes to ulcerations on the lower legs. Postphlebitic disease, chronic primary varicose veins, and extraluminal compression of veins are processes that are recognized to create venous hypertension.[36,43]

Adequate perfusion of local tissue becomes increasingly difficult in the presence of venous hypertension. Resulting pathologic changes include dilatation of blood vessels and increased intercellular capillary pore size, which permits the release of fibrinogen and other elements into pericapillary tissues. As fibrinogen is converted to fibrin, a layer of fibrin develops around the capillary and acts as a barrier to oxygen diffusion to surrounding tissue; these tissues now become vulnerable to incidental trauma.[14]

Venous ulcers are characterized as being (1) located in the gaiter area (midcalf to heel), (2) shallow, (3) irregularly shaped, and (4) painless to moderately painful. The lower leg is commonly edematous, and the surrounding skin may have a dry scaly dermatitis, a woody texture, and a reddish-brown discoloration. These pigmentation changes are attributed to the deposition of hemosiderin in the tissue. Management of venous hypertension to prevent ulceration requires reduction of edema by compression therapy, periodic elevation of the leg, and avoidance of mechanical trauma. A detailed discussion of the pathophysiologic process of venous ulcers, prevention, and management is presented in Chapter 6.

Diabetic. When ulcers occur on the foot of the patient with diabetes, it is commonly termed a diabetic ulcer. Such ulcers are extremely complex in cause, and this label does not indicate the factors precipitating the ulcer. A triad of contributing factors includes artial insufficiency, trauma, and peripheral neuropathy.[30] Arterial insufficiency may be precipitated by the increased prevalence of microvascular and macrovascular occlusions associated with diabetes mellitus. Ulcerations can also develop as a consequence of painless trauma in the presence of peripheral neuropathy. Repetitive stress or mechanical trauma can be caused by the pressure of an undetected pebble in the patient's shoe or friction of the shoe tongue against the dorsum of the foot. Neuropathy can also place the patient at increased risk for incurring thermal injury by such innocent actions as walking across a hot, sandy beach or soaking the foot in hot water. Diabetic ulcers may or may not be painful, tend to be polymicrobial, and are commonly associated with osteomyelitis.

Key preventive strategies strive to reduce the risk of injury in the neuropathic foot. For example, foot soaks are not recommended, well-fitting shoes should always be worn to protect the feet from trauma or thermal injury, and the skin should be kept well moisturized. Chapter 6 provides a comprehensive discussion of diabetic ulcers.

Infectious Factors

Many skin rashes or ulcers are indicative of an infectious process and can occur around wounds or be misinterpreted as a result of pressure, shear, friction, or chemical irritation. Candidiasis, herpes zoster, herpes simplex, and impetigo are infectious processes that should be familiar to the nurse.

Candidiasis. Cutaneous candidiasis represents an epidermal infection with *Candida* species, most commonly *Candida albicans* (Plate 24). Candidiasis is manifested by erythema, maceration, and pustules, which are abraded into papules. Solid placques of moist red areas may more accurately describe candidiasis when located in skin folds. Satellite pustular lesions (outside the advancing edge of candidiasis) are an important diagnostic feature of candidiasis.[20] Intact pustules are not always visible because they may be unroofed by apposing skin and clothing.[13]

Predisposing factors include the presence of a moist environment and antibiotic therapy. Damp surgical dressings, the perineum, the perineal area, and intertriginous areas (breast and inguinal skin folds) are typical moist areas. Antibiotics predispose the patient to develop candidiasis by altering the normal skin flora. Immunosuppressed patients and patients with diabetes, psoriasis, or atopic dermatitis are more vulnerable to candidiasis.[27]

Candidiasis is most often determined clinically by the signs, symptoms, and predisposing factors. Patients may also complain of pruritus or burning at the site. If a laboratory test is conducted, a potassium hydroxide preparation (KOH) of scrapings is the most relevant test. Scrapings from an intact pustule and the contents are needed to yield the best results. Because the skin can be colonized with *Candida albicans* but not infected, swab cultures for *Candida* are not informative; such cultures cannot distinguish between infection and colonization.[13]

Folliculitis and contact dermatitis can be confused with candidiasis and can be distinguished by the presence or absence of papules, pustules, or erythema. Folliculitis, the asymptomatic inflammation of a hair follicle, is characterized by isolated pustules with a hair central to each pustule; erythema and papules are atypical of folliculitis. Manifestations of contact dermatitis include erythema with papules; pustules would be observed only with candidiasis. Distribution can also help distinguish between contact dermatitis and candidiasis because a contact dermatitis will be limited to the area in contact with the irritant.

Candidiasis can be treated with a topical antifungal agent available as a cream, powder,

---

Box 1-3   STRATEGIES TO PREVENT MOISTURE BUILDUP

Dust intertriginous skin folds with absorbent powders such as cornstarch.

Separate intertriginous skin folds with skin sealants (spray or wipes) and soft gauze.

Use skin sealants or solid-wafer barriers underneath dressings and around wounds.

Change dressings before they become saturated.

Use a support surface (if needed) with air-vent capabilities.

---

or ointment. Antifungal powders are indicated when candidiasis develops in an adhesive field such as the peristomal skin. When creams are used, they should be applied sparingly to reduce moisture entrapment. Because ointments can further trap moisture and therefore exacerbate the candidiasis, they may not be preferred.

Prevention of moisture buildup is the single most important intervention to prevent candidiasis. Box 1-3 lists strategies to prevent moisture buildup.

Impetigo. Impetigo is most commonly seen in children and is caused by gram-positive bacteria (usually *Staphylococcus aureus*). The initial onset is a pustule with little or no surrounding erythema. Lesions quickly form a yellow-tan crust when disrupted. Beneath the crust is a superficial glistening base; ulcerations are not present because the infection is quite superficial and barely extends below the stratum corneum.[13] Impetigo can occur anywhere but is most common on the face.

It is most important to distinguish impetigo from a streptococcal infection and from herpes simplex. Streptococcal infections can be determined by culture and appearance. Clinically, streptococcal skin infections are deeper, extending through the epidermis so that an ulcer is seen when the crust is removed. Furthermore, streptococcal skin infections are commonly surrounded by erythema. Herpes simplex can be distinguished not only from impetigo by culture, but also by early manifestations; herpes simplex begins with grouped, clear vesicles that are uniform in size, and it recurs at the same site.[13,20]

Treatment involves topical or systemic antibiotics. Small limited lesions may be effectively managed with topical antibiotics with 7 to 10 days of either orally administered erythromycin or penicillin-resistant penicillins (such as dicloxacillin) are appropriate for systemic treatment.

Bullous Impetigo. Bullous impetigo is a *Staphylococcus aureus* infection of the epidermis with large, fragile clear or cloudy bullae (Plate 3). When these bullae rupture, a thin crust develops and a rim of the bulla roof often remains encircling the crust. Satellite lesions may develop by autoinoculation.[13] Common locations include the face, neck, and extremities and may be typified by pruritus. Predisposing factors include poor hygiene and inadequate attention to skin injury.

As with impetigo, dicloxacillin and erythromycin are preferred antibiotics for treatment of bullous impetigo. Spontaneous healing will occur without antibiotics over 3 to 6 weeks.

Herpes Simplex. Herpes simplex virus (HSV) infections of the epidermis is highly contagious and can be spread by direct contact. HSV is typically classified as either HSV-1 (oral herpes) or HSV-2 (genital herpes). However, genital lesions from HSV type 1 and oral lesions from HSV type 2 are becoming more common, a trend that may be a consequence of sexual freedom and ease of transmission. HSV lesions, however, are not limited to the lips and genital area and may occur anywhere on the skin.

HSV infections have two phases: primary infection and secondary phase. During the primary infection, the virus becomes established in a nerve ganglion; type 1 HSV most often occurs during childhood, whereas type 2 HSV commonly occurs after sexual contact in sexually active individuals.

Symptoms of the primary infection range from being undetectable to localized pain, headache, generalized aching, malaise, and tender regional adenopathy. Uniform, grouped vesicles develop on an erythematous base; the vesicles soon become pustules that erode, drain, and crust (Plate 4). Primary lesions last for 2 to 6 weeks and heal without scarring. As the lesion heals, the virus enters the skin nerve endings and ascends through peripheral nerves to the dorsal root ganglia where it remains in a latent stage.

Reactivation of the virus can occur in response to local trauma (abrasion) or systemic changes (such as stress, fatigue, compromised immune system). The virus then travels back down the peripheral nerve to the site of initial infection to trigger a recurrence. Prodromal symptoms of burning at the site may precede the onset of the erythematous base, papules, and vesicles. Crusts cover the eruptions within 2 to 4 days and are shed in approximately 8 days exposing a reepithelialized surface.

Clinical presentation of grouped vesicles on an erythematous base is a key indicator of herpes simplex and can be confirmed with a Tzanck smear. However, the reliability of the Tzanck smear is best when the lesion sampled is a vesicle and becomes less reliable with pustules, crusts, or ulcers.[20]

Antiviral medications (acyclovir) are effective in treating the HSV infection and are available in topical, oral, and intravenous administration. Acyclovir decreases healing time, viral shedding, and duration of pain.[13,20]

Nursing care should be directed at keeping the lesions dry, avoiding trauma, and providing comfort. Burow's solution (aluminum acetate) soaks and refrigerated hydrogel dressings can relieve the topical pain commonly associated with HSV lesions. When shedding HSV lesions are present, skin cleansing should be done cautiously so that spreading of the virus is avoided, particularly when the lesions are present on the buttocks.

Herpes Zoster. Herpes zoster, commonly referred to as shingles, is an infection within the epidermis that occurs along dermatome distribution (Fig. 1-5). Eruptions result from the reactivation of the varicella virus that entered the cutaneous nerves during a bout with chicken pox and has remained dormant in the dorsal root ganglia. Reactivation can occur as a result of immunosuppression, fatigue, and emotional trauma. The elderly may be predisposed to herpes zoster as a consequence of a potential decline in immunologic function.[13]

Herpes zoster eruptions are typically limited to a single dermatome (Plate 5). Eruptions begin with a red, swollen plaque (which may initially be interpreted as a macule) and spreads to involve part or all of a dermatome. Vesicles develop in clusters and vary in size. Over the next few days, vesicles become filled with purulent fluid (pustules) followed by rupturing and crusting. In some debilitated patients, the eruption may become more extensive and inflammatory, with necrosis or secondary infections developing.[13,20]

Treatment is quite similar to HSV with acyclovir and Burow's solution to act as an astringent on the lesions. Analgesics may be necessary to control the pain associated with herpes zoster.

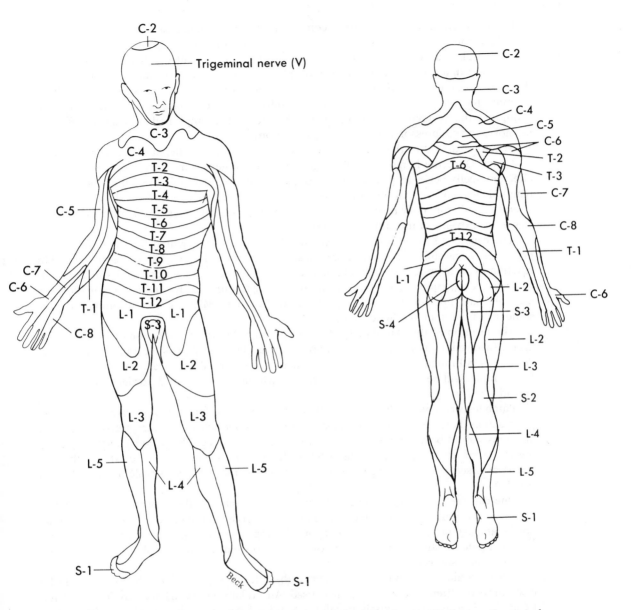

Fig. 1-5 Dermatome areas derived from spinal nerve distribution. Segments: *C*, cervical; *T*, thoracic; *L*, lumbar; *S*, sacral. (From Thibodeau G: Anthony's textbook of anatomy and physiology, ed 13, St. Louis, 1990, Mosby–Year Book, Inc.)

Allergic Factors

Numerous allergic responses, local and systemic, can be manifested on the skin. The concern of the nurse is of course to describe the manifestations accurately and report the assessment to the physician in a timely fashion. Those allergic responses that are localized reactions to such things as adhesives, wound care products, or solutions is the focus of this section. These types of skin damage are commonly called "allergic contact dermatitis."

Allergic contact dermatitis is an immunologic response that causes tissue inflammation and is often confused with irritant contact dermatitis. Clinical skin manifestations can include weeping epidermis, crusting, edema, erythema, and vesicles (Plate 6).

A true allergic dermatitis requires exposure to a contactant or allergen and has two phases. The first phase is the sensitization phase (exposure to a substance or chemical to the skin of a nonsensitized individual) and requires approximately 7 days to transpire. This chemical then attaches to an epidermal protein found on the surface of the Langerhans cell. From here the allergen is exposed to T-lymphocytes in the lymph node (the site of effector, memory, and suppressor T-lymphocyte production).[13,20]

When reexposed to the allergen, the second phase, called "elicitation," occurs within 1 to 2 days. Once the Langerhans T-cell delivers the antigen to memory T-cells in the skin, effector T-cells begin to produce lymphokines. Inflammatory cells are summoned by the lymphokines, and allergic manifestations can be observed. Suppressor T-cells are believed to end the inflammatory reaction. Clinical manifestations can range from erythema to vesicles to the extreme of moist desquamation.

The cause or source of the allergen may be obvious or obscured by other concurrent processes. A careful detailed assessment and interview is imperative to identify the skin reaction as an allergic response. Familiar causes of allergic contact dermatitis include poison ivy, nickel, rubber compounds, paraphenylenediamine (a dye used to color hair, for example) and ethylenediamine (a preservative found in Mycolog cream, aminophylline, some insecticides, or synthetic waxes).[13,20]

The location of the skin damage is an important clue to identification of the causative agent. Involved areas typically have sharp margins. The distribution of an allergic contact dermatitis is limited to the areas of contact. Therefore an allergic reaction to an adhesive, for example, will be the shape of the adhesive, will have well-defined borders, and will not spread.

Patch tests can be conducted to confirm the suspected offending agent causing the allergic reaction; however, these tests must be properly conducted and interpreted. Suspected allergens should be applied to the skin and secured with tape. The patient's back is usually the preferred site for patch testing. After 48 hours, the patches are removed and the test site is assessed for skin damage, which is graded using a standard scale as described in Box 1-4.[17]

One can prevent allergic contact dermatitis by simply avoiding contact with allergens. However, recognizing or identifying the potential allergen is the key to prevention and may not be an easy task. When a patient reports having "sensitive skin," prudence would indicate that patch testing of adhesives is valuable to prevent a potential skin reaction, which would complicate recovery.

When an allergic response is suspected, the offending product or chemical should be discontinued. Often a substitute can be used. Antiinflammatory agents may be warranted topically or systemically; this is usually determined based on the severity of the allergic reaction.

Miscellaneous Factors

Radiation. Radiotherapy triggers changes in the skin that may be sufficient to create ulcerations during therapy, immediately after therapy, or years after the completion of radiation therapy. Skin changes associated with radiotherapy includes erythema, dry desquamation, moist desquamation, tissue fibrosis, edema, and hypopigmentation or hyperpigmentation. Histologically, epidermal atrophy, scarring, loss of epidermal accessory

---

Box 1-4 SCALE FOR INTERPRETATION OF PATCH TEST RESULTS[13,20]
+1 = Macular erythema +2 = Papules and vesicles +3 = Bullae

structures, microvascular occlusions and the presence of large amounts of connective tissue have been reported. Reduced fibroblast proliferation and massive cellular damage to the cytoplasm and nucleus have been identified as the key processes responsible for skin changes in irradiated tissue and the subsequent abnormal wound healing.[28]

Radiation-induced lesions are initially shallow and may occur spontaneously or in response to trauma. The ulcer is often painful and progressively enlarges to the margins of the irradiated skin field despite optimum local treatment. Characteristically, the radiation ulcer has a shaggy border with nonviable tissue present in the base. Squamous cell cancer can develop at the site of an ulcer in irradiated tissue and should be evaluated by biopsy.[28] When it is feasible, radiation ulcers are best treated surgically with extensive débridement of irradiated tissue and a wide myocutaneous flap.

Current radiation techniques (higher voltage machines) are better able to spare the skin, but, irradiated tissue should always be considered extremely vulnerable and protected from unnecessary traumatic insults such as friction, shear, pressure, adhesives, or chemicals.

Extravasation. The administration or leakage of particular solutions into subcutaneous tissue (by intravenous infiltration or subcutaneous injection) can create chronic nonhealing ulcers. Harmful solutions include total parenteral nutrition, sodium bicarbonate, heparin, fat emulsion, vasoconstricting agents, and antineoplastic agents.[25,29] Depending on the solution, tissue damage may result from toxic cellular damage, vasoconstriction, or thrombocytopenia, which may lead to pain, vesiculation, induration, edema, and necrosis. Extent of tissue damage varies with type of solution and the concentration of the solution. The osmotic effects of parenteral nutrition solutions can also impair cellular function by disrupting the osmotic equilibrium between intracellular and extracellular fluids.

Treatment usually requires local excision and débridement. In the presence of extensive tissue damage, skin grafting may be warranted to achieve adequate coverage of the defect.

CONCLUSION

As the body's largest organ, the skin serves several complex functions: protection, thermoregulation, sensation, metabolism, and communication. Numerous factors influence the skin's ability to adequately provide these functions such as age, ultraviolet radiation exposure, hydration, medications, nutrition, and soaps. Likewise, the skin's integrity can be jeopardized by different types of damage.

Wound management must be grounded in a comprehensive knowledge base of the structure and function of the skin. Additionally, the nurse must be able to distinguish between different types of skin damage based on data collected from an astute assessment and patient interview. Only with this depth of information can the negative sequelae of each type of skin damage be understood and appropriate prevention and treatment interventions initiated.

SELF-EVALUATION

QUESTIONS

1. Explain why maintenance of skin integrity is vital to health and life.
2. Identify the two major layers of the skin.
3. Explain why the cells of the stratum corneum are called "keratinocytes."
4. The reproductive layer of the epidermis is known as:
   a. stratum lucidum.
   b. stratum granulosum.
   c. stratum germinativum, or basal layer.
   d. stratum spinosum, or prickly layer.
5. Define "rete ridges" and explain their significance.
6. The vessels of the papillary dermis are responsible for nourishing the epidermis, since the epidermis is an avascular layer.
   True
   False
7. Identify the two structural proteins found in the dermis that provide skin strength and elasticity.
8. List five major functions of the skin.
9. Identify at least two mechanisms by which the skin protects against pathogenic invasion.
10. Which of the following can be synthesized in the skin?
    a. Vitamin E
    b. Vitamin K
    c. Vitamin D
    d. Vitamin A
11. Describe the changes in the skin that occur with aging.
12. Identify changes that occur with excess exposure to ultraviolet radiation.
13. Excessive use of soaps or detergents may impair the bacterial resistance of the skin.
    True
    False
14. Which of the following is known to interfere with epidermal regeneration and collagen synthesis?
    a. Antibiotics
    b. Oral contraceptives
    c. Steroids
    d. Antihypertensives
15. List seven categories of factors known to damage the skin.
16. A lesion that is raised, solid, and less than 0.5 cm in diameter is a:
    a. macule.
    b. papule.
    c. pustule.
    d. nodule.
17. A blister that measures 1.5 cm in diameter may also be called a:
    a. bulla.

    b. pustule.

    c. vesicle.

    d. wheal.

18. Distinguish between erosion and ulcer according to depth of tissue damage.

19. List at least four interventions to reduce epidermal stripping.

20. List three treatment options to prevent chemical skin irritation in a patient with diarrhea.

21. Which of the following accurately characterizes chemical skin irritation?

    a. Erythema with satellite lesions

    b. Erythema and erosion of skin

    c. Ulcerations with necrotic tissue in wound bed

    d. Ulcerations with pustules

22. Neuropathic ulcers are also referred to as:

    a. arterial ulcers.

    b. diabetic ulcers.

    c. radiation ulcers.

    d. venous ulcers.

23. State the two phases of an allergic contact dermatitis.

24. Candidiasis can be described as a:

    a. macular rash with ulcerations.

    b. papular rash within the hair follicle.

    c. pustular erythematous rash.

    d. vesicular rash with placque formation.

25. Which of the following statements is true of herpes simplex lesions?

    a. Initially develop as papules.

    b. Distribution follows the dermatomes.

    c. Erythema signifies a secondary infection.

    d. Vesicles are uniformly shaped and grouped.

26. Ulcerations precipitated by radiation:

    a. are painless.

    b. can be prevented with good hygiene.

    c. develop within 18 months after irradiation.

    d. have shaggy margins.

SELF-EVALUATION

ANSWERS

  1. The skin serves as a protective barrier against the external environment and contributes to maintenance of a homeostatic internal environment.

  2. Epidermis and dermis.

  3. These cells are almost completely filled with keratin, which is a fibrous protein. Keratinocytes form a dry protective layer on the surface of the skin.

  4. c

  5. "Rete ridges" are the epidermal protrusions of the basal layer that point downward into the dermis; they help to anchor the epidermis, thus providing structural integrity.

6. True
7. Collagen and elastin.
8. Protection
   Thermoregulation
   Sensation
   Metabolism
   Communication
9. The keratinocytes of an intact stratum corneum provide a resistant barrier; the constant shedding of squames prevents entrenchment of microorganisms.

   The sebum secreted by the sebaceous glands maintains an acid pH (4.0 to 6.8), which inhibits growth of microorganisms.

   The normal skin flora provides bacterial interference to pathogens.

   The skin has an immune system: Langerhans cells in the epidermis: macrophages and mast cells in the dermis. Langerhans cells are antigen-presenting cells; macrophages phagocytize bacteria; mast cells contribute to the inflammatory response by release of histamine.

10. c
11. Epidermal turnover time is increased (21 days in young adults; doubled by 35 years of age)
    Reduced barrier function
    Diminished sensory perception
    Reduced vitamin D production
    Decreased number of Langerhans cells, increasing the risk of skin cancer and pathogenic invasion
    Reduced inflammatory response
    Reduced number of sweat glands
    Loss of subcutaneous fat
    Flattening of dermal papillae and rete ridges
    Diminished vascularity
    Changes in melanocytes, resulting in gray hair
    Wrinkling because of loss of underlying tissue
12. Visible signs include dryness, tough leathery skin, wrinkling, and irregular pigmentation.
    Damage to DNA results in transformation of cells and increased risk of basal or squamous cell carcinoma and malignant melanoma.
    Thickening of epidermal cells.
    Changes in dermal vessels (become dilated and tortuous).
    Reduced number of Langerhans cells, thereby reducing immunocompetence of skin.
13. True
14. c
15. Mechanical, chemical, vascular, allergic, infectious, radiation, thermal, and extravasation
16. b
17. a
18. *Ulcers* involve the loss of epidermis and dermis. Healing occurs by scar formation.

Erosion involves partial loss of epidermis; tissue loss does not extend below the epidermis. Healing occurs without scarring.
19. Do not apply tape under tension.
    Remove tape slowly by peeling skin away.
    Use porous adhesives
    Use skin sealants or solid-wafer barriers under adhesives.
    Avoid use of tapes by using roll gauze, or self-adherent tape.
    Use Montgomery straps.
20. Apply moisture barrier ointments after each stool.
    Apply rectal pouch if stooling more than 3 times per 8 hours.
    Apply ointment pastes if moisture-barrier ointment is ineffective.
21. b
22. b
23. Sensitization phase and elicitation phase
24. c
25. d
26. d

REFERENCES

1. Alterescu V and Alterescu K: Etiology and treatment of pressure ulcers, Decubitus 1(1):28, 1988.
2. Auger MJ: Mononuclear phagocytes, Br Med J 298:546, 1989.
3. Benyon RC: The human skin mast cell, Clin Exp Allergy 19:375, 1989.
4. Bergstrom N: Lecture presented at "Prediction, Prevention and Early Treatment of Pressure Ulcers"; National Pressure Ulcer Advisory Panel meeting, March 1991, Washington DC.
5. Bernstein NR: Appearance: concepts of perception and disfigurement (Chapter 1), Body and face images: personality and self-representation (Chapter 2), and Disfigurement and personality development (Chapter 3). In Emotional care of the facially burned and disfigured, Boston, 1976, Little, Brown & Co.
6. Bettley FR: Some effects of soap on the skin, Br Med J 1:1675, 1960.
7. Council on Scientific Affairs: Harmful effects of ultraviolet radiation, JAMA 262:380, 1989.
8. Bryant RA: Saving the skin from tape injuries, AJN 88(2):189, 1988.
9. Braden B and Bergstrom N: A conceptual schema for the study and etiology of pressure sores, Rehabil Nurs 12(1):8+, 1987.
10. Ehrlich HP and Hunt TK: Effects of cortisone and vitamin A on wound healing, Ann Surg 167:324, 1968.
11. Gay S and Miller S: Collagen in the physiology and pathology of connective tissue, Stuttgart, 1978, Gustav Fischer Verlag.
12. Gilchrest BA: Skin aging and photoaging, J Am Acad Dermatol 21:610, 1989.
13. Habif TP: Clinical dermatology: a color guide to diagnosis and therapy, ed 2, St. Louis, 1990, Mosby–Year Book, Inc.
14. Husni EA: Skin ulcers secondary to arterial and venous disease. In Rudolph R and Noe JM, editors: Chronic problem wounds, Boston, 1983, Little, Brown & Co.
15. Jacob SW, Francone CA, and Lossow WJ: Structure and function in man, ed 5, Philadelphia, 1982, WB Saunders.
16. Kuller JM: Part I: Skin development and function, Neonatal Network 3:18-23, 1984.
17. Lehninger AL: Principles of biochemistry, New York, 1982, Worth Publishers, Inc.
18. Lober CW and Fenske NA: Photoaging and the skin: differentiation and clinical response, Geriatrics 45:36, 1990.
19. Longaker MT and others: Studies in fetal wound healing, VI. Second and early third trimester fetal wounds demonstrate rapid collagen deposition without scar formation, J Pediatr Surg 25:63, Jan 1990.

20. Lookingbill OP and Marks JG: Principles of dermatology, Philadelphia, 1986, WB Saunders Co.
21. Millington PF and Wilkinson R: Skin, Cambridge, Engl, 1983, Cambridge University Press.
22. Noble WC: Microbial skin disease: its epidemiology, London, 1983, Edward Arnold.
23. Pollack SV: Systemic medications and wound healing, Int J Dermatol 21:489, 1982.
24. Potts JF: Sunlight, sunburn, and sunscreens, Postgrad Med 87:52, June 1990.
25. Renfro L, Moy J, and Sanchez M: Cutaneous ulcers caused by drugs, Wounds: a Compendium of Clinical Research and Practice 2(6):236, 1990.
26. Roe DA: Nutrition and the skin, New York, 1986, Alan R Liss, Inc.
27. Roth RR and James WD: Microbial ecology of the skin, Annu Rev Microbiol 42:441, 1988.
28. Rudolph R: Radiation ulcers. In Rudolph R and Noe JM, editors: Chronic problem wounds, Boston, 1983, Little, Brown & Co.
29. Rudolph R: Toxic drug ulcer. In Rudolph R and Noe JM, editors: Chronic problem wounds, Boston, 1983, Little, Brown & Co.
30. Rudolph R and Noe JM: Other leg ulcers. In Rudolph R and Noe JM, editors: Chronic problem wounds, Boston, 1983, Little, Brown & Co.
31. Rudowski W: Burn therapy and research, Baltimore, 1976, Johns Hopkins University Press.
32. Sams WM: Structure and function of the skin. In Sams WM and Lynch PJ, editors: Principles and practice of dermatology, New York, 1990, Churchill Livingstone.
33. Shuster S, Fisher GH, Harris E, and Binnell D: The effect of skin disease on self image, Br J Dermatol 90(suppl 16):18, 1978.
34. Siebert JW and others: Fetal wound healing: a biochemical study of scarless healing, Plast Reconstr Surg 85:495, 1990.
35. Silverberg N and Silverberg L: Aging and the skin, Postgrad Med 86:131, 1989.
36. Skillman JJ: Venous leg ulcers. In Rudolph R and Noe JM, editors: Chronic problem wounds, Boston, 1983, Little, Brown & Co.
37. Solomons B: Lecture notes on dermatology, ed 5, Oxford, 1983, Blackwell Scientific Publications.
38. Spince AP and Mason EB: Human anatomy and physiology, Menlo Park, Calif, 1987, The Benjamin/Cummings Publishing Co, Inc.
39. Stender IM, Blichmann C, and Serup J: Effects of oil and water baths on the hydration state of the epidermis, Clin Exp Dermatol 15:206, 1990.
40. Stryer L: Biochemistry, ed 3, New York, 1988, WH Freeman & Co.
41. Weinberg AN and Swartz MN: General considerations of bacterial diseases. In Fitzpatrick TB and others, editors: Dermatology in general medicine: textbook and atlas, New York, 1987, McGraw-Hill Book Co.
42. Thelan LA, Davie JK, and Urden LD: Textbook of critical care nursing: diagnosis and management, St. Louis, 1990, Mosby–Year Book, Inc.
43. Tretbar L: Chronic venous insufficiency of the legs: pathogenesis of venous ulcers, J Enterostom Ther 14:105+, 1987.
44. Wheater PR, Burkitt, HG, and Daniels, VG: Functional histology, ed 2, Edinburgh, 1987, Churchill Livingstone.
45. White MI, Jenkinson DM, and Lloyd DH: The effect of washing on the thickness of the stratum corneum in normal and atopic individuals, Br J Dermatol 116:525, 1987.
46. Wolff K and Stingl G: The Langerhans cell, J Invest Dermatol 80:17s, 1983.
47. Woodburne RT and Burkel WE: Essentials of human anatomy, New York, 1988, Oxford University Press.

2 Principles of Wound Healing and Wound Management

DOROTHY B. DOUGHTY

OBJECTIVES

1. Define the terms in relation to wounds and wound healing: primary intention, secondary intention, tertiary intention, partial-thickness wound, full-thickness wound.

2. Identify the key components and usual time frame for partial-thickness wound repair.

3. Explain why a moist wound surface enhances the repair process.

4. Describe the three major phases of full-thickness wound repair to include key events for each phase and the wound appearance in each phase.

5. Explain the role of the following cells in the wound-healing process: platelets, polymorphonuclear leukocytes, macrophages, and fibroblasts.

6. Explain why large full-thickness wounds may require skin grafting to complete epithelialization whereas large partial-thickness wounds can spontaneously reepithelialize.

7. Describe the impact of the following factors on wound healing, and identify nursing implications:
   - Tissue perfusion and oxygenation
   - Nutritional status
   - Presence or absence of infection
   - Diabetes mellitus
   - Corticosteroid administration
   - Immunosuppression
   - Aging
   - Disease processes
   - Topical therapy

8. Identify three priorities in effective wound management.

9. Identify seven principles underlying appropriate topical therapy and the rationale for each.

10. Differentiate between appropriate cleansing techniques and solutions for a clean proliferating wound and an infected or necrotic wound.

11. Identify clinical features, indications, contraindications, and guidelines for use for each of the following:
    - Transparent adhesive dressings
    - Hydrocolloid wafer dressings
    - Nonadhesive semipermeable polyurethane foam dressings
    - Absorption dressings
    - Gauze dressings
    - Gel dressings
    - Synthetic barrier dressings

12. Identify indications and guidelines for use of topical preparations.

13. Utilize wound-healing principles and knowledge of available products to identify appropriate dressings or preparations for each of the following wounds:
    - Full-thickness wounds with necrosis
    - Full-thickness wounds with exudate or dead space, or both
    - Full-thickness wounds that are clean and proliferating
    - Partial-thickness wounds

14. Identify factors that may contribute to a nonhealing wound.

Nurses play a vital role in wound management. They are responsible for dressing and monitoring acute wounds such as surgical incisions and are frequently asked to establish management protocols for chronic wounds such as pressure ulcers or vascular ulcers. Nursing interventions can either enhance or delay the wound-healing process; thus nurses must be knowledgeable regarding the wound-healing process and the implications for wound management.

For centuries wound healing was regarded as a rather mysterious process, with wound management based on practitioner preference as opposed to scientific principles. Recent research has contributed much knowledge regarding the wound-healing process and the factors that facilitate this process; today's nurses must base their care on these research-based principles and must stay abreast of new findings if they are to provide appropriate wound care. In this chapter the normal process of wound healing is reviewed and the implications for wound management are discussed.

PHYSIOLOGY OF WOUND HEALING

The ability to repair tissue damage is an important survival tool for any living organism. Regardless of the type or severity of the injury, there are only two mechanisms by which repair occurs: regeneration, or replacement of the damaged or lost tissue with "more of the same," or connective tissue repair, in which the damaged or lost tissue is replaced by scar formation. The type of repair is determined by the tissue involved in the injury and its ability to regenerate; tissues that are capable of regeneration do so, whereas those incapable of regeneration must produce connective tissue to fill the defect or knit tissues back together.[12,33]

Thus the mechanism of repair for any wound is dependent on the tissue layer or layers involved and their capacity for regeneration. This means that wounds confined to the epidermal and dermal layers will heal by regeneration; the reason is that epithelial, endothelial, and connective tissue can be reproduced. In contrast, wounds extending *through* the dermis heal by scar formation because most of the deeper structures (hair follicles, sweat glands, sebaceous glands, subcutaneous tissue, and muscle) do not regenerate.[12] Injuries to bone, such as fractures, heal by regeneration; however, chronic or necrotic processes usually require resection of the involved bone to eliminate infection and promote healing.[31] Skeletal muscle may regenerate if innervation and vascularization are maintained or reestablished *and* if reproductive muscle cells are present in the remaining muscle; however, most wounds involving muscle loss fail to meet these criteria and heal by scar formation.[40]

Types of Wound Healing

Wound healing may be said to occur by "primary, secondary, or tertiary intention."[62] This classification separates wounds based on the amount of primary closure; the degree of closure determines the amount of connective tissue (scar) required to repair the defect and also reflects the wound's susceptibility to infection.

A wound healing by primary intention is one that is surgically closed, thus minimizing the tissue defect and the potential for infection. These wounds usually heal quickly, with minimal scar formation, so long as infection and secondary breakdown are prevented. A surgical incision is an example of a wound healing by primary intention.[62]

A wound heals by secondary intention when it is left open and allowed to heal by production of connective tissue (scar). These wounds require a longer time to heal because of the amount of connective tissue required to fill the defect and are more subject to infection, since they lack the epidermal barrier to microorganisms. Examples of wounds healing by secondary intention are pressure ulcers and abdominal wounds that are left open to the fascia layer.[62]

Wounds are said to heal by tertiary intention when there is a delay between injury and closure. These wounds require more connective tissue (scar) than wounds that are primarily closed, but less than those that heal completely by scar formation (secondary intention). An example of a wound healing by tertiary intention is an abdominal wound that is initially left open for drainage but later closed.[62]

Another way to classify wounds is by depth, that is, tissue layers involved. Partial-thickness wounds are those that are confined to the skin layers (epidermis and dermis); these wounds are expected to heal by regeneration. Full-thickness wounds are those involving total loss of the skin layers (epidermis and dermis) and extending into the subcutaneous and possibly the muscle and bone layers; these wounds require connective tissue repair.[23]

The Wound Healing Process

For many years wound healing was a mysterious process, always hoped for but poorly understood and therefore poorly managed. As research provides new insight into the repair process, we are provided with the principles of wound management.

Wound healing is best understood as a cascade of events. Injury sets into motion a series of physiologic responses that are coordinated and sequenced and, in a healthy host, invariably result in healing.[33] Appropriate wound management is dependent on an understanding of the normal repair process, the factors affecting this process, and the interventions that can impact either positively or negatively on the outcome.

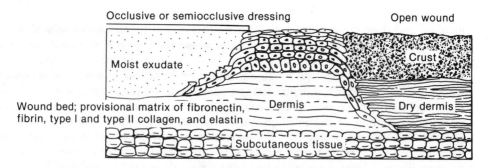

Fig. 2-1   Diagram of migration of epidermal cells in moist environment and dry environment. (Modified from Goslen JB: J Dermatol Surg Oncol 14:962, 1988.)

Partial-Thickness Wound Healing. Partial-thickness wounds are shallow wounds involving less than total loss of the skin layers; these wounds are moist and painful because of the loss of the epidermal covering and exposure of the nerve endings.[23] When the wound involves loss of the epidermis with exposure of the basement membrane, the wound base appears bright pink-red. When there is partial dermal loss, the wound base usually appears pale pink with distinct red "islets" (Plate 7); these islets represent the basement membrane of the epidermis, which "dips down" into the dermis to line the epidermal appendages (Fig. 2-1). These islands of epidermal basement membrane are important in partial-thickness wound healing; all epidermal cells are capable of regeneration, and each islet will serve as a source of new epithelium.[61]

The major components of partial-thickness repair are an initial inflammatory response, epithelial proliferation and migration (resurfacing), and reestablishment of the epidermal layers with resumption of normal cellular functions.[48,61] If the wound involves dermal loss, connective tissue repair will proceed concurrently with the epithelial repair (Table 2-1).

Epidermal repair. Tissue trauma triggers an acute inflammatory response; this causes some edema of the injured area and produces a serous exudate containing leukocytes. (In the past this exudate was allowed to dry on the wound surface, creating a scab.) In partial-thickness wounds the inflammatory response is a limited one, subsiding in less than 24 hours.[61] Epidermal cells throughout the wound bed begin to proliferate and migrate across the wound bed within 24 hours; in wounds that are kept moist, this migration may begin as early as 8 hours after injury. The new epidermis originates from the epidermal cells at the wound margins and from epidermal cells lining the epidermal appendages; thus the wound rapidly resurfaces. In wounds left open to air, resurfacing is usually complete within 6 to 7 days; in wounds that are kept moist, resurfacing proceeds more rapidly and is usually complete within 4 days.[61] The reason is that epidermal cells can migrate only across a moist surface; in a dry wound, the epidermal cells must tunnel down to a moist level and must secrete collagenase to lift the scab away from the wound surface in order to migrate (Fig. 2-1). The migrating epidermis is only a few cells thick; once the wound surface is covered, the epidermal cells in that area cease lateral migration (a process known as "contact inhibition") and begin upward (rather than lateral) migration, so that stratification of cells is reestablished.[61] The new epidermis appears pink and dry. As the epidermal cells resume their normal functions, the epidermis will gradually repigment to match the person's normal skin tone.

Table 2-1   Key events and mediators in wound healing

Tissue layers involved	Repair process	Key mediators	Critical events in repair process
PARTIAL-THICKNESS Epidermis; may involve dermis	Regeneration	Epithelial cells (keratinocytes)	• Epithelial proliferation and lateral migration (resurfacing) • Reestablishment of normal skin layers and function
NOTE: If dermis is involved, collagen repair proceeds concurrently with epithelialization.			

FULL-THICKNESS
 Complete loss of epidermis and dermis
 Subcutaneous tissue involved
 May involve muscle, bone, and joint
	Scar formation (connective tissue repair)	Platelets
		 Macrophages
			• Defensive (inflammatory) phase
			    Hemostasis
			    Inflammation
			 • Proliferative (fibroblastic) phase
			    Granulation
			    Epithelialization
			    Contraction (open wounds only)
			 • Maturation (remodeling) phase
			    Collagen lysis
			    Collagen synthesis

Dermal repair. In wounds involving both dermal and epidermal loss, dermal repair proceeds concurrently with reepithelialization. New blood vessels begin to sprout and fibroblasts become plentiful by about 7 days after the injury; collagen fibers are visible in the wound bed by the ninth day, and collagen synthesis continues until about 10 to 15 days after the injury. This new connective tissue then gradually contracts. In wounds that are kept moist, connective tissue repair begins about 3 days earlier (2 to 3 days after the injury); the reason is probably that new connective tissue forms only in the presence of suitable exudate. In a wound left open to air, a moist environment is not established until the epidermis has migrated across the wound bed, lifting the scab and providing protection from dehydration.[61]

Full-Thickness Wound Healing. Full-thickness wounds, by definition, involve total loss of the epidermal and dermal layers; these lesions extend at least to the subcutaneous tissue layer and may involve the fascia and muscle layer and even the bone and joint capsule.[23] These lesions present as craters, with the depth determined by tissue layers involved and the patient's body build (Plate 8). They may involve necrotic tissue or infection, and they are frequently associated with extensive tissue damage, such as sinus tract formation or undermining (tissue defects extending out under wound edges).[23]

In discussing the normal repair process for full-thickness wounds, it is important to note that the model for full-thickness repair is the acute wound, such as a surgically induced wound; these wounds have been studied extensively under laboratory conditions. It has been well established that in a relatively healthy host, an acute wound will heal fairly quickly; this is attributable to the cascade phenomenon, which tends to keep a wound on

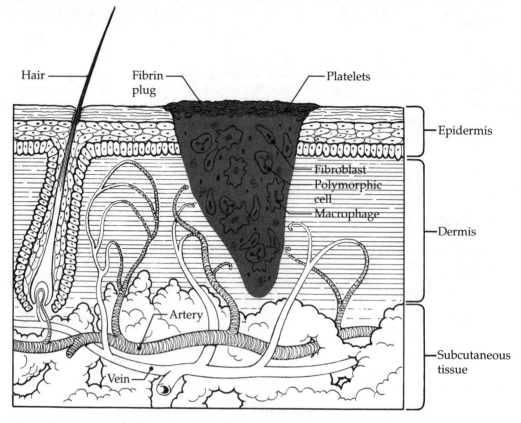

Fig. 2-2 Diagram of inflammatory phase of wound repair in full-thickness wound.

the "healing track."[33] In clinical practice, however, nurses are frequently dealing with chronic wounds such as pressure ulcers or vascular ulcers; these wounds behave quite differently. In this section, the normal repair process is described, and differences between acute and chronic wounds are then addressed.

Full-thickness tissue repair proceeds through three phases: the defensive, or inflammatory, phase; the proliferative, or fibroblastic, phase; and the remodeling, or maturation, phase. These phases do not occur in isolation; overlap between phases exists. The platelets and the macrophages appear to be the principal mediators for full-thickness repair[10,24] (Table 2-1).

Defensive Phase. The defensive phase is the body's immediate response to injury. The major events during this phase are hemostasis and inflammation (Fig. 2-2).

HEMOSTASIS. Hemostasis is a complex phenomenon involving several interrelated factors and several coagulation "pathways." Tissue injury serves to initiate the clotting process; cellular and vascular disruption exposes blood to collagen, which activates coagulation factors and causes platelet aggregation.[10] The result is fibrin clot formation, which provides initial wound closure as well as preventing excessive loss of blood and body fluids. Recent research has identified another aspect of this process; the platelets release several growth factors, which attract the cells and chemical substances needed for wound repair.[10,24] Thus hemostasis, which is the body's normal response to tissue injury, actually initiates the entire wound-healing cascade (Fig. 2-3).

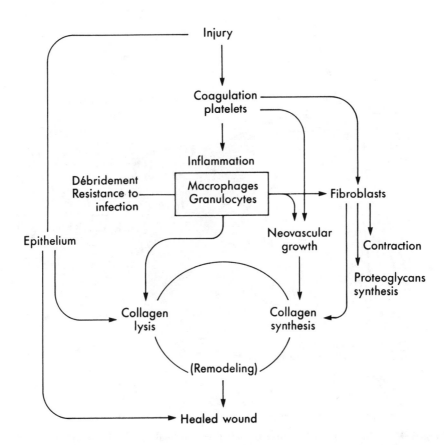

Fig. 2-3 Schema demonstrating that coagulation triggers the wound-healing cascade. (From Levenson S, Seiffer E, and Van Winkle E, Jr.: Nutrition. In Hunt TK and Dunphy JE, editors: Fundamentals of wound management, New York, 1979, Appleton-Century-Crofts.)

INFLAMMATION. The second major event in the defensive phase is inflammation (Fig. 2-2). Tissue injury and activation of clotting factors stimulate the release of vasoactive substances, such as histamine, which cause the surrounding vessels to dilate and to become more permeable.[10] This results in vasocongestion and in leakage of serous fluid into the wound bed, which causes the wound to appear erythematous, edematous, and warm, with varying amounts of exudate. Chemoattractants produced by the platelets, activated clotting factors, and fibrin breakdown products attract leukocytes into the wound bed.[10] Polymorphonuclear leukocytes (PMNs) are the first white blood cells to enter the wound, arriving within 6 hours; although they have a short life span, they provide initial protection against bacterial invasion.[12] Within about 4 days after injury, macrophages arrive in the wound bed and gradually replace the leukocytes. Both the leukocytes and the macrophages act as the body's defenders, phagocytizing bacteria and breaking down necrotic tissue.[10,62] However, the macrophage, which is derived from a monocyte, plays a much broader role. Evidence indicates that the macrophage assumes the "director" role throughout the wound-

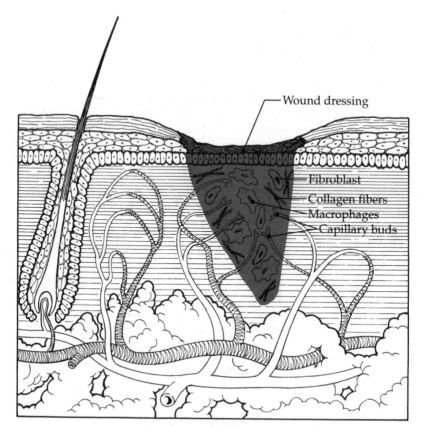

Fig. 2-4   Schema of proliferative phase of wound healing in full-thickness wound. Notice extension of capillary buds into wound.

healing process.[44] Studies have shown that macrophages are normally present during all phases of wound healing and that elimination of macrophages significantly impairs wound healing.[33,44] In addition to their phagocytic and débridement functions, macrophages produce chemoattractants and growth factors; these substances attract cells needed for tissue repair and control various wound-healing processes. In addition, macrophages convert macromolecules into the amino acids and sugars needed for wound healing and secrete lactate, which stimulates collagen synthesis.[33,44]

The overall result of the defensive phase of wound healing is control of bleeding and establishment of a clean wound bed. In a clean wound, the inflammatory phase lasts approximately 3 days; in necrotic and infected wounds, the inflammatory phase is prolonged and wound healing is delayed.

Proliferative Phase. The second phase of full-thickness wound healing is the *proliferative phase;* in this phase the defect is filled with new connective tissue, and the wound is covered with new epithelium. The major components of this phase are *granulation* and *epithelialization;* in wounds healing by secondary intention, contraction also occurs and serves to reduce the size of the defect[48,62] (Fig. 2-4).

GRANULATION. Granulation refers to the formation of new connective tissue (scar) to fill the defect; this involves neoangiogenesis and synthesis of various connective tissue substances. New capillary networks must be established to provide the oxygen and nutrients needed for synthesis of collagen and other connective tissues, and these fragile new capillary networks require the support of collagen fibers. Thus collagen synthesis and capillary proliferation occur simultaneously in a codependent fashion.[10,20]

Neoangiogenesis. Neoangiogenesis is stimulated by the hypoxia that results from disruption of vascular pathways; hypoxia is believed to be the stimulus that turns wound healing "on" and "off."[20] Capillary proliferation occurs in response to the oxygen gradient that exists between the vascularized periphery of the wound and its hypoxic center. In addition, hypoxia stimulates the release of angiogenesis factors by macrophages; these factors are chemoattractants for endothelial cells. The new endothelial cells seem to sprout from blood vessels at the edge of the wound; the new capillary loops advance toward the center of the wound and eventually connect with loops advancing from the other direction, or with adjacent loops.[20,24]

Collagen synthesis. Neoangiogenesis occurs concurrently with collagen synthesis, which is the second component of the granulation process.[10] Actually the term "collagen synthesis" represents an oversimplification of the process. Formation of scar tissue involves multiple phases and synthesis of many connective tissue substances. Recent studies indicate that fibronectin and hyaluronic acid are the major components of the initial granulation tissue; these substances provide a matrix for collagen fiber deposition and cell migration. These substances are gradually replaced by immature collagen fibers (type III collagen) and proteoglycans, which provide tensile strength and resilience. The matrix composition continues to change with maturation. The final scar is composed primarily of mature collagen fibers, or type I collagen, which is the type normally found in dermal tissue.[10]

The *fibroblasts* are the cells responsible for synthesis of collagen and other connective tissue substances and are therefore critical to the repair process.[10] Fibroblasts seem to originate from perivascular cells;[20] they begin to appear in the wound bed toward the end of the inflammatory phase. Fibroblast migration and proliferation occur in response to chemoattractants and growth factors produced by platelets, macrophages, and inflammatory substances.[36] Macrophages seem to be a particularly important stimulus; on contact with hypoxic tissue, they release growth factors that stimulate fibroblast replication.[20,37]

Fibroblast migration and proliferation does not ensure connective tissue synthesis. It appears that fibroblasts must be stimulated to synthesize collagen and other repair substances. The primary stimulants for connective tissue synthesis appear to be lactate and ascorbate (the reduced form of ascorbic acid); these substances activate the enzymes needed for collagen synthesis. Both lactate and ascorbate are present in significant levels in the hypoxic wound bed; thus the wound environment itself provides the stimulants needed for tissue repair.[20,33] In summary, fibroblasts are attracted to the wound bed, encouraged to reproduce, and finally directed to produce connective tissue, a well-ordered sequential process controlled by various growth factors.

Collagen synthesis is a complex production. Within the cell, collagen peptides are assembled and hydroxylation reactions, which render the collagen less susceptible to breakdown, occur. The immature collagen fibrils are then secreted into the extracellular space; at this point they have a gel-like consistency and provide no tensile strength to the wound, though they do support the advancing capillary networks. The collagen fibers then develop intermolecular "cross-links," which gradually mature and provide tensile strength.[20,33] Eventually the collagen fibers become completely insoluble.

In wounds healing by primary intention, collagen synthesis usually peaks at about the sixth or seventh day, though collagen production continues for weeks or even months. In wounds healing by secondary intention, this proliferative phase may be prolonged.[42,62] Each phase of collagen production has specific oxygen and nutrient requirements; thus the patient's ability to heal is very dependent on his vascular and nutritional status, as is discussed later in this chapter.[20]

In sutured wounds, only a small amount of collagen is needed to mend the defect, and collagen synthesis occurs concurrently with epidermal migration. Incisional status can be observed and monitored, but granulation occurs at a deeper level and is not visible. In open wounds, however, granulation tissue is visible and presents as a red, very vascular, granular wound bed (Plate 9). This appearance is attributable to the numerous capillary loops in combination with collagen fibers. This extremely vascular granulation tissue actually matures into a relatively avascular scar; once the repair process is complete the need for oxygen and nutrients is reduced, and many of the vessels regress.[10,42,62]

CONTRACTION. In open wounds, formation of granulation tissue occurs concurrently with wound *contraction;* the tissue and skin surrounding the defect are mobilized and pulled together, thus reducing the size of the defect (Fig. 2-5). Contraction does not occur in sutured wounds, where there is minimal tissue defect;[62] however, it can play a significant role in wounds healing by secondary intention. Contraction speeds the healing process because it reduces the amount of scar tissue (collagen) required for repair. Contraction is mediated by myofibroblasts; these actin-rich cells synthesize collagen and appear to pull the collagen fibers toward the cell body by extension and retraction of pseudopodia.[10,48] The degree of contraction is limited by the mobility of the surrounding tissue. Sacral and abdominal wounds are located in mobile areas and can contract significantly, whereas a wound overlying a bony prominence (such as the trochanter) has limited potential for contraction and therefore will require more granulation tissue to fill the defect. Contraction is considered undesirable in some wounds, since it can cause cosmetic deformities or flexion contractures of joints.[42]

EPITHELIALIZATION. The final component of the proliferative phase is epithelialization; this involves migration of epithelial cells from the wound edges to resurface the defect. In wounds with minimal tissue defects, such as surgical incisions, epithelial migration occurs concurrently with collagen synthesis;[62] in open wounds, epithelialization is delayed until a bed of granulation tissue is established. The reason is that epithelial cells will not migrate across a dry surface or across necrotic tissue.[20,33]

Large wounds healing by secondary intention may require skin grafting because there is a limit to epidermal migration, usually about 3 cm from the point of origin.[9] In a full-thickness wound epidermal cells are present only at the wound margin, since epithelial cells normally present in the lining of the hair follicles and the sweat glands have been destroyed.[42] Grafting may also be required if there is no "free border" of epithelial cells at the periphery; this may occur in wounds healing by secondary intention if the border epidermis rolls under itself, creating a closed, nonproliferative wound edge.

Maturation phase. The final phase in full-thickness wound healing is the maturation, or remodeling, phase. This phase begins when the wound has been closed by connective tissue synthesis and epithelialization and continues for up to a year or even longer.[37,42] Remodeling involves the simultaneous processes of collagen lysis and collagen synthesis

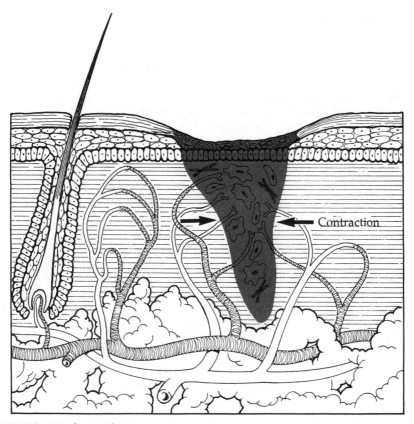

Fig. 2-5   Schema of wound contraction.

and appears to be mediated by macrophages.[44] Disorganized collagen fibers are removed from the wound by collagenase and are replaced with newly synthesized fibers oriented along the lines of mechanical stress. Thus remodeling normally provides a scar with maximum tensile strength.[37,42]

An imbalance between the dual processes of collagen lysis and synthesis can complicate wound healing. For example, hypertrophic scarring and keloid formation are believed to be caused by an imbalance in which collagen synthesis exceeds collagen lysis. On the other hand, hypoxia or malnutrition significantly reduces the rate of collagen synthesis and may result in wound breakdown.[37,42] At best, the tensile strength of scar tissue is never more than 80% of the tensile strength in nonwounded tissue.[12] Wounds healing by primary intention demonstrate 30% normal tensile strength at 3 weeks and 80% (maximal level) at 60 days.[12]

Acute versus Chronic Wounds. As described above, the normal repair process is an exquisitely coordinated cascade that virtually ensures wound healing in a relatively healthy host. Yet nurses are frequently confronted with nonhealing wounds such as pressure ulcers, venous stasis ulcers, or ischemic ulcers. How do these chronic wounds differ from acute wounds such as incisions? There is much left to learn about chronic wounds. We do know, however, that chronic wounds usually result from an underlying process such as vascular insufficiency,[2] whereas acute wounds begin with an injury that disrupts vasculature and initiates hemostasis. Since hemostasis is the initiator for the wound-healing cascade, absence of this event may help explain the static nature of chronic wounds. In addition, chronic wounds frequently occur in compromised patients;[2] the impact of host factors on wound healing is discussed in the next section.

FACTORS IMPACTING ON WOUND HEALING

Wound healing is a *systemic* process and is therefore significantly affected by systemic conditions. Research into the wound-healing process has clearly identified many systemic factors that affect a person's ability to heal (Box 2-1).

Tissue Perfusion and Oxygenation

Oxygen fuels the cellular functions essential to the repair process; therefore the ability to perfuse the tissues with adequate amounts of oxygenated blood is critical to wound healing.[7,20,60,62] Although hypoxia in the wound bed serves as a *stimulus* to endothelial and fibroblast replication, the desired *response* to this stimulus is dependent on adequate oxygenation at the wound periphery.[20,43] Tissue hypoxia adversely affects wound healing in the following ways:[7,20]

- Impaired collagen synthesis. The rate of collagen synthesis is dependent on oxygen availability; there are several stages in collagen production that cannot be completed without adequate levels of oxygen.[7,20] Tissue Po_2 of about 40 mm Hg is needed to support fibroblast proliferation and collagen synthesis.[20]
- Decreased epithelial proliferation and migration.[7,20]
- Reduced tissue resistance to infection. Leukocytes can migrate and ingest bacteria in hypoxic environments; however, their ability to kill bacteria is largely oxygen dependent. This oxidative killing pathway is particularly significant in wounds contaminated or infected with *Staphylococcus aureus, Proteus vulgaris, Klebsiella pneumoniae, Escherichia coli,* and *Salmonella typhimurium,* as well as wounds contaminated with anaerobes. The critical oxygen level appears to be 30 mm Hg.[20,60]

It is obvious that hypoxic cells are unable to carry out the functions essential to tissue defense and wound healing and that any patient who has compromised pulmonary or cardiovascular function is at risk for delayed wound healing and wound infection. This includes patients who are hypotensive, hypovolemic, or hypoxic because of trauma, sepsis, or impaired cardiac or pulmonary function. It also includes patients with damaged vessels limiting tissue perfusion. Radiation, diabetic angiopathy, and peripheral vascular disease can cause enough damage to the capillary basement membrane to severely impair or even prevent wound healing. Thus support for wound healing must include measures to improve tissue perfusion and oxygenation: for example, nasal oxygen for patients who are hypoxic;[43] maintenance of hydration, which has been shown to significantly affect tissue Po_2 by increasing blood volume and decreasing blood viscosity;[43] management of edema by elevation or compression, or both; and referrals as indicated for further evaluation and management of vascular status. Hyperbaric oxygen may be of benefit in some situations and is discussed later in this text.

> ## Box 2-1   FACTORS AFFECTING WOUND HEALING
>
> - Tissue perfusion and oxygenation
> - Nutritional status
> - Infection
> - Systemic states affecting wound healing
>   Diabetes mellitus
>   Hematopoietic abnormalities
>   (thrombocytopenia, neutropenia,
>   anemia)
>   Renal failure
>   Immunosuppression
>
> - Corticosteroid administration
> - Aging
> - Topical therapy

Nutritional Status

Of equal importance is the person's nutritional status.[7,30] Nutrients provide the raw materials needed for wound repair and prevention of infection; the following nutrients have been identified as critical to the wound healing process.

- Adequate protein stores are required for collagen synthesis and epidermal proliferation and for immunocompetence and prevention of infection. The average young adult requires 0.8 to 0.9 g/kg/day for maintenance; higher amounts are needed in older patients and patients with significant wounds or infection.[25,29,38,53]
- Calories are needed to provide energy for tissue defense and wound repair. Usual caloric needs for the adult average between 1500 and 3500 calories/day; however, infection or tissue damage increases caloric demands significantly.[17,29,30,51,53,54]
- Vitamin C is an essential cofactor for collagen synthesis and is also needed to maintain capillary wall integrity. The Recommended Daily Allowance for vitamin C is 60 mg; however, some studies have indicated significant losses of vitamin C from severe wounds. Supplementation with 250 to 500 mg/day has been recommended.[8,12,21,53]
- Vitamin A is indicated for patients receiving corticosteroids. Vitamin A serves to partially counteract the adverse effects of steroids on wound healing; it restores the local inflammatory response and the stimulus to epithelial migration.[12] Recommended dosage is 20,000 to 25,000 International units/day for 10 days, or topical application of vitamin A three times a day.[17,52] However, excessive vitamin A can exacerbate the inflammatory response and cause damage to the wound.
- B complex vitamins are required for effective cross-linking of collagen fibers.[8,20]
- Iron is required to support oxygen transport and is also a cofactor needed for collagen synthesis.[20]
- Copper is needed to support the cross-linking of collagen fibers.[8,20]
- Zinc is a necessary cofactor for collagen formation and protein synthesis. Stress and weight loss will deplete zinc stores. Chronic steroid administration is also known to depress serum zinc levels. Although supplemental zinc is necessary to correct deficiencies, the benefits of zinc supplements for patients with normal zinc levels is controversial.[12,17,30]

Since wound healing is clearly dependent on availability of essential nutrients, nursing management must include assessment of nutritional status and nutrient intake, coupled with appropriate intervention.

Presence or Absence of Infection

A third factor of importance in wound healing is the presence or absence of infection. Wound infection prolongs the inflammatory stage, induces additional tissue destruction, delays collagen synthesis, and prevents epithelialization.[2,45] Thus it is important to treat infections aggressively and appropriately.

It is important to recognize that although all dermal wounds are contaminated not all wounds are infected. Clinical infection is determined by the colony count, which represents the balance between the bacterial load and the host's resistance.[45] Either heavy bacterial contamination or compromised host resistance can result in a colony count of more than 100,000 organisms/ml, which is considered indicative of clinical infection. This is based on studies showing that wounds with more than 100,000 organisms/ml (10^5) do not heal, whereas wounds with less than 100,000 organisms/ml will heal normally.[45] It should be noted that this guideline does not hold true for the B-hemolytic streptococcus; this organism can impair or prevent healing with colony counts of *less* than 100,000/ml.[45]

Since infection is a significant deterrent to wound healing, nurses need to be astute in their wound assessment and accurate in their culture technique. Wound culture and sensitivity is indicated for any of the following:[2,3,19,31,55]

- Signs of local infection (erythema, edema, induration, purulent or very foul-smelling drainage, pain, crepitance)
- Signs of systemic infection (fever, leukocytosis)
- Bone involvement (because of risk for osteomyelitis)
- Nonhealing wound. Failure of the wound to progress may be the only indication of "silent" infection; one study found that 34% of the wounds clinically judged to be free of infection had colony counts greater than 100,000 organisms/ml.[45] Alvarez suggests that these silent infections may cause the hypertrophic granulation tissue sometimes seen in wounds managed with moist wound healing; infection delays epithelial migration.[1,45] Thus any wound that fails to improve with appropriate management should be evaluated for occult infection.[2,45]

To obtain an accurate culture, the nurse must (1) obtain appropriate cultures, that is, aerobic and anaerobic cultures in wounds with necrotic tissue or sinus tracts, but aerobic culture only in open viable wounds,[50] and (2) use correct technique to minimize risk of contamination; that is, flush the wound with saline, utilize a calcium alginate swab, and swab the wound edges and the wound base using a 10-point coverage technique[2] (Fig. 2-6). Eschar should not be cultured. Culture results should then be used to obtain appropriate physician orders for antibiotics.

Diabetes Mellitus

It has been well established that wound healing is impaired in the patient with diabetes mellitus; since approximately 11 million Americans have diabetes, this is quite significant. Studies indicate that the patient with diabetes experiences reduced collagen synthesis, impaired wound contraction, and delayed epidermal migration.[34,48,53] This delay in wound repair has been attributed to angiopathic changes in both large and small vessels that result in impaired perfusion. An increased incidence of infections in the patient with diabetes may

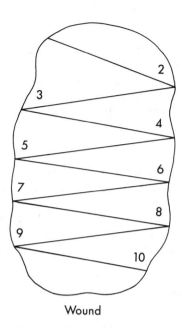

Wound

Fig. 2-6 Ten-point coverage technique for wound culture. (From Alvarez O, Robert J, and Wiseman D: Wound 1(1):35-51, 1989.)

also contribute to impaired wound healing. Hyperglycemia-induced leukocyte dysfunction and vascular insufficiency are believed to be possible causes for this increased infection rate.[34,48,53] (A more detailed discussion of the pathophysiologic changes that occur in the patient with diabetes can be found in Chapter 6.) Management of wounds in patients with diabetes must therefore include measures to maximize tissue perfusion as well as strict control of blood glucose levels.

Corticosteroid Administration

Another factor impinging on wound healing is administration of corticosteroids. Steroids are known to inhibit epithelial proliferation and to exert powerful antiinflammatory effects.[49] It is this impaired inflammatory response that significantly retards wound healing. The normal migration of neutrophils and macrophages into the wound bed is inhibited. Such inhibition increases the wound's vulnerability to infection and interrupts the healing cascade. Reduced migration of macrophages is particularly significant, since it is the macrophage that produces chemoattractants and growth factors, which drive collagen synthesis and wound contraction.[7,12,17,53]

One way in which steroids exert their antiinflammatory effect is by stabilization of lysosomal membranes; lysosomes are cellular components whose activity is required for breakdown of phagocytized material within the macrophage. This breakdown process is critical to macrophage function; it also produces lactate as a byproduct, which stimulates collagen synthesis. As mentioned earlier, vitamin A can partially counteract the effects of corticosteroids; it appears to do so by its labilizing (as opposed to stabilizing) effect on lysosomal membranes.[12,17,53]

Immunosuppression

Any disease process or medication that suppresses the immune system can delay wound healing. This is attributable primarily to impairment of the inflammatory process, which increases susceptibility to infection and delays the healing process.[53] It should be noted that although neutropenia increases the risk of wound infection neutropenia alone will not significantly impair wound healing.[21] Studies have shown that both débridement and granulation can occur in the absence of neutrophils.[57]

Aging

The aging process produces many changes in the skin and underlying tissues that render a person more susceptible to injury and less able to heal. Changes that affect wound healing include a delayed inflammatory response, increased capillary fragility, reduced collagen synthesis and neoangiogenesis, and slower epithelialization.[14,16,27,53] Aging cannot be prevented; to maximize healing in the older patient, it is important to provide optimal systemic and topical support and to eliminate any correctable impediments.

Other Systemic Factors

In addition to the specific conditions noted above, any systemic condition that adversely affects health status can negatively affect wound healing. Renal and hepatic disease, malignancy, and sepsis are among these factors. Hematopoietic abnormalities can impair wound healing because red blood cells are needed for oxygen transport, and platelets are necessary for hemostasis and for initiation of the wound-healing cascade. Studies have recently addressed the impact of sleep and stress on wound healing also.[30,53] Thus, to maximize wound healing, the nurse must maintain a holistic perspective and must strive to enhance the patient's overall health status.

Topical Therapy

While wounds heal from "the inside out," topical therapy significantly affects the wound's surface environment and can therefore either facilitate or impair the healing process. Principles underlying appropriate topical therapy are discussed later in this chapter.

PRINCIPLES OF WOUND MANAGEMENT

Effective wound management depends on elimination or control of causative factors, provision of systemic support, and implementation of appropriate topical therapy. These aspects are appropriately considered wound management priorities (Box 2-2). Each of these priorities requires nursing interventions based on careful assessment.

Reduce or Eliminate Causative Factors

The first treatment priority is elimination of causative factors; thus assessment focuses initially on determination of wound origin. This applies primarily to chronic wounds; the cause of acute wounds is usually known and irreversible, such as surgical incisions or accidental injuries.

In addition to evaluating the patient's general risk factors (such as overall health status, mobility, sensory status, nutritional status, continence status), the nurse should look for specific clues to the cause of the wound. These may be derived from wound location or wound characteristics. Additional clues that reveal the origin of the wound are listed in Table 1-1.

Box 2-2   WOUND MANAGEMENT PRIORITIES

1. Reduce or eliminate causative factors: pressure, shear, friction, moisture, circulatory impairment, neuropathy
2. Provide systemic support for wound healing
   - Nutritional and fluid support
   - Control of systemic conditions affecting wound healing
3. Apply appropriate topical therapy
   - Remove necrotic tissue
   - Identify and eliminate infection
   - Obliterate dead space
   - Absorb excess exudate
   - Maintain moist wound surface
   - Provide thermal insulation
   - Protect the healing wound

Having identified causative factors, the nurse must intervene to eliminate or control these factors. This may involve:

- Selection of an appropriate support surface, for reduction of pressure, shear, friction, or moisture[39]
- Implementation of a turning schedule
- Implementation of measures to reduce shear and friction, such as use of a turn sheet or trapeze, socks or heel protectors, use of knee gatch when head is elevated, light dusting of powder or cornstarch on sheets
- Incontinence management, such as bowel training or prompted voiding programs, external collection devices, skin care
- Use of elevation or compression therapy to reduce venous hypertension.
- Measures to promote blood flow to ischemic areas, such as hydration, elimination of nicotine and caffeine, avoidance of cold
- Orthotics and patient education for patient with neuropathy

The importance of these familiar nursing interventions cannot be emphasized too strongly. *Failure to address cause will result in a nonhealing wound, despite appropriate systemic and topical therapy.* There is no dressing available that can compensate for an uncorrected pathologic condition.[5]

Provide Systemic Support

The second treatment priority is provision of systemic support. As outlined in the discussion on wound-healing physiology, the complex phenomenon of repair occurs only in the presence of adequate oxygen and nutrients and in the absence of deterrents.[53] Thus nursing assessment must include evaluation of the patient's cardiovascular and pulmonary function, nutritional and fluid status, and conditions or factors affecting the wound-healing process. Assessment factors may include:

- Cardiovascular and pulmonary function, such as blood pressure, pulse and respiratory rates, distal pulses, capillary refill, presence or absence of edema, pallor, temperature changes, Po_2[23]
- Nutritional and fluid status, such as actual weight as compared to ideal weight; laboratory indicators of visceral protein status such as albumin, transferrin, and prealbumin; current total intake of calories and protein to include oral, enteral, and parenteral routes; clinical indicators of malnutrition such as joint edema, sparse hair, dry skin, lethargy[23]

- Conditions or factors known to deter wound healing, such as diabetes, steroid administration, immunosuppression[23]

Having assessed the patient for evidence of systemic support for wound healing, the nurse must intervene to correct any host deficiencies. This may involve:

- Measures to support tissue oxygenation, such as hydration, elevation of edematous extremities, administration of nasal oxygen to patient with low Po_2
- Measures to correct nutritional deficiencies, such as dietary or nutritional support consultation; provision of oral, enteral, or parenteral support; provision of vitamin and mineral supplements
- Measures to control wound healing deterrents, such as blood glucose control and administration of vitamin A for patient on steroids.

Apply Appropriate Topical Therapy

The third priority in wound management is implementation of appropriate topical therapy. The goal of topical therapy is to create a local wound environment that supports and facilitates the repair process.

Principles. Principles of topical therapy are derived from scientific studies of the wound-healing process and include the following.

1. *Remove necrotic tissue and foreign bodies or particles.*[15,31,52] Necrotic tissue prolongs the inflammatory process and serves as a medium for bacterial growth. Thus the first objective in management of a necrotic wound is débridement. The one exception to this rule is the ischemic wound with dry eschar; in these patients, the dry eschar provides a barrier to infection. Removal of this eschar converts the wound to an open lesion, which is extremely vulnerable to overwhelming infection; because the ischemic tissue is unable to provide the oxygen needed for infection control and wound healing, the result may be amputation. In this situation, the recommended management is use of topical antibiotic solutions (such as povidone-iodine complex) and dry dressings to reduce bacterial growth and maintain the closed dry wound.[35]

2. *Identify and eliminate infection.* Wound infection prolongs the inflammatory phase, delays collagen synthesis, inhibits epidermal migration, and induces additional tissue damage because the bacteria compete with the fibroblasts and other repair cells for oxygen.[2,45] Wounds should be carefully assessed for any evidence of infection and cultured when appropriate. Treatment of wound infections should be culture specific.[50]

    Wounds involving necrotic tissue frequently involve both aerobic and anaerobic infection; *Bacteroides* is the most common anaerobe. Wounds without necrotic tissue involve only aerobes, with *Pseudomonas aeruginosa* and *Staphylococcus aureus* being the most common.[50] When the infection invades viable tissue surrounding the wound, systemic antibiotics should be considered so that blood and tissue antibiotic levels adequate for infection control can be achieved.[4] The role of topical antibiotics has not been clearly established.[4] Though they may be effective in reducing the number of bacteria on the surface of the wound bed, topical antibiotics do not penetrate nonviable tissue.

3. *Obliterate dead space.* The term "dead space" refers to areas of tissue destruction underlying intact surface tissues, such as sinus tract formation. Such areas provide a fluid medium for bacterial growth and can contribute to abscess formation. If the

wound is granulating and contracting, sinus tracts also pose the risk of superficial wound closure over a fluid-filled defect. Thus the dead space should be obliterated by light packing.[23,52]

4. *Absorb excess exudate.* Large amounts of exudate can macerate surrounding skin and dilute the wound-healing factors and nutrients at the wound surface. In addition, bacterial toxins in the exudate may inhibit the wound repair process.[9,23,59]

5. *Maintain a moist wound surface.* A moist wound surface prevents desiccation and cell death, enhances epidermal migration, and promotes angiogenesis and connective tissue synthesis. A moist wound surface also supports autolysis by rehydration of desiccated tissue, enhanced migration of leukocytes into the wound bed, and accumulation of enzymes.[2,3,58,59,61]

6. *Provide thermal insulation.* Insulation maintains normal tissue temperature; this improves blood flow to the wound bed and enhances epidermal migration.[41,59]

7. *Protect the healing wound from trauma and bacterial invasion.*[59] Trauma disrupts newly formed vessels, connective tissue, and epidermis, thus delaying the healing process. Open wounds are subject to infection, which causes additional tissue destruction and delays wound healing.

Wound Assessment. Effective topical therapy is governed by the principles listed above and is based on assessment of the wound itself. Assessment parameters include wound depth, or stage, wound characteristics, and characteristics of the surrounding tissue. This is discussed in Chapter 3.

Topical Therapy: an Overview. Nurses are frequently charged with implementing an agency-wide program for prevention and management of skin breakdown. Establishment of such a program involves updating both written protocols and staff members' knowledge and beliefs regarding wound care. Although the principles of moist wound healing have been well documented for many years, the historical focus in wound care has been on the prevention of infection. This focus is the basis for wound care practices such as aggressive cleansing, nonselective use of antiseptics, air exposure, and dry dressings.[33] The belief that wounds must be kept dry to prevent infection is widespread; thus dissemination of current research findings is critical to the establishment of appropriate wound care practices.

Wound coverings have been used on wounds for a very long time and have evolved from "natural" coverings, such as feathers and leaves, to gauze, to more sophisticated dressings based on current research findings.[2] In recent years there has been a proliferation of wound dressings designed to promote moist wound healing. These dressings can be categorized as either passive or interactive. Passive dressings are those that provide wound protection and maintain a moist environment, thus facilitating the repair process. Interactive dressings represent another advance in wound coverings; these are dressings that interact with substances in the wound bed to actually *enhance* the wound-healing process.[5] Current research focuses on interactive wound products and the possibility of actively manipulating the healing process, as through topical application of wound healing factors.[24,28]

Topical Therapy: Principles, Products, and Procedures. Optimal wound management is dependent on careful wound assessment and on appropriate use of products based on wound-healing principles, as outlined above. In this section, procedures and products for wound care are discussed in light of these principles.

Wound cleansing. The goals of wound cleansing are (1) removal of bacteria and surface contaminants, such as slough, foreign bodies, purulent exudate, and (2) protection of the healing wound. Thus cleansing procedures and solutions for infected or necrotic wounds differ from those that are appropriate for clean proliferating wounds.

CLEAN PROLIFERATING WOUNDS. Guidelines for cleansing noninfected proliferating wounds include the following:

- Gentle flushing of wound surface to minimize disruption of the proliferative layer, as with a piston syringe and low force (no needle). Some practitioners recommend cleansing only the surrounding skin and leaving the wound surface undisturbed, since the film of exudate on the wound surface contains growth factors, nutrients, and proliferating cells.[2,9] Hydrotherapy, high-pressure irrigation, and mechanical scrubs are all contraindicated, since they remove the proliferative substances on the wound surface and may damage fragile new tissue.[47]
- Use of noncytotoxic solutions, such as saline solution or Pluronic F68.[46] Antiseptics commonly used in wound care (such as povidone-iodine, chlorhexidine, acetic acid, hydrogen peroxide, and hypochlorite solutions) are *contraindicated* in the management of clean proliferating wounds because they damage or destroy the cells required for tissue repair.[32,46]

INFECTED OR NECROTIC WOUNDS. Guidelines for cleansing infected, heavily contaminated, or necrotic wounds are as follows:

- Thorough irrigation of the wound surface to remove avascular debris and bacteria. Optimal irrigation force can be obtained with a 35 ml syringe and a 19-gauge needle; this maximizes bacterial removal while minimizing tissue trauma.[47] Hydrotherapy may also be used.
- Use of surfactant cleansers, or saline, *or* selective use of topical antiseptics. In making a decision regarding use of antiseptics, the nurse should be aware that antiseptics exert their effects by damaging cell membranes, and multiple studies have confirmed that commonly used antiseptics are deleterious to fibroblasts and other cells needed for wound repair. Thus their use is justified only when one is managing a heavily contaminated wound. Some practitioners argue that antiseptics are *never* indicated, since they may impair the body's own defenses against infection.[13,32,46]
- If commercial cleansers or antiseptics are used, the nurse must be knowledgeable regarding the characteristics of the individual agent so that the most appropriate agent is selected.[11,23] (See Table 2-2 for actions and considerations with commonly used antiseptics.)

Wound dressings. Effective topical therapy requires selection and application of an appropriate dressing. It must be emphasized that there is no one right dressing for each wound; rather, there is available a variety of dressings that the nurse can utilize to implement the wound healing principles discussed previously (Table 2-3). Dressing selection is focused initially on *therapeutic efficacy* and is based on wound assessment. Does the wound require débridement? Does it appear infected? Are there sinus tracts that need to be packed? How much exudate is present? *All* wounds require a moist wound surface, insulation, and protection from trauma and bacterial invasion.[23] Dressing selection also involves usage considerations, such as frequency of dressing change, ease or difficulty of dressing application, and cost or reimbursement factors.

To correctly select a dressing, the nurse must be knowledgeable of available products and appropriate utilization.[6] In this section commonly used dressings are described in

Table 2-2   Antiseptic solutions

Solution	Actions	Considerations
Hypochlorite solutions Dakin's solution Chlorpactin	Effective against *Staphylococcus, Streptococcus* Dissolves necrotic tissue Controls odors	Toxic to fibroblasts in normal dilutions Must protect intact skin around wound to prevent breakdown
Povidone-iodine preparations	Broad-spectrum effectiveness when used on intact skin or small relatively clean wounds	Toxic to fibroblasts in normal dilutions Questionable effectiveness in infected wounds May cause iodine toxicity when used in large wounds over prolonged period of time
Acetic acid	Effective against *Pseudomonas aeruginosa* in superficial wounds	Toxic to fibroblasts in standard dilutions Changes color of exudate and so may provide false assurance for elimination of infection
Hydrogen peroxide	Provides mechanical cleansing and some débridement by effervescent action	Can cause ulceration of newly formed tissue Toxic to fibroblasts Should never be used to pack sinus tracts; can cause air embolism Should not be used for forceful irrigation; can cause subcutaneous emphysema, which mimics gas gangrene

Data from Cooper D: Fundamental products and their usage. In Guide to wound care, Chicago, 1983, Hollister, Inc., and from Lineaweaver W, Howard R, Soucy D, et al: Arch Surg 120:267-270, 1985.

terms of characteristics, indications, contraindications, and guidelines for usage.

TRANSPARENT ADHESIVE DRESSINGS. Transparent adhesive dressings were the first dressings to become available to foster moist wound healing. These dressings are semipermeable membranes; they permit gaseous exchange between the wound bed and the environment but prevent bacterial invasion because of pore size. Gas permeability allows water vapor to pass from the wound surface out, which helps prevent maceration of the surrounding skin, and allows atmospheric oxygen to diffuse into the wound bed, though diffusion is limited by the volume of exudate covering the wound surface. These dressings are nonabsorptive, and so they rapidly create a fluid environment in the presence of exudate.[59] Critical clinical features, indications, contraindications, and guidelines for use are outlined in Box 2-3.

Table 2-3 Wound dressings

Dressing type	Debride	Absorb	Fill dead space	Protect from trauma	Protect from infection	Insulate	Keep moist	Examples
Transparent adhesive	+ A			+	+	+	+	OpSite, Bioclusive, Tegaderm, Polyskin, AcuDerm, Blisterfilm, Ensure-it
Hydrocolloid wafer dressings	+ A	+		+	+	+	+	DuoDerm, Restore, Intact, Intrasite, Tegasorb, Ultec, Comfeel Ulcer Dressing, Hydrapad, J&J Ulcer Dressing
Semipermeable polyurethane foam	+ A	+		+		+	+	Allevyn, Lyofoam, Synthaderm, Epilock
Absorption dressings	+ A	+	+	+			+	Bard Absorption Dressing, Hydragran, Sorbsan, Kaltostat, DuoDerm Paste and Granules, Comfeel Ulcus paste and powder, Debrisan,
Gauze	+ A*	+	+					Gauze dressings, Mesalt
Synthetic barrier dressing	+ A	+		+		+	+	Hydron
Gel dressings	+ A	+ G	+ G	+			+	Vigilon, ElastoGel, Intrasite Gel, Geliperm

A, Autolytic; *G*, granulate form.
*If kept moist.

HYDROCOLLOID WAFER DRESSINGS. Hydrocolloid wafer dressings are adhesive wafers that contain hydroactive particles. They are moldable and easy to apply and have a repellent surface.[2,59]

Most hydrocolloid dressings are occlusive; they do not permit oxygen to diffuse from the atmosphere into the wound bed. It has been well documented that a hypoxic wound bed stimulates neoangiogenesis and fibroblast proliferation so long as the wound periphery provides enough oxygen to support endothelial and fibroblast replication. In addition, the gel produced by some hydrocolloid dressings has been shown to have fibrinolytic properties; fibrin-breakdown products then act as chemoattractants for endothelial cells. Thus occlusion does not interfere with wound healing and may actually promote full-thickness repair.[5]

Occlusion has been theorized to pose increased risk of wound infection, since the environment that fosters proliferation of fibroblasts, endothelial cells, and epithelial cells may also foster growth of microorganisms. It is true that occlusive dressings are not recommended for wounds that are infected; however, recent data indicate that occlusion may actually *protect* clean wounds from secondary infection. Hutchinson reported on 70 studies of wound infections under conventional and occlusive dressings; infection rates under occlusive dressings averaged 2.6% as compared to 7.1% under conventional dressings. In addition, occlusion was associated with elimination of certain organisms, such as *Pseudomonas.* Hydrocolloid dressings were shown superior to gauze and transparent adhesive dressings in preventing secondary infection.[22]

Critical clinical features, indications, contraindications, and guidelines for use of hydrocolloid dressings are outlined in Box 2-4.

NONADHESIVE SEMIPERMEABLE POLYURETHANE FOAM DRESSINGS. These foam dressings are nonadherent wafers that have absorptive capacity and a repellent hydrophobic surface; they have limited permeability but are not totally occlusive.[2] See Box 2-5 for clinical features, indications, contraindications, and guidelines for use.

ABSORPTION DRESSINGS. The category absorption dressings includes dextranomer beads, copolymer starch dressings, and calcium alginate dressings; these dressings are designed to handle large amounts of exudate. Because they are placed *into* the wound, they also obliterate dead space.[2,23,56] Clinical features, indications, contraindications, and guidelines for use are outlined in Box 2-6.

GAUZE DRESSINGS. Gauze dressings are standard in many settings; they create a dry as opposed to a moist environment and so are contraindicated unless modified. Gauze dressings can be used very effectively to absorb exudate and to fill sinus tracts. In addition, they can be used to deliver topical agents to the wound bed. See Box 2-7 for clinical features, indications, contraindications, and guidelines for use.

GEL DRESSINGS. Gel dressings vary in composition (from about 94% water to 96% glycerin) and in form; they are available as sheet dressings and as granulates. All gel dressings help to maintain a moist wound surface.[2,59] Clinical features, indications, contraindications, and guidelines for use are outlined in Box 2-8.

SYNTHETIC BARRIER DRESSING. The synthetic barrier dressing was designed to prevent wound dehydration while providing exudate management. When mixed, it forms a paste that conforms to the wound bed and maintains a moist surface; pores in the dressing allow excess exudate to pass through for absorption by a secondary dressing. The dressing is semipermeable and nonadhesive.[23] Clinical features, indications, contraindications, and guidelines for use are listed in Box 2-9.

COMBINATION DRESSINGS. There are now available many combination dressings that

Box 2-3 TRANSPARENT ADHESIVE DRESSINGS: CRITICAL CLINICAL FEATURES

- Support autolytic débridement of wounds with dry eschar
- Help prevent infection because of hydrophobic outer surface. Studies have shown that bacteria do not penetrate the membrane; however, bacteria may migrate into the wound from the surrounding skin.[22]
- Maintain moist wound surface
- Provide some degree of insulation because of the fluid layer retained next to the wound surface
- Provides a nonadherent surface against wound bed and so does not traumatize the wound with removal; adhesives may damage fragile intact skin surrounding wound with removal

INDICATIONS FOR USE
- Partial-thickness wounds
- Dry necrotic wounds requiring débridement

CONTRAINDICATIONS TO USE
- Exudative wounds
- Wounds with sinus tracts (unless used with packing)
- Friable skin surrounding the lesion

GUIDELINES FOR USE
- Must have border of intact dry skin; shaving and defatting of skin improves seal
- Frequency of change based on exudate accumulation or loss of secure seal

Box 2-4 HYDROCOLLOID WAFER DRESSING: CRITICAL CLINICAL FEATURES

- Support autolytic débridement, especially for wounds with slough or a combination of necrosis and exudate
- Prevent secondary infection; reduce infection rates as compared to conventional dressings
- Provide limited to moderate absorption, depending on thickness and formula of specific dressing
- Maintain moist wound surface
- Provide insulation of wound
- Do not adhere to wound bed and so protect from traumatic removal; may traumatize fragile surrounding skin and so must be carefully removed

INDICATIONS FOR USE
- Partial-thickness wounds (stage II)
- Shallow full-thickness wounds (stage III). Considered the dressing of choice for venous ulcers, in conjunction with compression
- Granulating stage IV ulcers with minimal-moderate exudate

CONTRAINDICATIONS TO USE
- Heavily exudative wounds
- Wounds with undermining or sinus tracts, unless used with some type of packing
- Infected wound
- Fragile surrounding skin

GUIDELINES FOR USE
- Edges need to be secured with tape
- Frequency of change based on amount of exudate; typical frequency every 3 to 5 days. Dressing should be changed for wrinkling, or if edges loosen or dressing leaks.
- Yellowish odorous exudate is normal when dressing is removed.

Box 2-5 NONADHESIVE SEMIPERMEABLE POLYURETHANE FOAM DRESSINGS: CRITICAL CLINICAL FEATURES

- Support autolytic débridement in exudative wounds but not in dry wounds
- Provide minimal to moderate absorption of wound exudate
- Maintain moist wound surface
- Insulate wound surface
- Nonadherent surface provides atraumatic removal

INDICATIONS FOR USE

- Full-thickness wounds with moderate amounts of exudate (stage III or granulating stage IV). For wounds with depth or dead space, use with packing.
- As secondary dressing to provide additional absorption and some protection against contaminants, because of repellent surface

CONTRAINDICATIONS TO USE

- Partial-thickness wounds with no exudate
- Full-thickness wounds with dry eschar
- Wounds with sinus tracts, unless used with packing

GUIDELINES FOR USE

- May need to protect intact skin around wound from maceration with skin sealant, for example.
- Must secure wafer with elastic bandage, wrap bandage, or tape. More difficult to use in sacral area.
- Dressing change frequency is dependent on exudate; typical frequency is every 2 to 5 days.

---

combine features of the dressings already discussed. In evaluating any dressing, the nurse needs to study the clinical characteristics of the dressing to determine appropriate usage.

TOPICAL PREPARATIONS. The category topical preparations includes simple emollient preparations as well as preparations delivering active agents to the wound bed. Emollient preparations, that is, sprays, creams, and ointments, function primarily to maintain a moist wound surface; some also contain ingredients designed to enhance wound healing.[18]

Antibiotic preparations may be indicated for heavy contamination, which interferes with wound healing. The following topical antibiotics do not exert cytotoxic effects: Silvadene (silver sulfadiazine), Polysporin (polymyxin B–bacitracin), Neosporin (polymixin B sulfate–neomycin sulfate–gramicidin), benzoyl peroxide, bacitracin zinc, and J&J First Aid Cream.[2]

Liquid gel preparations must be used with moisture-retentive dressings. Some gels have been found in the laboratory setting to stimulate fibroblast activity; these preparations would be most appropriate for proliferating full-thickness wounds.[26]

All topical preparations require use of secondary dressings for absorption of exudate, obliteration of dead space, and protection of the wound bed, and most topical preparations require reapplication several times daily.

BIOLOGIC DRESSINGS. Biologic dressings include pigskin grafts and amnion dressings; these dressings are used to provide temporary wound coverage, a moist healing environment, and protection from bacterial invasion.

Box 2-6   ABSORPTION DRESSINGS: CRITICAL CLINICAL FEATURES

- Support autolytic débridement as long as moist wound surface is maintained
- Absorb large volumes of exudate, up to 20 times weight of each dressing
- Eliminate dead space
- Maintain moist wound surface when used correctly

INDICATIONS FOR USE

- Wounds with moderate to large amounts of exudate (stages III and IV)
- Wounds with sinus tracts. NOTE: Narrow sinus tracts are probably best managed with ribbon gauze packing.
- Wounds with a combination of necrosis and exudate

CONTRAINDICATIONS TO USE

- Wounds with minimal exudate. NOTE: Absorption dressings that are placed in the wound in a *moist* state may be used for wounds with minimal exudate that require packing.
- Wounds covered with dry eschar; these wounds must be debrided before a filler dressing can be used.
- Partial-thickness wounds (stage II)

GUIDELINES FOR USE

- *Copolymer starch dressings* are applied to the wound in moist form, and so they may be used for wounds with minimal exudate as well as for wounds with large amounts of exudate. They are usually changed daily; the wound is flushed and then lightly packed with the dressing.
- *Dextranomer bead dressings* are applied to the wound in dry or paste form, and so they are appropriate only for exudative wounds. The frequency of dressing change is dependent on amount of exudate but is usually once or twice a day. Tight packing of the wound is contraindicated because dressings are designed to swell with exudate.
- *Calcium alginate dressings* are applied to the wound in dry form, and so they are appropriate only for exudative wounds; if used for less exudative wounds, they should be moistened with saline. These dressings are available in standard-size dressings as well as ribbons for packing sinus tracts. They are effective for shallow exudative wounds as well as for deep wounds.[56]
- All dressings require a *cover dressing*. The cover dressing provides protection from environmental contaminants and some degree of insulation; the cover dressing should be selected based on wound location and amount of protection needed. For example, a gauze cover dressing may be sufficient for a trochanteric ulcer, whereas a sacral ulcer in an incontinent patient may require a waterproof secondary dressing such as transparent adhesive dressings or semipermeable polyurethane foam dressings with waterproof tape.

Topical Therapy: Matching Wounds to Principles and Products. The last section of this chapter addresses clinical decision making relative to topical wound care. Various types of wounds are discussed in terms of wound characteristics, wound-healing principles are applied, and appropriate dressings are identified. Wounds are categorized as full thickness with necrosis, full thickness with exudate or dead space, full thickness that are clean and proliferating, and partial thickness.

Full-thickness wounds with necrosis (Plates 10 and 11). Full-thickness wounds, as described previously, involve the subcutaneous tissue and may involve muscle or bone and joint. These wounds may involve necrotic tissue; in this case, the initial treatment goal is débridement. Débridement options and considerations are as follows:

Box 2-7   GAUZE DRESSINGS: CRITICAL CLINICAL FEATURES

- Support autolytic débridement if applied moist and kept moist
- Provide absorption of exudate
- Can be used as filler dressing to pack sinus tracts
- Must be used with appropriate solutions or gels to maintain moist wound surface

INDICATIONS FOR USE
- Exudative wounds
- Wounds with dead space or sinus tracts
- Wounds with combination of exudate and necrotic tissue

CONTRAINDICATIONS TO USE
- Partial-thickness wounds, unless used with topical agent that maintains moist wound surface
- Dry wounds covered with necrotic tissue, unless used with debriding agents or solutions

GUIDELINES FOR USE
- Mesh gauze should be used against the wound surface, as opposed to cotton-filled sponges. Fine mesh is recommended as opposed to coarse mesh because fine mesh is less likely to damage the wound with removal.
- Wounds should be packed lightly; tight packing compromises blood flow, may be painful, and delays wound closure.
- Narrow sinus tracts are best managed with narrow ribbon gauze.
- Moisturizing agents must be added to the gauze to prevent trauma and promote healing; the one exception is hypertonic saline gauze, which is intended for heavily exudative wounds and is placed into the wound dry.
- Topical agents used with gauze should be selected based on assessment of wound status; for example, noncytotoxic agents should be used for clean proliferating wounds.
- Frequency of dressing change is dependent on the amount of exudate.
- Moist gauze is placed *into* the wound but kept off the surrounding skin to prevent maceration.

- Surgical débridement is often the best option if the patient is a surgical candidate, because it is rapid and effective and may convert the chronic wound to an acute wound. Some patients are considered poor candidates because of the surgical and anesthetic risks. Laser débridement is becoming more familiar to surgeons and has advantages over surgical débridement such as instant hemostasis and sterilization of the wound. Many leg and foot lesions can be done on an outpatient basis.
- Conservative instrumental débridement involves removal of loose avascular tissue with sterile instruments; it may be done by the physician or by nurses who have been taught the procedure and have obtained institutional and physician clearance. Indications, contraindications, and guidelines are listed in Box 2-10.
- Enzymatic débridement involves use of enzymatic ointments or solutions. A physician's order is required, and manufacturers' guidelines must be carefully followed. It should be noted that enzymatic preparations are *not* active in a dry environment and are not intended for use on dry eschar. Therefore any eschar must be crosshatched with a scalpel, and the wound surface must be kept moist.[23]
- Autolysis. Autolysis refers to breakdown of necrotic tissue provided by the body's own white blood cells. Autolysis can be accomplished with use of any moisture-retentive

Box 2-8   GEL DRESSINGS: CRITICAL CLINICAL FEATURES

- Support autolytic débridement because of moisturizing effects
- Granulate form can be used to fill dead space
- Provide limited absorption of exudate
- Maintain moist wound surface
- Nonadherent surface provides atraumatic removal

INDICATIONS FOR USE

- Partial-thickness wounds, best managed with sheet form
- Full-thickness wounds, usually best managed with granulate form
- Can be used to support autolytic débridement

CONTRAINDICATIONS TO USE

- No contraindications; must match appropriate form of gel dressing to wound

GUIDELINES FOR USE

- *Granulate form* is used to lightly pack full-thickness wound. Provides minimal to moderate absorption; frequency of dressing change is dependent on the amount of exudate. Usual frequency is once or twice a day.
- *Sheet form* is most appropriate for partial-thickness wounds. Sheet gels made primarily of water can macerate the surrounding skin, and so they should be cut to fit the lesion. Frequency of dressing change is usually every other day, depending on the volume of exudate. Sheet gels made primarily of water must be monitored carefully and changed frequently enough to prevent dehydration of the dressing. When these dressings are used to support autolytic débridement of eschar, more frequent dressing changes are usually required.
- Cover dressings are selected based on the amount of protection needed.

Box 2-9   SYNTHETIC BARRIER DRESSING: CRITICAL CLINICAL FEATURES

- Provides for absorption of exudate
- Maintains moist wound surface
- Provides some degree of insulation
- Provides for atraumatic removal

INDICATIONS FOR USE

- Partial-thickness wounds, with tape or secondary dressing for security
- Full-thickness wounds with exudate

CONTRAINDICATIONS TO USE

- Wounds with dry eschar
- Wounds with sinus tracts

GUIDELINES FOR USE

- Secondary dressing is changed as needed, depending on the volume of exudate
- Synthetic barrier dressing is changed once or twice a week

Box 2-10   CONSERVATIVE INSTRUMENTAL DÉBRIDEMENT

INDICATIONS
- Dermal ulcer (pressure ulcer, diabetic ulcer, vascular ulcer) with loose necrotic tissue.

CONTRAINDICATIONS
- Densely adherent necrotic tissue when interface between viable and nonviable tissue cannot be clearly identified.
- Patient with impaired clotting mechanism and increased risk of bleeding.
- Noninfected ischemic ulcer covered with dry eschar when tissue oxygenation is insufficient to support infection control and wound healing (examples: arterial ulcers, diabetic ulcers with dry gangrene).

GUIDELINES
- Utilize sterile instruments.
- Clearly identify tissue to be removed as avascular; grasp avascular tissue and hold it taut so that line of demarcation is clearly visualized.
- Avoid all vascular structures and any structures or tissue not clearly identified as avascular.
- Utilize particular caution at periphery of wound; center of wound usually represents area of greatest depth, and periphery represents most superficial area.
- Err on the conservative side.
- Flush the wound with sterile saline after debriding.
- Control minor bleeding with pressure or silver nitrate ($AgNO_3$) sticks, or both.

---

dressing; the moist wound surface helps promote rehydration of the avascular tissue, and the wound fluid contains white blood cells and enzymes that break down the necrotic tissue.[2] The type of dressing selected is influenced by the amount of wound exudate, the presence or absence of wound infection, and the patient's immune status. Transparent adhesive dressings may be the best choice for wounds covered with dry eschar because they are nonabsorptive, rapidly create a fluid environment, and permit monitoring of the wound. Hydrocolloid dressings have been shown to be effective in providing autolysis for moist wounds with necrotic tissue; they maintain a fluid environment while absorbing excess exudate.[2] Gel dressings and moist absorption dressings also promote autolysis because they add moisture to the wound surface. If the wound is covered with dry eschar, crosshatching facilitates the autolytic process.

Time frames for autolysis vary; however, significant progress is usually seen within 96 hours.[2]
- Mechanical débridement. Wound irrigations (that is, with a syringe and needle) and hydrotherapy are beneficial in removal of loose avascular tissue. Hydrotherapy is advantageous with large gaping wounds but commonly dehydrates the skin.

Full-thickness wounds with exudate or dead space (Plates 12 and 13). Full-thickness wounds with exudate or dead space require packing for obliteration of the dead space or sinus tracts, absorption of excess exudate, elimination of any infection, maintenance of a moist wound surface, insulation, and protection. The nurse must first assess for signs of infection and obtain a culture if indicated. Dressing options include:
- Synthetic absorption dressings (copolymer starch dressings, dextranomer beads, calci-

um alginate dressings, and absorptive pastes, powders, or granules).
- Gauze moistened with appropriate solution or gel and lightly packed into the wound. Clean wounds should be managed with noncytotoxic solutions; if antiseptics are used for infected wounds, they should be discontinued as soon as the wound is clean.
- Secondary dressing based on amount of protection needed.

Full-thickness wounds that are clean and proliferating (Plates 12 and 13). These wounds have no necrotic tissue, no infection, minimal or no dead space, and minimal to moderate amounts of exudate. They require variable amounts of absorption, maintenance of a moist wound surface, insulation, and protection. Dressing options include:
- Absorption dressing, that is, synthetic absorption dressing or gauze dressings with noncytotoxic solutions or gels. As exudate decreases, only *moist* absorption dressings should be used to prevent desiccation and trauma.
- Hydrocolloid dressings, with the addition of pastes, granules, or powders if additional absorption is needed.
- Semipermeable polyurethane foam dressings, with the addition of pastes, granules, or powders if additional absorption is needed.
- Granulate gel dressings.
- Synthetic barrier dressing.

Partial-thickness wounds (Plate 7). Partial-thickness wounds are superficial and primarily require maintenance of a moist wound surface, insulation, and protection, with absorption of minimal to moderate amounts of exudate. Appropriate dressings include:
- Hydrocolloid dressings.
- Transparent adhesive dressings.
- Sheet form of gel dressings.
- Synthetic barrier dressing.
- Emollient dressings with nonadherent secondary dressing.

Decision Making Regarding Topical Therapy. In selecting a dressing for a particular wound, the nurse must assess the wound, determine its needs in terms of the principles for topical therapy, and then identify dressings that are therapeutically appropriate. The decision regarding *which* of the appropriate dressings to use is based on practical considerations such as frequency of dressing change, difficulty of dressing change procedure, cost, and reimbursement. The challenge is to optimize the healing environment while minimizing cost and time expenditures.

Wound management is an evolving discipline. Research is ongoing, and new products are developed in response to research findings. In addition, new knowledge regarding efficacy of existing products permits the informed nurse to make ever better clinical decisions regarding wound management. Product decisions should always be made on the basis of current knowledge and research results; thus the nurse involved in wound management must carefully review current publications and product literature and must remain open to new ideas and new developments.

Wound Management: Additional Options. This discussion has focused on conservative wound management, that is, nursing interventions and topical therapy that promote wound healing. Some patients will benefit from more aggressive therapy, such as surgical intervention, hyperbaric oxygen, electrical stimulation, or topical application of wound-healing factors. The nurse should remain constantly aware of these alternatives and should make appropriate referrals for patients who may benefit from these treatment modalities. These treatment options are discussed in later chapters.

It should be noted that some patients should be promptly referred for surgical evaluation, even if their wounds seem to be progressing well with conservative therapy. These are the patients with full-thickness breakdown over bony prominences who will be at high risk for repeat breakdown, such as a paraplegic who is wheelchair bound and who has ischial ulcers. Healing by secondary intention will produce a bony prominence covered with scar tissue, which is *less* resistant to breakdown than the original tissue. This patient would probably benefit from a flap procedure in which the bony prominence is shaved (if indicated) and well-vascularized muscle is rotated into the defect to cover the bony prominence.[31,55]

SUMMARY

A frequently asked question in wound care is, "What should I do if the wound doesn't progress? Should I select another dressing?" The answer to this question provides an excellent summary for this chapter. The nurse must always remember that wound healing occurs from the *inside out;* that is, it is a systemic process. If the wound fails to heal, the nurse must reassess the management plan in terms of:

- Causative factors. Have the etiologic factors been identified and controlled?
- Systemic (host) factors. Is tissue perfusion adequate in the area? Is the patient hypoxic? Is the patient malnourished? Is the patient on steroids? These factors *must* be controlled if healing is to occur.
- Local (wound environment) factors. Is topical therapy appropriate? Is the wound free of necrotic tissue? Has infection been ruled out? (Occult infection is a common cause of failure to heal.[1]) Is excess exudate being absorbed? Is the wound bed moist and protected? So long as topical therapy is principle-and-research based, it is appropriate. The nurse must remember that it is not the *dressing* that heals the wound; rather, the wound heals by a systemic process that is facilitated by an appropriate local environment. Thus it is inappropriate to constantly modify topical therapy; modifications are indicated only when assessment indicates that the wound characteristics have changed and that a different dressing will better meet the wound's changing needs.

In summary, the nurse must remember what topical therapy can and cannot do. It *can* promote healing by providing a favorable local environment; it *cannot* compensate for an underlying pathologic condition or host deficiencies. To effectively manage wounds, the nurse must always address all three priorities: causative factors, host factors affecting wound repair, and topical therapy.

SELF-EVALUATION

QUESTIONS AND PROBLEMS

1. Explain why wounds confined to the epidermal and dermal layers heal by regeneration, whereas wounds extending *through* the dermal layer into the subcutaneous tissue or fascia or muscle layer must heal by scar formation.
2. Explain what is meant by primary, secondary, and tertiary intentions.
3. Identify the major components of partial-thickness repair.
4. Explain why epidermal resurfacing and dermal repair proceed more rapidly when the wound surface is kept moist.
5. List the three major phases of full-thickness wound repair (in order).
6. Which of the following appear to be the principal mediators for full-thickness wound repair?
   a. Endothelial cells and fibroblasts
   b. Neutrophils and platelets
   c. Fibroblasts and neutrophils
   d. Platelets and macrophages
7. Describe the defensive (inflammatory) phase of full-thickness wound healing to include key events, mediating cells, result, and wound appearance.
8. Differentiate between the terms "granulation" and "epithelialization."
9. Explain the significance of the fibroblast in wound healing.
10. It is well known that adequate tissue perfusion and oxygenation are required for wound healing, yet recent research into occlusive dressings has indicated that hypoxia is the stimulus that turns wound healing on and off. Explain how both hypoxia and oxygenation can be critical to the repair process.
11. Contraction plays an important role in wound healing for:
    a. wounds healing by primary intention.
    b. wounds healing by secondary intention.
    c. superficial abrasions.
    d. all wounds.
12. Explain why large wounds healing by secondary intention may require skin grafting, whereas large partial-thickness wounds will epithelialize.
13. Identify the two components of the maturation phase and the desired outcome.
14. Identify two factors that may explain why chronic wounds are "indolent" as compared to acute wounds.
15. List at least six factors that affect wound healing.
16. Identify key nutrients needed for wound repair.
17. Which of the following reports indicates wound infection?
    a. Colony count of more than 10,000 organisms/ml
    b. Colony count of more than 50,000 organisms/ml
    c. Colony count of more than 100,000 organisms/ml
    d. Colony count of more than 1,000,000 organisms/ml
18. Identify indications and guidelines for wound culture.
19. Explain why vitamin A may be indicated for the patient on corticosteroids.
20. Identify three priorities for effective wound management.
21. Identify seven principles for appropriate topical therapy, and briefly state the rationale.

22. Compare and contrast appropriate cleansing techniques and solutions for noninfected proliferating wounds versus infected or necrotic wounds.
23. Explain why many commonly used antiseptics are *contraindicated* for use in proliferating wounds.
24. Occlusion promotes wound infection.
    True
    False
25. Identify management and dressing options for each of the following:
    a. Full-thickness wounds with necrosis
    b. Full-thickness wounds with exudate or dead space, or both
    c. Full-thickness wounds that are clean and proliferating
    d. Partial-thickness wounds

SELF-EVALUATION

ANSWERS

1. Wounds involving only the epidermis and dermis heal relatively quickly because epithelial, endothelial, and connective tissue can be reproduced. Wounds extending through the dermis and involving deeper structures must heal by scar formation because the deep dermal structures, subcutaneous tissue, and muscle do not regenerate.
2. Wounds that are well approximated with minimal tissue defect are said to heal by primary intention.
   Wounds that are left open and allowed to heal by production of granulation tissue are said to heal by secondary intention.
   Wounds are said to heal by tertiary intention when there is a delay between injury and closure.
3. Brief inflammatory response
   Epithelial proliferation and migration (resurfacing)
   Reestablishment of epidermal layers
   If dermis involved, connective tissue repair proceeds concurrently with reepithelialization.
4. A moist wound surface facilitates epidermal migration because epidermal cells can migrate only across a moist surface; in a dry wound, epidermal cells must tunnel down to a moist level and must secrete collagenase to lift the scab away from the wound surface in order to migrate.
   Connective tissue repair begins earlier when the wound surface is kept moist because new connective tissue forms only in the presence of suitable exudate.
5. Defensive (inflammatory) phase
   Proliferative (fibroblastic) phase
   Maturation phase
6. d
7. Key events are (1) hemostasis, mediated by clotting factors and platelets, and (2) inflammation, mediated by neutrophils and macrophages. The overall result of this phase is control of bleeding and establishment of a clean wound bed.
   Characteristics of wounds in the inflammatory phase are erythema, edema, pain, and exudate.

8. Granulation refers to the formation of new connective tissue (scar tissue) to *fill* a defect and involves neoangiogenesis and collagen synthesis. Granulation tissue appears very red, moist, and granular. Epithelialization refers to the migration of epithelial cells to *resurface* a defect. New epithelial tissue initially appears pink and dry and then gradually repigments to match the person's skin tone.

9. The fibroblast synthesizes the new connective tissue that fills the defect; wound healing cannot take place without normal fibroblast function.

10. The hypoxia resulting from disruption of vascular pathways creates an oxygen "gradient" between the vascularized periphery of the wound and its hypoxic center; this gradient stimulates capillary proliferation. Hypoxia also stimulates the release of angiogenesis factors by macrophages, which "attract" endothelial cells. Hypoxia also results in lactate production, which stimulates fibroblasts to synthesize collagen.

    Thus hypoxia in the wound center helps to *drive* tissue repair.

    Oxygen is required for cellular proliferation and migration and for immune system function. Therefore the ability to *respond* to the hypoxic stimulus with capillary proliferation, the ability to synthesize collagen, and the ability to control bacterial proliferation are all dependent on adequate oxygen levels at the advancing wound edge.

11. b

12. There is a limit to epidermal cell migration, and in full-thickness wounds epidermal cells are present only at the wound margins. In partial-thickness wounds, epidermal cells are present in the lining of the hair follicles and sweat glands as well as the wound periphery.

13. The two components are collagen lysis and collagen synthesis. The desired outcome is a well-organized scar with maximum tensile strength (80% that of nonwounded tissue).

14. They are likely to begin with circulatory compromise, as opposed to injury. Injury initiates hemostasis, which triggers the wound-healing cascade; circulatory compromise does not trigger the wound-healing cascade.

    They frequently occur in compromised hosts.

15. Tissue perfusion and oxygenation
    Nutritional status
    Infection
    Diabetes mellitus
    Corticosteroid administration
    Immunosuppression
    Aging
    Systemic factors include renal or hepatic disease, malignancy, sepsis, hematopoietic abnormalities, sleep, and stress
    Topical therapy

16. Proteins
    Calories
    Vitamins C, A, and B complex
    Iron, copper, and zinc

17. c

18. *Indications:*
   Signs of local infection
   Signs of systemic infection
   Bone involvement
   Nonhealing wound
   Guidelines:
   Wounds with necrosis or sinus tracts: aerobic and anaerobic cultures
   Open viable wounds: aerobic culture only
   Flush wound with saline
   Use calcium alginate swab
   Swab wound edges and wound base
   Transport to laboratory promptly
19. Vitamin A partially counteracts the adverse effects of steroids on wound healing.
20. Elimination or control of causative factors
   Provision of systemic support
   Appropriate topical therapy
21. Remove necrotic tissue; necrosis serves as a medium for bacterial growth and prolongs the inflammatory phase.
   Identify and eliminate infection; infection prolongs the inflammatory phase, delays collagen synthesis and epidermal migration, and induces additional tissue damage.
   Obliterate dead space; dead space provides a fluid medium for bacterial growth and contributes to abscess formation. In granulating wounds, dead space poses a risk of premature closure over a fluid-filled defect.
   Absorb excess exudate; excessive exudate can macerate the surrounding skin and dilute the wound healing factors and nutrients at the wound surface.
   Maintain a moist wound surface to prevent desiccation and cell death and to enhance cellular migration.
   Provide thermal insulation to enhance blood flow and epidermal migration.
   Protect the healing wound from trauma and bacterial invasion.
22. Clean proliferating wounds by gently flushing with *noncytotoxic* solutions to *minimize* disruption of wound surface.
   For infected and necrotic wounds, thoroughly irrigate using a 35 ml syringe with a 19-gauge needle; use surfactant cleansers or saline *or* selectively use antiseptics to remove bacteria and avascular debris from wound surface.
23. They are cytotoxic, damaging fibroblasts and other cells critical to the repair process.
24. False
25. *Full-thickness wounds with necrosis*
   Surgical débridement
   Conservative instrumental débridement
   Enzymatic débridement
   Autolysis: using moisture-retentive dressings, such as transparent adhesive dressings or gel dressings for dry eschar, hydrocolloid dressings or moist absorption dressings for moist wounds with necrosis.
   Full-thickness wounds with exudate or dead space, or both
   Absorption dressings

Gauze moistened with appropriate solution or gel
Secondary dressing selected based on amount of protection needed
Full-thickness wounds that are clean and proliferating
Absorption dressings
Hydrocolloid dressings
Semipermeable polyurethane foam dressings
Granulate gel dressings
Synthetic barrier dressing
Partial-thickness wounds
Hydrocolloid dressings
Transparent adhesive dressings
Sheet form of gel dressings
Synthetic barrier dressing
Emollient dressing with nonadherent secondary dressing

REFERENCES

1. Alvarez O: Controversies in wound management, Presented at Southeast Region IAET (International Association for Enterostomal Therapy) Conference, Charleston, SC, Nov 9, 1989.
2. Alvarez O, Rozint J, and Wiseman D: Moist environment: matching the dressing to the wound, Wounds 1(1):35-51, 1989.
3. Baxter C and Mertz P: Local factors that affect wound healing. In Eaglstein W, Baxter C, Mertz P, et al, editors: New directions in wound healing, Princeton, NJ, 1990, ER Squibb & Sons.
4. Baxter C and Rodeheaver G: Wound assessment and categorization. In Eaglstein W, Baxter C, Mertz P, et al, editors: New directions in wound healing, Princeton, NJ, 1990, ER Squibb & Sons.
5. Bolton L, Pirone L, Chen J, and Lydon M: Dressings' effects on wound healing, Wounds 2(4):126-134, 1990.
6. Braden BJ and Bryant R: Innovations to prevent and treat pressure ulcers, Geriatr Nurs 11(4):182-186, 1990.
7. Bryant R: Wound repair: a review, J Enterostom Ther 14: 262-266, 1987.
8. Caldwell MD and Kennedy-Caldwell C: Micronutrients and enteral nutrition. In Rombeau JL and Caldwell MD, editors: Enteral and tube feeding, vol 1, Philadelphia, 1984, WB Saunders Co.
9. Carpenter R: The microenvironment of the healing wound, Presented at International Association for Enterostomal Therapy annual conference, Washington, DC, June 10, 1989.
10. Clark R: Overview and general considerations of wound repair. In Clark R and Henson P, editors: The molecular and cellular biology of wound repair, New York, 1988, Plenum Press.
11. Cooper D: Fundamental products and their usage. In Cooper D, Watt R, and Alterescu V (major contributors): Guide to wound care, Chicago, 1983, Hollister, Inc.
12. Cuono C: Physiology of wound healing. In Dagher F, editor: Cutaneous wounds, Mt. Kisco, NY, 1985, Futura Publishing Co.
13. Duncan J, White A, Wood B, and Moore E: Physical and physiological properties of an effective wound cleanser, monograph, Irving, Texas, 1989, Carrington Laboratories.
14. Ebersole P and Hess P: Toward healthy aging: human needs and nursing response, ed 3, St. Louis, 1990, Mosby–Year Book, Inc.
15. Garrigues N: Pressure ulcers, Curr Concepts Wound Care 10(1):4-10, 1987.
16. Giorilla C and Bevil CW: Nursing care of the aging client: promoting healthy adaptation, Norwalk, Conn, 1985, Appleton-Century-Crofts.
17. Goodson WH and Hunt TK: Wound healing. In Kinney JM, Jeejeebhoy KN, Hill GL, and Owen OE, editors: Nutrition and metabolism in patient care, Philadelphia, 1988, WB Saunders Co.
18. Guthrie M, Diakiw J, Zaydon A, et al: A randomized double-blind clinical study of Dermagran Dual Therapeutic System in the treatment of decubitus ulcers, Wounds 1(3):142-154, 1989.
19. Harding K: Wound care: putting theory into clinical practice, Wounds 2(1):21-32, 1990.

20. Hunt TK: The physiology of wound healing, Ann Emerg Med 17(12):2-10, 1988.

21. Hunt TK and Van Winkle W Jr: Normal repair. In Hunt TK and Dunphy JE, editors: Fundamentals of wound management, New York, 1979, Appleton-Century-Crofts.

22. Hutchinson J: Prevalence of wound infection under occlusive dressings: a collective survey of reported research, Wounds 1(2):123-133, 1989.

23. International Association for Enterostomal Therapy: Standards of care for dermal wounds: pressure ulcers, revised ed, Irvine, Calif, 1991, IAET.

24. Jackson D and Rovee D: Current concepts in wound healing; research and theory, J Enterostom Ther 15(3):133-137, 1988.

25. Jeejeebhoy KN: Nutrient metabolism. In Kinney JM, Jeejeebhoy KN, Hill GL, and Owen OE, editors: Nutrition and metabolism in patient care, Philadelphia, 1988, WB Saunders Co.

26. Johnson A, White A, and McAnalley B: Comparison of comomon topical agents for wound treatment: cytotoxicity for human fibroblasts in culture, Wounds 1(3):186-192, 1989.

27. Kligman A: Skin care of the nursing home resident, monograph, New Brunswick, NJ 1985, Johnson & Johnson.

28. Knighton D, Fiegel V, Doucette M, et al: The use of topically applied platelet growth factors in chronic nonhealing wounds: a review, Wounds 1(1):71-78, 1989.

29. Lang CE and Schulte CV: The adult patient. In Lang CE, editor: Nutritional support in critical care, Rockville, Md, 1987, Aspen Publishers, Inc.

30. Lee KA and Stotts NA: Support of the growth hormone–somatomedin system to facilitate healing, Heart Lung 19(2):157-163, 1990.

31. Linder R and Morris D: The surgical management of pressure ulcers: a systematic approach based on staging, Decubitus 3(2):32-38, 1990.

32. Lineaweaver W, Howard R, Soucy D, et al: Topical antimicrobial toxicity, Arch Surg 120:267-270, March 1985.

33. Maibach H and Rovee D, editors: Epidermal wound healing, Chicago, 1971, Mosby–Year Book, pp 4 to 42.

34. Marzella L, Sengottuvelu S, Mason P, and Myers R: Mechanisms of impaired cutaneous wound healing in obese diabetic mice, Wounds 2(4):135-147, 1990.

35. McAnaw M, Troyer-Caudle J, Heath P, et al: Development of a multidisciplinary dysvascular and insensitive foot clinic, Wounds 2(1):7-17, 1990.

36. McCarthy JB, Sas DF, and Furcht LT: Mechanisms of parenchymal cell migration into wounds. In Clark R and Henson P, editors: The molecular and cellular biology of wound repair, New York, 1988, Plenum Press.

37. McPherson J and Piez K: Collagen in dermal wound repair. In Clark R and Henson P, editors: The molecular and cellular biology of wound repair, New York, 1988, Plenum Press.

38. Munro HN: Aging. In Kinney JM, Jeejeebhoy KN, Hill GL, and Owen OE, editors: Nutrition and metabolism in patient care, Philadelphia, 1988, WB Saunders Co.

39. National Pressure Ulcer Advisory Panel: Pressure ulcers: prevalence, cost, and risk assessment, Consensus Development Conference Statement, Decubitus 2:24-28, 1989.

40. Phillips G and Knighton D: Skeletal muscle regenerates, Wounds 2(2):82-94, 1990.

41. Pollack S: Wound healing: a review. II. Environmental factors affecting wound healing, J Enterostom Ther 9:14-16, 35, 1982.

42. Pollack S: Wound healing: a review. I. The biology of wound healing, J Enterostom Ther 8(6):16-21, 39, 1981.

43. Rabkin J and Hunt T: Infection and oxygen. In Davis J and Hunt T, editors: Problem wounds: the role of oxygen, New York, 1988, Elsevier Science Publishing Co.

44. Riches D: The multiple roles of macrophages in wound healing. In Clark R and Henson P, editors: The molecular and cellular biology of wound repair, New York, 1988, Plenum Press.

45. Robson MC: Disturbances of wound healing, Ann Emerg Med 17(12):1274-1278, 1988.

46. Rodeheaver G: Controversies in topical wound managment, Wounds 1(1):19-34, 1989.

47. Rogness H: High-pressure wound irrigation, J Enterostom Ther 12:27-28, 1985.

48. Rudolph R: Natural wound healing process. In Rudolph R and Noe JM, editors: Chronic problem wounds, Boston, 1983, Little, Brown & Co.

49. Rudolph R: Ulcers in patients taking glucocorticoids (steroids). In Rudolph R and Noe JM, editors, Chronic problem wounds, Boston 1983, Little, Brown & Co.

50. Salzberg C, Gray B, Petro J, and Salisbury R: The perioperative antimicrobial management of pressure ulcers, Decubitus 3(2):24-26, 1990.

51. Selivanov V and Sheldon GF: Enteral nutrition and sepsis. In Rombeau JL and Caldwell MD, editors: Enteral and tube feeding, vol 1, Philadelphia, 1984, WB Saunders Co.

52. Shack R and Manson P: Traumatic wounds. In Dagher F, editor: Cutaneous wounds, Mt. Kisco, NY, 1985, Futura Publishing Co.

53. Silane M and Oot-Giromini B: Systemic and other factors that affect wound healing. In Eaglstein W, Baxter C, Mertz P, et al, editors: New directions in wound healing, Princeton, NJ, 1990, ER Squibb & Sons.

54. Stein TP and Levine GM; Human macronutrient requirements. In Rombeau JL and Caldwell MD, editors: Enteral and tube feeding, vol 1, Philadelphia, 1984, WB Saunders Co.

55. Steuber K and Spence R: Pressure sores. In Dagher F, editor: Cutaneous wounds, Mt. Kisco, NY, 1985, Futura Publishing Co.

56. Tintle T and Jeter K: Early experience with a calcium alginate dressing, Ostomy/Wound Management 28:74-81, May-June 1990.

57. Tonnesen M, Worthen GS, and Johnston R: Neutrophil emigration, activation, and tissue damage. In Clark R and Henson P, editors: The molecular and cellular biology of wound repair, New York, 1988, Plenum Press.

58. Turner-Beatty M, Grotewiel M, Fosha-Dolezal S, et al: Biochemical and histologic changes due to moisturization during wound healing, Wounds 2(4):156-161, 1990.

59. Turner T: Semiocclusive and occlusive dressings. In Ryan T, editor: An environment for healing: the role of occlusion, London, 1985, The Royal Society of Medicine.

60. Whitney J: Physiologic effects of tissue oxygenation on wound healing, Heart Lung 18(5):466-476, 1989.

61. Winter G: Epidermal regeneration studied in the domestic pig. In Hunt TK and Dunphy JE, editors: Fundamentals of wound management, New York, 1979, Appleton-Century-Crofts.

62. Wysocki A: Surgical wound healing: a review for perioperative nurses, AORN J 49(2):502-518, 1989.

3 Wound Assessment and Evaluation of Healing

DIANE M. COOPER

OBJECTIVES

1. Describe four methods of categorizing wound evaluation instruments and include two examples of each category.
2. State the definition of each stage of tissue loss in the classification system proposed by the IAET and NPUAP.
3. Differentiate between partial thickness and full thickness.
4. Describe at least three advantages and disadvantages of each category of wound evaluation instruments.
5. Identify the indication for using two-dimensional measures and three-dimensional measures.
6. Describe four methods of two-dimensional and three-dimensional measures.
7. Describe 11 macroscopic indices of healing.
8. Discuss recommendations for the frequency of documenting wound status.
9. Describe the limitations of the current status of wound assessment modalities.
10. Identify five conditions that are necessary before a systematic approach for the evaluation of wound healing can be developed.

Accurate and regular assessments of the wound and surrounding skin should be critical underpinnings of any wound care plan. These assessments need to drive treatment decisions (that is, type of dressing, method of débridement, and frequency of dressing change). Such wound assessments should also provide the base-line data from which one could evaluate the repair that has occurred within the wound, thus, again, influencing the treatment decisions.

Unfortunately the reality is that most clinicians do not make regular systematic wound assessments. When regular assessments are obtained, they are largely subjective and have poor reliability (that is, consistency between clinicians when repeated over time) and validity (that is, actually measure what they propose to measure). As a result, our ability to track or monitor tissue healing objectively is severely curtailed.

This chapter (1) describes the instruments currently available for assessing wound status clinically and evaluating the process of healing, (2) describes some of the readily identifiable macroscopic indices of healing, (3) suggests documentation guidelines, and (4) presents recommendations for the future of clinical assessment and measurement of wounds.

WOUND EVALUATION

The longer and more intently one cares for human wounds, the more complex the concept "wound" becomes. Wounds can be divided, as they are throughout this book, into acute and chronic states. Wounds can be further classified according to cause (such as venous ulcer, pressure ulcer, arterial ulcer), depth (partial thickness or full thickness), closure (approximated or open), and other characteristics. Because wounds are complex phenomena, it would be naïve to believe that ultimately, or optimally, a single approach to wound evaluation for all types of wounds is appropriate. Actually, few pathologic conditions are evaluated with a single instrument or parameter. In fact, the more intricate the process, such as congestive heart failure, the more clinicians rely on several measures (such as radiologic examination, physical examination, pulse, and hematocrit) to capture accurately the extent of the condition.

In recognition of the complexity of the healing process as well as the uniqueness of various types of wounds, evaluation of wound status and healing, once viewed as basic and easy to accomplish, is being exposed for its inherent difficulty and demand for rigor. Therefore the clinician should be familiar with the strengths and limitations of several methods currently available to assess wound status. In addition, the clinician must develop an appreciation for the need to use a combination of evaluative modalities that would allow one to evaluate wound status accurately and infer the quality of repair in relation to the normal healing trajectory.

Unfortunately, reliable and valid instruments to measure clinically the reparative process are currently lacking. Ideally, such instruments should be clinically useful and theory based and provide a mechanism that systematically and objectively monitors the status of tissue healing. This paucity of valid wound healing assessment tools can be attributed to several factors[9]; three factors are particularly relevant for nursing. First, the importance of nursing interventions in supporting wound healing has been clearly articulated relatively recently. Levine has described healing activities as being "central" to nursing practice.[33-36] This recognition has facilitated a more active rather than a passive approach to wound management by nurses. Before this heightened awareness of the impact of nursing interventions on wound repair, the inadequacy of wound evaluation was not fully appreciated. Nurses are now struggling with the need for terms and tools to use to accurately evaluate wounds and the healing process.[10,11] Second, despite the recent explosion in scientific or basic science-related knowledge regarding the intricacies of the healing process, little agreement exists, even among noted authorities, about which indices of wound healing are most appropriate to evaluate clinically. Finally, and perhaps most germane, many clinicians lack adequate knowledge regarding the science of instrument development, most particularly the development of valid and reliable, clinically useful instruments.[49]

Table 3-1   Schema of noninvasive instruments for clinical evaluation of wound status and healing

Category	Instrument	Goal
Prediction	Norton scale	Pressure ulcer risk
	Gosnell scale	Pressure ulcer risk
	Braden scale	Pressure ulcer risk
	SENIC	Risk of postoperative infection
Classification	Red, Yellow, Black	Describe wound status
	Wound Severity Score	Describe wound status
	Wells incisional category	Grades incision
	Staging	Level of tissue damage
	Burn area	Amount of tissue injured
Measurement	Linear	Area of wound and contraction
	Photography	Area of wound and contraction
	Wound tracings	Area of wound and contraction
	Planimetry	Area of wound and contraction
	Kundin Wound Gauge	Area of wound and contraction
	Molds	Area of wound and contraction
	Foam	Area and contraction
	Water instillation	Area and contraction
Assessment of wound status	Red, Yellow, Black	Describe surface tissue status
	Wound Assessment Inventory	Assess inflammation
	Wound Characteristics Instrument	Assess essential wound characteristics

Despite this set of circumstances, there are several ways to cluster currently available approaches to the evaluation of tissue repair: invasive and noninvasive instruments, research-appropriate instruments, clinically "user-friendly" approaches, instruments that provide readily usable information, and those that require skillful interpretation of the data obtained. However, the clinically based practitioner needs readily usable tools to measure the complex wound repair process. Furthermore, these tools need to provide theoretically based information so that appropriate and timely interventions can be derived. Therefore this chapter focuses on the clinically useful yet noninvasive approaches to the assessment of wound status.

Most instruments appropriate for evaluating wounds noninvasively in the clinical setting can be clustered under four broad categories: (1) prediction of wound development, (2) classification of existing wound, (3) measurement of existing wound, and (4) assessment of wound status (Table 3-1).

Prediction of Wound Development

Instruments have been developed to be used to determine a patient's risk for developing a wound, specifically a pressure ulcer. Such tools include the Norton scale,[40,41] Gosnell

---

Box 3-1   STAGING SYSTEMS FOR BREAKDOWN*

STAGE 1
Nonblanchable erythema of intact skin; the
heralding lesion of skin ulceration

STAGE 2
Partial-thickness skin loss involving epidermis
or dermis, or both. The ulcer is superficial
and presents clinically as an abrasion,
blister, or shallow crater.

STAGE 3
Full-thickness skin loss involving damage or
necrosis of subcutaneous tissue, which may
extend down to but not through underlying

fascia. The ulcer presents clinically as a deep
crater with or without undermining of
adjacent tissue.

STAGE 4
Full-thickness skin loss with extensive
destruction, tissue necrosis, or damage to
muscle bone or supporting structures (such
as tendon, joint capsule)

NOTE: If the wound involves necrotic tissue,
staging cannot be confirmed until the wound
base is viable.

---

*Intervention may prevent progression; or a stage 1 lesion may be the first clinical indicator of deep tissue damage, which is irreversible.

scale, [21,22] and Braden scale[2,3,6] and are discussed in detail in Chapter 5. Although more commonly associated with risk assessment, many of the parameters measured by these tools are pertinent to impaired wound healing and can therefore provide data regarding a patient's healing potential, should a wound occur. A patient's risk for developing a surgical wound infection can also be anticipated with instruments as described by Haley and colleagues.[24]

Classification of Wounds

Several methods exist to classify wounds.[15,18,29,39,42,50] Such classification can be done according to the involved tissue layers or the color of the wound bed. Unfortunately, many inconsistencies exist in the terminology of the classification systems, creating confusion among practitioners; validity and reliability data are also lacking for most of these tools.

Tissue Layers

Staging. Shea [47] first described a method for classifying wounds according to tissue layers. This has subsequently been modified.[23,28,29,39,42] Consequently, much confusion currently exists about staging systems between institutions and clinicians. Some of these instruments are designed for specific ulcers such as pressure or diabetic ulcers.

A four-stage classification scheme has been advanced by the International Association of Enterostomal Therapy, Inc (1986)[28] and National Pressure Ulcer Advisory Panel (1989)[39] as described in Box 3-1. Although this system is often used in connection with pressure-induced ulcers, it can be used with wounds of any cause.

Accurate staging requires knowledge of the anatomy of skin and deeper tissue layers, the ability to recognize these tissues, and the ability to differentiate between these tissues. Careful evaluation of the wound bed facilitates accurate staging. Staging wounds is a complex skill that takes time to develop; it is often easier, more accurate, and more reliable for novice wound care clinicians to describe the wound according to other macroscopic observations while learning to recognize the specific tissue layers.

Although staging terms describe the type of tissue involved, additional important wound characteristics are not revealed, such as depth of the wound, topography of the wound, exudate, condition of the wound bed, and condition of the surrounding skin. Furthermore, because the staging system is based upon recognition of the predominant wound bed tissue such as dermis, epidermis, muscle, or tendon, a wound that is healing optimally may manifest tissue that is difficult to classify. Therefore it is unclear how to stage a healing wound where granulation tissue, scar tissue, or both, have filled the wound bed. It is also important to remember that because the staging system is based upon the ability to assess the type of tissue in the wound bed, a wound bed covered with necrotic tissue cannot be accurately staged. In such situations, staging must be deferred. Despite these flaws, staging tissue layers does provide (1) increased uniformity of language and (2) a beginning basis for evaluation of protocols. Nurses need to adopt agreed-upon terms and discontinue use of many differing categories. Of course, reliability and validity studies are also needed for these staging systems. Plates 7, 8, 12, 14, 15, and 18 are examples of each stage of ulcer.

Partial thickness versus full thickness. The terms "partial-thickness" and "full-thickness wounds" can also be used to describe the extent of tissue damage. These terms pertain strictly to the amount of true skin injured. For example, a full-thickness wound indicates that the dermis and epidermis have been damaged; tissue loss extends below the dermis (Plates 8 and 13). Wound repair then will occur by neovascularization, fibroplasia, and contraction. A partial-thickness wound is confined to the skin layers; damage does not penetrate below the dermis and may in fact be limited to the epidermal layers only (Plates 2 and 7). These wounds heal by reepithelialization primarily.

Unfortunately, "partial thickness" and "full thickness" are imprecise terms when describing the specific type of tissue present in the wound bed. For example, a full-thickness wound may expose subcutaneous tissue, muscle, tendon, or bone. Furthermore these terms fail to convey the depth of the wound, the condition of the surrounding skin, presence of exudate, and the topography. Partial-thickness and full-thickness terminology is more commonly utilized in burn therapy. (Burn wounds are not addressed in this text.)

Color. The Red, Yellow, Black (RYB)[15] color concept is another suggested wound classification method. This technique directs the clinician to assess the surface of the open wound (regardless of origin) and to categorize it as falling within one of the three color categories. The red wound is viewed as healthy, whereas the black wound is obviously worrisome. The yellow wound lies somewhere in between, with the goal of therapy being the removal of the yellow surface and exposure of the underlying healthy red tissue. This system was developed originally by industry and has not undergone testing for reliability and validity.

Although the system is salutory in that it offers clinicians clear categories by which to classify wounds, directs them to look at wounds more closely, and focuses them toward a system of treatment, it also has the potential of oversimplifying the complexity of the healing process. To encourage clinicians to think that healing can be evaluated by a single variable is, in many ways, to trivialize the healing process.

Additionally, because of the ease with which clinicians can assess wounds using this system, it erroneously allows some to believe they have fully assessed a wound as a result of making a single observation. Finally, the conclusion that all red wounds are healthy should be rejected; healthy and unhealthy shades of red exists. The RYB system should not be considered to be an adequate evaluation of the status of a wound. Certainly, incorporation of the color concept into a system where other essential manifestations of wound healing were present would be of value in wound assessment.

Measurement of Wounds

Many of the current approaches to wound evaluation commonly focus on wound measurement and may involve either two-dimensional or three-dimensional measurements.

Two-Dimensional Measurements. In clinical practice, two-dimensional measurements are one of the simplest and most widely used approaches to wound measurement. Linear measurement, wound tracings, and wound photographs are examples of commonly used two-dimensional measurements. Unfortunately, these types of measures used in isolation do not provide information about the depth of a wound. Planimetry may be used with wound tracings or wound photographs to document the surface area of shallow wounds and wounds with depth.

Linear measurements. Increasingly, clinicians have begun to routinely record the size of the wound or extent of tissue injury by measuring the involved area. Although in most cases these measurements are imprecise, linear measurements do provide an objective basis for evaluating the overall dimensions of a wound. Paper or plastic rulers can be used and are commercially available from many companies. Measurements, recorded in centimeters or millimeters, should describe the length and width of an open wound and the extent of ecchymosis or erythema surrounding the wound. Such measurements are inexpensive, readily available, and easily accomplished by most clinicians and cause little discomfort to the patient.

To strengthen the value and accuracy of linear measurements, one should take measurements in a consistent manner and record them in such a way that communicates the specific aspects of the wound used as landmarks. For example, numerical readings may be accompanied by arrows to clearly indicate the direction of the measurements relative to the position of the wound on the body; north-south measurements would be indicated by an arrow drawn vertically (↑), whereas measurements for the east-west axis would be depicted by horizontal arrows (→). Such an approach decreases confusion and allows the measurement to be repeated with some degree of consistency.

Although linear measurements provide greater objectivity than subjective appraisals of wound size, they are not without problems. Because the perimeter of open wounds is often irregular, it can be difficult to determine the best position on the wound surface from which to obtain the readings. Furthermore, two-dimensional measurements are unable to account for variations in irregular wounds or wounds with depth; for such wounds, two-dimensional measurements can be essentially meaningless. Certainly, the rigor with which the measurement is obtained influences the results, and the reliability of such measures is low. However, when repeated over time, linear measures of wounds without depth do provide gross information regarding the trend of the wound repair process.

Wound tracings. Another approach to open wound measurement is tracing the external surface or perimeter of the wound using transparent paper or transparent acetate and a marking pen. This approach received attention as early as 1937 when Lecomte du Nouy,[32] using this technique, defined the "index of cicatrization" (that is, the index of scar tissue formation) after taking serial tracings of hundreds of wounds. As with rulers, the use of a transparent medium to record the external shape of the wound is inexpensive and easily accomplished and produces minimal discomfort for the patient.

Numerous wound care products are now packaged in transparent wrappings making such tracing material readily accessible; some manufacturers have incorporated rulers or concentric circles on their packaging to facilitate both tracings and linear measurements. The sterile side of such packaging can be placed over the wound and the perimeter can be easily traced; both tracing and linear appraisal of a wound should be obtained at the time of the dressing change.

Although obtaining such measurements is certainly better than not, the consistency with which these measurements are taken affects reliability of the measures. Some wounds may be difficult to trace because of their position on the body; in addition, measurements obtained with the patient lying in different positions or by the use of different landmarks cannot be considered reliable. Finally, clinicians may experience difficulty in determining what constitutes the wound edge.

Wound tracings can be used to generate two-dimensional measurements but can also be used to calculate the surface area of the wound. Unfortunately, when Bohannon and Pfaller[4] studied the practicality and accuracy of various techniques to determine the area of a wound, they concluded that "the greatest source of error in tracing wounds may be in the tracing itself rather than the determination of the area traced." Therefore it is imperative to use rigor and precision when one is tracing the wound to increase the reliability of the measures.

More often, however, wound tracings are used as a pattern against which subsequent tracings can be compared; this is best accomplished if each pattern is dated. In this way, multiple clinicians have a rough, visual estimate of the size of the external wound opening and can determine if the size or shape of the wound is changing.

Wound photography. Wound photographs can be used along with linear measurements to provide a two-dimensional approach that facilitates both wound measurement and wound assessment. Whether pictures of a wound are taken with an exquisite camera or an "instantaneous" Polaroid, the resulting image provides a template against which changes in wound status can be observed and compared. The use of such pictures can reveal much about the course of healing over time: the relative size of the wound, the color of the tissue, the amount of exudate, and the condition of the surrounding skin. Serial photographs should be taken from the same distance so that changes in the course of healing become apparent. In this way changes can be evaluated quickly even by clinicians who are less familiar with the patient.

Certainly, photographs that can be viewed in a timely manner are superior to those that require a lapse before developing. However, the quality of the image from an instamatic camera may not be ideal. Additionally, the camera may not adequately capture the three-dimensional wound thus leaving the clinician in doubt about the depth of the wound, the character of the exudate, or the topography of the wound.

The color of tissue within the wound or exudate on the surface of the wound can also be greatly modified as a consequence of the developing process. It is not unusual for a wound photograph to reflect an image vastly different in color from that of the actual wound. For this and other reasons, wound photographs, though certainly helpful in some situations, may not prove reliable. Additionally, in most clinical settings, an expensive camera and a person skilled in its use may not be a realistic approach for bedside clinicians.

Planimetry. As noted previously, wound tracings can be used to calculate the surface area of the wound. This involves planimetry, a method that requires careful counting of the number of squares on a metric graph paper that lie within a wound tracing or photograph

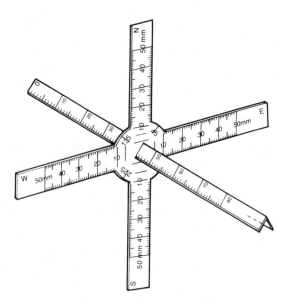

Fig. 3-1   Kundin Wound Gauge. (Courtesy Pacific Technologies and Development Corporation, San Mateo, Calif.)

placed over that paper. Once determined, the resulting number gives a precise indication of the area of the wound (as reflected in the tracing or photograph) in square centimeters. Computer-aided planimeters have expedited the tedious manual process. Such technology is understandably expensive, and the process still somewhat time consuming.

Either approach to surface-area measurement (that is, manual or computer assisted), however precise, hardly seems realistic for use by the bedside clinician. Additionally, although planimetry is generally accurate when used on flat wounds, it ceases to provide a complete picture of the wound in the case of full-thickness or deep wounds. Because of the time and precision involved, it is not surprising that this method has been employed more by researchers than by practicing clinicians.

Three-Dimensional Measurements. Two-dimensional measurements are relatively simple to use; however, they do not accurately describe wounds with depth. Accurate measurement of full-thickness wounds requires a three-dimensional approach. Such approaches include linear measurements, wound molds, foam dressings, and fluid instillation.

Linear measurements. To obtain the three dimensions of the wound, one must measure the depth of the wound in addition to the length and width. The most common method of obtaining wound depth is by insertion of a cotton-tipped applicator into the wound bed and placement of a mark on the applicator to indicate the level of the skin. This mark is often simply the examiner's thumb and index finger, but it may also be an ink mark. The cotton-tipped applicator is then held against a metric ruler to determine the depth of the wound. Although this technique is inherently imprecise (particularly with irregularly shaped wound beds), serial measurements provide a trend of measurements that one can only hope will reflect a tendency toward healing.

Aware of the lack of clinically useful ways to measure "irregular structures on the human body with or without depth," Kundin[30,31] developed the "wound gauge," or Kundin Wound Gauge (Fig. 3-1). This instrument, composed of three rulers placed at right angles, provides the clinician with a user-friendly device by which the length, width, and depth (in the case of "crater" wounds) of the wound are measured. By then using a specific mathematical formula or formulas one can ascertain the area of a surface lesion or the volume of wounds with depth.

Although clinically useful, this instrument presents problems with reliability when used by different clinicians. To obtain and compare serial measures, it is essential that the instrument be consistently placed over the same location of the open wound bed. Such placement can be challenging in the presence of a wound with a greatly irregular base or when the readings are being collected by different clinicians. Furthermore, if it is used correctly, attempts to account for the extent of undermining in a pressure ulcer, for example, must be consistent between clinicians.

Interestingly, Thomas and Wysocki[48] demonstrated that, although the Kundin gauge was equally reliable to photographs and acetate tracings in the evaluation of small wounds, it consistently produced data that indicated underestimation of wound area in larger and irregularly shaped wounds. Unfortunately, it is these wounds that are most in need of accurate measurement. These investigators showed that when photographs, acetate tracings, and the Kundin gauge were compared the three measures were highly correlated ($r = 0.93$), though correlation between acetate and photographs were the highest ($r = 0.99$). However, it is important to recognize that Thomas and Wysocki's findings were obtained by using two nurses specifically trained to use these instruments and to identify wound landmarks. The reliability of such measurement devices when used by multiple nurses with varying skill levels is not known but would probably be lower.

An additional concern with the use of the wound gauge as a clinical measurement tool is cost. Each gauge costs approximately $2.00 and should not be reused. In these times of cost containment a financial outlay of this magnitude to monitor a patient's wound over time may be unacceptable.

Wound molds. In 1966, Pories and his colleagues[44] reported the use of molds to assess the volume of open wounds. Studying eight servicemen undergoing excision of pilonidal cysts, the investigators instilled alginate (a substance used to make dental impressions) into the open wounds each day after surgery to monitor the course of healing. Once placed in the wound, the initially liquid medium thickens and can then be removed easily from the wound and subsequently placed in a liquid beaker (or weighed). By calculating the amount of fluid displaced over a series of molds, one can assess the status of the wound repair process.

Other investigators have used this wound mold approach to evaluate healing, particularly in pressure ulcers.[45] The ability of several trained individuals to instill this material in the same manner has been reported to be high.

Reports indicate that placement of molding medium in wounds does not appear to injure granulating wounds, nor has it been reported to cause patient discomfort. Additionally, properly stored wound molds (that is, in air-sealed bags to avoid desiccation) provide a permanent reflection of the course of healing, a quality that few other approaches to wound evaluation possess. Realistically, however, it is difficult to imagine that the instillation of the mold medium would be practical in most clinical settings as an everyday method of evaluating wounds by bedside clinicians.

Foam dressings. More recently, various dressing materials (such as silicone elastomer, Silastic) that serve not only to provide local wound care therapy, but also simultaneously to provide information about progress in healing have been described.[20,27,55] So far, these dressings have not been approved for use in the United States. This approach should afford another source of information about wound volume. If these dressings could be retained and reviewed serially, they, like the alginate molds, could provide more objective evidence of the course of the healing process. In addition to ease of application, these materials could be particularly beneficial when monitoring wound healing in patients in the community.

Fluid instillation. One final way of measuring wound volume, albeit imprecise, is to instill a known quantity of solution (such as sterile water or saline) into the wound cavity, allowing it to fill to the perimeter. The fluid is then extracted by syringe or suction and the amount recorded. When carried out serially, with the patient in the same position each time the measurement is taken, changes in the size of the wound cavity could be determined. This approach appears more feasible in the clinical setting than perhaps the use of alginate molds. Problems can arise, however, in situations where, because of the position of the wound on the body, instillation and brief retention of the fluid by the wound crater are difficult to accomplish.

Several two- and three-dimensional methods for wound measurements exist. Although linear measurements are the most commonly employed clinically, reliability is lacking. Because such measurements are frequently used as indices of progression in healing or as reflections of the effectiveness of a particular therapy, caution should be exercised in accepting all readings as accurate. Clinicians must use accuracy and precision when obtaining measurements. Furthermore, wound landmarks from which the measurements are obtained must be clearly documented and communicated to subsequent caregivers.

In addition to measurement of the length, width, and depth of wounds, there are several techniques that can be used to calculate the area of the wound. Such calculations can be done from linear measurements or wound photographs with linear measurements or by using wound molds, foam dressings, or fluid instillation. Acetate tracings of the wound perimeter are reportedly more accurate in determining actual wound area than either wound photographs or calculations with the Kundin three-dimensional wound gauge.[48]

Assessment of Wound Status

Although most clinicians can easily identify a "healed" or "unhealed" wound, many would be hard pressed to delineate the subtle changes *within* a wound that indicate that healing is occurring (that is, the status of the wound). Detailing the minute changes that occur in the healing process has been viewed as being of marginal importance. However, with the changes in health care and an increasing number of chronic wounds, knowledge of macroscopic changes in a wound becomes more valued. The ability to assess the status of the wound over time and to monitor its progress relative to known markers becomes desirable. Much as a patient's temperature is taken at a single time and evaluated in relation to the trend of multiple readings taken over time, so too the assessment of wound status can serve as a barometer of the wound's health status. These markers, however are not randomly selected but, rather, are theory-based macroscopic reflections of the wound. Over time, the collection of numerous wound status reports could serve to reveal the actual course of healing. Instruments currently used for assessment of wound status can be classified according to those that assess closed wounds and open wounds.

Closed Wounds. Two instruments currently reported in the literature are designed specifically to assess incisional wounds or wounds closed by primary intention: the ASEP-SIS[8,53] and the Wound Assessment Inventory (WAI).[26] When measures are repeated over time, a trend in the healing process is revealed. Each of these approaches to wound assessment has undergone varying degrees of testing for reliability and validity and should be thoroughly evaluated before use with patients. These instruments are described briefly in Chapter 4.

Open Wounds. Two instruments, the Wound Characteristics Instruments (WCI)[14] and the Red, Yellow, Black system (RYB)[15] are reported for use in the assessment of open wounds or wounds healing by secondary intention. The WCI asks the clinician to assess the "essential" characteristics of postsurgical wounds at a single point in time, but serially, so that trends and patterns in the status of the wound may be identified. The latter system (that is, RYB) directs the clinician to assess visually the surface of the wound and to use that assessment to select specific products for topical wound management. Again, if the RYB system is repeated over time, a trend in the wound color would be identified.

The Wound Characteristics Instrument. The WCI,[14] a criterion-referenced measurement, is a 17-item rating scale designed for use by clinicians evaluating the macroscopic, and thus visible to the naked eye, characteristics of open, soft-tissue, postsurgical wounds. In addition to encouraging the use of a common vocabulary among clinicians when open wounds are being discussed, this instrument directs the clinician to complete a wound assessment in a systematic manner. A systematic and consistent wound evaluation technique is essential to capture the subtle changes within a wound that can be otherwise easily overlooked.

The clinician using the WCI is directed to assess essential components or generic characteristics within the specific regions of the wound. For example, Plates 16 and 17 demonstrate the contrast in the presence of epithelial tissue at the rim of two wounds. These observations are then ranked along a continuum from the optimal to the worst manifestations of that state.

The WCI has undergone reliability testing and both content and construct validity testing. Content validity scores by surgeon experts indicated a high level of agreement regarding the structural and generic characteristics of the open wound with an average congruency percentage at 90%. Construct validity and reliability testing by registered nurses indicated a range of difficulty scores among the items. The WCI continues to undergo testing for reliability and validity.

The Red, Yellow, Black system. Although the Red, Yellow, Black system[15] is discussed as a method of classifying wounds (Table 3-1), it may also be considered an assessment tool for healing status because it involves observation and assessment before classification and can be conducted serially. The limitations of this system have been previously addressed.

Several tools are available to enable the clinician to predict wounds to develop, classify existing wounds, measure existing wounds, and assess the status of a wound. Unfortunately, these methods have undergone varying degrees of rigorous testing and vary in reliability and validity. When selecting a tool, the clinician must first determine the parameters to be assessed. Once this determination is made, a decision can be made regarding which tool is most appropriate for the situation. Finally, the clinician must keep in mind that it is unrealistic to expect one instrument to be an adequate gauge of wound status. One tool will

Table 3-2   Grading system for vascular wounds on extremities

Grade	Characteristics

0	Preulcerative lesion
	    Healed ulcers
	    Presence of bony deformity

1	Superficial ulcer without subcutaneous tissue involvement
2	Penetration through the subcutaneous tissue; may expose bone, tendon, ligament, or joint capsule
3	Osteitis, abscess, or osteomyelitis
4	Gangrene of digit
5	Gangrene of foot requiring disarticulation

From Glugla M and Mulder GD: The diabetic foot: medical management of foot ulcers. In Krasner D, editor: Chronic wound care: a clinical source book for healthcare professionals, King of Prussia, Penn, 1990, Health Management Publication, Inc.

not capture all the information necessary to adequately describe and evaluate the dynamic nature of a wound. Often, for example, wounds that are classified as stage 3, or full thickness, require additional descriptions of wound parameters. Such macroscopic indices of healing are discussed next.

MACROSCOPIC INDICES OF HEALING

Several wound parameters that serve as a macroscopic index of healing can be assessed clinically with the naked eye. The parameters that are presented are those that (1) are based on current understanding of wound-healing physiology, (2) have a range of manifestations, and (3) have the potential of being manipulated by the clinician. Each parameter gains clinical significance when described with precision. Because a discussion of assessment of wounds closed by primary intention is presented in Chapter 4 in this chapter, only those pertaining to wounds healing by secondary intention are discussed.

Size

Determination of the size of the wound is a basic assessment parameter; its significance is demonstrated by the inclusion of this parameter in many of the evaluation tools and clinical practice. Although the clinician cannot directly control the size of a wound, ensuring that the patient's nutritional needs are met will influence the quality of healing and the ability of the open wound to contract, hence affecting the size of the wound. Nursing interventions that support the delivery of nutrients (such as oxygen, vitamins, and micronutrients) to the wound, in essence, support the wound to decrease in size and heal.[43,51,52] For example, the fibroblast requires nutrients to synthesize hydroxyproline and, ultimately, collagen; as collagen remodels in the third stage of healing, wound contraction occurs. In a starved environment, this will not proceed effectively and contraction will be thwarted.

Evaluating the size of a wound is perhaps then one of the first local measurements the clinician should obtain and should be repeated at intervals. Wound-size determinations are recorded in centimeters or millimeters and include the width, length, and depth of the wound. Irregularly shaped wounds may require several measures of each dimension (length, width, or depth) to adequately capture the size of the wound. Locations from which measurements were obtained can be indicated with an ink mark on the surrounding intact skin or recorded in the care plan.

Extent of Tissue Involvement

Obviously the larger or deeper the wound, the greater is the potential for secondary problems (such as infections) and prolonged healing. Any injury involving vessel interruption institutes the healing trajectory and therefore elicits a systemic response. Therefore assessing a wound to determine the extent of tissue involvement is an essential aspect of wound evaluation. The extent of tissue damage guides the selection of interventions appropriate to restore tissue integrity and also provides some information about the length of time the healing process may require.

Several methods are available to describe the extent of tissue damage. These include partial thickness, full thickness and, with pressure ulcers, staging (Table 3-1). In the case of burn wounds, the classical estimation of area of the burn can be used.[37] A specific ulcer-grading system for vascular wounds on the extremities has also been described[23] (Table 3-2). Increasingly, these systems are being related to algorithms, or plans, of care. However, such protocols need to be researched to determine effectiveness; a process that will require sound methods of assessing and measuring wound-healing progress.

Presence of Undermining or Tracts

Full-thickness wounds must be carefully evaluated for evidence of undermining or sinus tract formation as demonstrated in Plates 8 and 15. Undermining most often occurs with pressure-induced ulcers that are complicated by shear force, whereas tracts can be expected in dehisced wounds and ulcers caused by a combination of neuropathy and arterial insufficiency.

Location and extent of undermining or sinus tracts must be accurately documented so that progress in wound healing and effectiveness at eliminating or reducing the cause can be evaluated. For example, extension of tissue damage by continued shear will be evidenced by enlargement of the undermined area. Gentle probing of the wound bed with a cotton-tipped applicator will reveal undermined tissue or tracts as demonstrated in Plate 15.

Anatomic Location

The anatomic location of the wound or skin damage is also important to document. Descriptors are used to convey which bony prominence the lesion lies over or the specific body locations. For example, a pressure ulcer may develop on the right calcaneous or left ischial tuberosity; a shear injury may be located in the gluteal fold; a venous ulcer may develop on the medial aspect of the right lower leg.

Location is significant not only because of the need to communicate accurately with colleagues, but also because location influences healing potential. The closer the wound is to the upper region of the body, the greater the likelihood of healing. Extremity wounds in the elderly, therefore, are often slow to heal, not simply because of underlying conditions that thwart healing, but also because they are distant from the upper body regions.

Type of Tissue in Wound Base

The type of tissue that can be present in the wound bed can range from viable tissue to nonviable tissue. Viable tissue (granulation, epithelialization, muscle, subcutaneous tissue, and so on) must be distinguished from nonviable tissue. This determination is most commonly made by observation of the color of the tissue in the wound. The presence of nonviable tissue (or necrotic tissue) in the wound is cause for concern because it is associated with altered tissue oxygenation or wound desiccation. Because wound healing is greatly compromised in the midst of necrotic tissue,[25] prompt removal of necrotic tissue from wounds must be a common goal of the multidisciplinary health care team. Débridement options are discussed in Chapter 2.

Color

Color, as has been noted before, is another important index of healing. Typically, clean, granular wounds are described as being red; yellow, tan, and black may be used to describe the presence of necrotic tissue or desiccated tissue such as tendon. In reality, these colors are inadequate in truly reflecting the many colors that can accompany a wound. For example, a wound may be pink, as shown in Plate 16, pale red as shown in Plate 18, or intensely red as shown in Plates 9 and 17. This range of just the color red portrays the continuum of healing from optimal to suboptimal. The Wound Characteristics Instrument is an attempt to capture the range of color states that reflect optimal to worst healing within and surrounding the wound; it is still under investigation, however. Therefore it is important to closely observe and precisely describe the color of the wound tissue, wound exudate, and changes in the skin surrounding the wound.

Terminology should be standardized to accurately describe optimal and suboptimal wound colors. For example, healthy granulation tissue is characteristically described as "beefy, red, and shiny" (Plate 9). Deviations from this optimal state should be described carefully and correlated with conditions that may account for the abnormality.

Suboptimal wound colors may be an indication of physiologic abnormalities such as those in the patient's fluid status, serum hemoglobin level, or nutritional status as shown in Plate 18.[38,46] Fluid status, as reflected by hematocrit, indicates adequacy of tissue hydration and tissue oxygenation potential; both hydration and oxygenation affect new vessel formation, which can be inferred macroscopically in the color and sheen of granulation tissue. Likewise, vitamin and mineral intake (vitamin C and iron specifically) affect collagen synthesis, new vessel formation, capillary stability, and hemoglobin formation and are therefore potentially reflected in tissue color.

Exudate

Exudate within the wound should be assessed for many characteristics: volume, color, consistency, and odor. Exudate characteristics may vary with the type of wound present. For example, a venous ulcer may produce more exudate than an arterial ulcer. Odor and color of exudate offer information that may be indicative of a wound infection. Extremely odorous, purulent exudate is frequently suggestive of an anaerobic infection.

Edge of the Open Wound

The rim, or the edge of the open wound, should be assessed as an integral part of wound evaluation. Plate 16 reveals the presence of new epithelial tissue at the wound edge; this is in contrast to the absence of epithelial tissue at the wound edge as shown in Plate 17. New epithelial tissue will not grow into a wound covered with necrotic debris or deprived of oxygen; many chronic wounds attest to that. Instead, these wounds demonstrate persistently gnarled edges with little to no evidence of new tissue growth at the wound rim. The clinician should observe closely for the appearance of new tissue at the wound edges. Unfortunately, assessment of the edge of the open wound is commonly overlooked and unappreciated. This situation underscores the need for a systematic approach to evaluate key landmarks within the open wound and the need for formal instruction regarding the structural components of the open wound.[14]

Interventions that could facilitate the appearance of new tissue at the rim of the wound are similar to those that influence the size of the wound: improved nutrition, supporting wound (tissue) oxygenation, and effective removal of necrotic tissue. Appropriate use of dressings that incorporate the principles of moist healing can also greatly facilitate epithelial migration.[1,54]

Presence of Foreign Bodies

Certainly the presence of foreign bodies (such as suture material) within an open wound should be assessed. Although quite routine in the care of an acute wound, suture material always presents a challenge to the healing process. The integrity of an approximated incision is threatened when an excessive number of sutures are used, when sutures are placed under tension, and when sutures are knotted numerous times. Timely removal of any foreign bodies in wounds closed by primary or secondary intention can enhance wound repair and conserve the patient's energy.

Condition of Surrounding Skin

Evaluation of the skin adjacent to the wound should also be a part of wound assessment because it reveals much about the patient's age, health status, and, at times, medications (such as steroids) they may be taking. Assessment of the skin surrounding a wound may provide an indication of the adequacy of the wound dressing's ability to absorb and contain exudate. Maceration of surrounding skin will occur when exudate pools onto intact skin for prolonged periods of time or gauze is inappropriately applied and overlaps onto intact skin. The following assessments of the skin surrounding the wound are essential: discoloration such as erythema or paleness, hematoma formation, interruptions in integrity (such as denudation, erosion, papules, pustules), maceration, or desiccation. The surrounding skin should also be palpated for the presence or absence of induration, which in selected cases may be an indication of deeper tissue damage. These assessments must be routine and regular.

Duration of Wound

Although seldom regarded a priority, the time since wounding, or "age" of the wound, is, in fact, a macroscopic parameter that deserves careful consideration. Given a clear understanding of healing, the 7-day-old surgical wound that shows no signs of inflammation is worrisome for different reasons from those for the venous ulcer that has persisted for several years. Both wounds are out of synchronization and need to be evaluated in light of what mechanisms might have altered the normal course of the healing trajectory. The fact that the surgical incision closed by primary intention is most likely to dehisce between day 5 and day 12 after surgery, or that a healing ridge should be apparent by approximately day 7 postoperatively can be evaluated knowledgeably only when the time span since wounding is used as a guidepost. Postoperatively, surgical patients should be observed for the presence or absence of such key time-related manifestations of optimal healing. With changing practices such as early discharge to home, astute wound assessments become increasingly important for home care nurses and long-term care nurses.

DOCUMENTATION GUIDELINES

As with any clinical condition, the nurse who provides wound care requires a thorough understanding of the normal physiologic process, evaluation of underlying conditions that might alter the optimal course, coordination of an outcome-driven plan used knowledgeably, and consistent evaluation of those outcomes at regularly prescribed intervals. Thus the importance of documentation and frequent evaluation becomes evident. Evaluation of outcomes and consistency of care are possible only when observations and interventions are documented. In the open, soft-tissue wound, documentation of the following macroscopic indices of wound healing is a nursing responsibility: anatomic location of the wound, dimensions and depth of wound (in centimeters), stage of wound, characteristics of wound base, presence or absence of undermining or sinus tract formation, exudate, condition of surrounding skin, and presence or absence of new epithelium at the rim.

One wound assessment tool cannot provide all of these data; a combination of many tools is often necessary for a comprehensive and accurate reflection of the status of the wound and the healing trend. For example, the classification system of staging should be used in combination with descriptive terminology to capture the color and size of the wound and type of tissue in the wound bed. Regular and routine wound evaluations collected at intervals over time should provide the information necessary to reflect the healing status of the wound. From this, the effectiveness of the plan of care (topical and systemic) can then be evaluated and revised as needed.

It is difficult to stipulate the appropriate frequency for wound assessment; no research to provide this information has been reported. Additionally, multiple variables influence the manner in which different types of wounds heal. Furthermore, healing will vary from one person to another.

Given these constraints, it becomes necessary to suggest frequency intervals for wound assessment based strictly on clinical experience. Certainly, acute wound situations (such as a wound infection or recent dehiscence) require close monitoring; thus assessments may be conducted as often as every 2 to 4 hours.

Although chronicity in a wound is not a reason to become any less vigilant, assessments may be conducted less frequently. For example, in the acute care setting, wound assessments may be documented with every dressing change but do not need to exceed once per day. In the home care and long-term care setting, twice-weekly wound assessments may be more practical and informative in terms of identifying any trend in the wound repair process. When assessment and measurement trends fail to indicate a movement toward healing in the wound, reevaluation of the treatment plan, treatment goals, causative factors, and institution of new therapies are warranted and essential.

RECOMMENDATIONS FOR MORE ACCURATE WOUND ASSESSMENT

Because so little has been documented about specific macroscopic indices of healing, it is imperative for clinicians to accept the responsibility and challenge to work at systematically recording and testing visible observations believed to reflect optimal and suboptimal healing. This is a particularly important activity given the increasing number of wound-care products that flood the market, the potential for enhancing or accelerating healing with substances as growth factors, the trend toward earlier patient discharge, and the advancing age of the population.

Nurses are critical participants in the process of developing a systematic approach for evaluating the healing wound. Unfortunately, many issues have delayed the development of such tools, and most of those are issues that nursing can control. To facilitate the development of a systematic approach to evaluating wound healing, five conditions seem necessary. First, clinicians must recognize the value and merit of the process of observation as an assessment methodology. Although in the early days of health care, observation was considered to be one of the finest forms of patient assessment, in recent times observation has been relegated to a position of lesser value. Instruments and machines are now viewed as superior, more objective, and of greater value.

Second, clinicians must document and describe the manner in which the wound was observed and exactly what was observed. Restoration of stature to observational activities will be incomplete if clinicians fail to share or communicate these observations. This provides the "data base" needed from which a consensus on terminology can be derived; hence the components of an evaluation instrument become apparent.

Third, clinicians need to acknowledge the difference between simply measuring the dimensions of a wound and the more complex process of assessing the status of the wound's multiple components and healing status. It is the experienced clinician who recognizes that wound assessment is a process that involves critical thinking skills and correlation of observations to potential causes. Wound assessment requires a comprehensive examination of the wound. The clinician must examine the wound not only for current observations, but also in comparison to past observations. These observations are then pondered in light of the patient's indicators for healing potential (that is, health status, nutritional status, and perfusion). Attention to detail is imperative. The data a careful wound assessment provides are not duplicated by any other tests or methods. The inadequacy of linear wound measurements or serial tracings alone, for example, become apparent; these methods present an incomplete picture. To accurately describe the wound one must assess it using additional parameters that go along with linear measurements. As the second condition is fulfilled and documentation of wound observations becomes more readily available in the literature, the parameters needed to comprehensively describe the wound will emerge.

A fourth condition is that the terms used to describe wounds must be standardized. By adopting a common vocabulary, an accurate description of the wound can be reliably conveyed to individuals and groups (such as institutions). Furthermore, testing of wound therapies is facilitated because the observations can now be clearly shared and understood between all involved health care providers. Although an organized vocabulary is yet to emerge, numerous terms have been defined and should be critiqued and adopted as appropriate.[5,14,28,39] For example, as a result of a consensus panel conference, the National Pressure Ulcer Advisory Panel recommends that "pressure ulcer" be the term by which clinicians refer to lesions otherwise known as "bedsores," "pressure sores," and even "decubitus ulcers." Such a recommendation greatly streamlines clinical vocabulary and begins to standarize the way clinicians speak about wounds. Clinicians interested in rectifying the confusion surrounding wounds should adopt the language suggested by this panel as a first step toward increasing the likelihood that order will evolve out of confusion.

Finally, clinicians must employ clinically useful evaluation tools with demonstrated reliability and validity. Support should be provided to those researchers who have developed clinically useful wound-evaluation tools. Continuing to use ill-defined methods of assessing patients when sound instruments exist is to perpetuate the problem.

Obviously, selected tools are more appropriate for certain types of wounds. Therefore nurses must describe and isolate the various tools available and critique them carefully for their merits or drawbacks in particular healing situations.

SUMMARY

In 1973 Levine[35] stated that "every healing process, regardless of its nature, occurs over a period of time. The success of the ultimate healing depends in large measure on what happens to the individual during that time. The nurse is the person on the health team who shares the most time with the patient, and thus no worker can influence the success of the healing process more than the nurse. Nursing processes of every kind are dedicated to the promotion of healing."

Despite the emphasis on the "wound" throughout this chapter, there needs to be an increased realization that evaluating wounds as if they exist separately from the patient is not only inadequate, but also inconsistent with the practice of nursing. Wound evaluation is in fact patient evaluation. With the increased realization of the complexity of healing comes the obligation to know all one can about the healing milieu (physiologic, psychologic, biochemical, and so forth). Careful accurate wound assessments are critical and guide decisions for wound care. However, providing care to the wound in isolation or evaluating the wound in isolation belies the fundamental holism of nursing.[33,34]

SELF-EVALUATION

QUESTIONS AND PROBLEMS

1. Distinguish between measurement of an existing wound and assessment of the wound status.
2. Which of the following methods is an example of categorizing a wound by classification?
   a. Linear measurements
   b. Photographs
   c. Staging
   d. Wound molds
3. Blisters are an example of which stage of tissue loss (according to the IAET and NPUAP)?
   a. Stage 1
   b. Stage 2
   c. Stage 3
   d. Stage 4
4. Define partial thickness and full thickness.
5. Describe three limitations associated with using only linear measurements to evaluate the wound and to assess wound status.
6. List the 11 macroscopic indices of wound healing that should be assessed and recorded.
7. Describe the following terms:
   Nonviable
   Eschar
   Granulation
   Epithelialization

SELF-EVALUATION

ANSWERS

1. *Measurement of existing wound:* The focus of measurement is to determine the size of the wound either with linear measurements, fluid instillation, wound molds, photographs, planimetry, or foam. Measurement captures only one aspect of the wound.
   Assessment of wound healing status: The focus is to delineate the subtle changes within the wound that indicate healing is occurring. Known markers would be used as barometers of the wound's health status. Ideally, repeated assessment of wound status would also reveal the wound's healing trajectory. The Wound Characteristics Instrument (WCI) is an instrument that is currently under investigation and contains 17 items that provide a framework to complete a systematic evaluation of the status of an open, soft-tissue postsurgical wound.
2. c
3. b
4. *Partial thickness:* tissue loss that is limited to the epidermal or dermal layers of the skin; damage does not penetrate below the dermis.

Full thickness: tissue loss that extends below the dermis. Unfortunately the exposed tissue may be subcutaneous tissue, muscle, tendon, or bone. The phrase does not indicate the extent of the full-thickness damage.

5. 1. Reliability of the measurements obtained can be quite varied, and so inconsistent linear measures may be reported.
  2. Quality of the tissue in the wound or presence of granulation, epithelial tissue, or nonviable tissue is not reflected in the measurement.
  3. Condition of the surrounding skin (such as erythema, induration, maceration) is not captured by the terminology.
  4. The presence of odor or exudate is not indicated.
  5. The fact that wounds are irregularly shaped makes it difficult to get accurate reflection of the size; most commonly, the clinician measures each axis only by the widest dimension.

6. Size, extent of wound, presence of undermining or tracts, anatomic location, type of tissue in wound base, color, exudate (amount, consistency, odor), edge of open wound, presence of foreign bodies, condition of the surrounding skin, and duration of the wound.

7. *Nonviable:* tissue that is not healthy or living; may also be more specific to state that it is eschar, adherent, slough, or other descriptive terms.
  Eschar: thick, leathery, black necrotic tissue.
  Granulation: establishment of capillaries and collagen in a full-thickness wound; appearance is beefy red, granular, and moist.
  Epithelialization: process of epithelial cells resurfacing a full- or partial-thickness wound.

REFERENCES

1. Alvarez O, Rozint J, and Wiseman D: Moist environment for healing: matching the dressing to the wound, Wounds 1(1):35-51, 1989.
2. Bergstrom N, Braden BJ, Laguzza A, and Holman V: The Braden scale for predicting pressure sore risk, Nurs Res 36:205-210, 1987.
3. Bergstrom N, Demuth PJ, and Braden B: A clinical trial of the Braden scale for predicting pressure sore risk, Nurs Clin North Am 22:417-418, 1987.
4. Bohannon RW and Pfaller BA: Documentation of wound surface area from tracings of wound perimeters, Phys Ther 63:1622-1624, 1983.
5. Boarini JH, Bryant R, and Zink M: Achieving autolysis with transparent dressings, St. Paul, Minn, 1987, Medical-Surgical Division: 3M Health Care.
6. Braden BJ and Bergstrom N: Clinical utility of the Braden scale for predicting pressure sore risk, Decubitus 2(3):44-51, 1989.
7. Bulstrode DJ, Goode AW, and Scott PJ: Stereophotogrammetry for measuring rates of cutaneous healing: a comparison with conventional techniques, Clin Sci 71:437-443, 1986.
8. Byrne DJ, Napier A, and Cuschieri A: Validation of the ASEPSIS method of wound scoring in patients undergoing general surgical operation, J R Coll Surg Edinb 33:154-155, 1988.
9. Cooper DM: Clinical assessment/measurement of healing: evolution and status, Clin Materials. (In press.)
10. Cooper DM: Optimizing wound healing: a practice within nursing's domain, Nurs Clin North Am 25:165-180, 1990.
11. Cooper DM: (Preface), Nurs Clin North Am 25:163-164, 1990.
12. Cooper DM: Challenge of open wound assessment in the home setting, Progressions 2(3):11-18, 1990.
13. Cooper DM: Human wound assessment: status report and implications for clinicians, AACN Clin Issues in Crit Care Nurs 1(3):533-563, 1990.

14. Cooper DM: Development and testing of an instrument to assess the visual characteristics of open, soft tissue wounds, doctoral dissertation, Philadelphia, 1990, University of Pennsylvania.
15. Cuzzell J: The new RYB color code, Am J Nurs 88:1342-1346, 1988.
16. Fawcett J and Downs FS: The relationship of theory and research, Norwalk, Conn, 1986, Appleton-Century-Crofts.
17. Forrest RD and Gamborg-Nielsen P: Wound assessment in clinical practice, Acta Med Scand, suppl 687:69-74, 1984.
18. Fylling CP: A comprehensive wound management protocol including topical growth factors, Wounds 1:79-86, 1989.
19. Gilman TH: Parameter for measurement of wound closure, Wounds 2(3):95, 1990.
20. Gledhill T and Waterfall WE: Silastic foam: a new material for dressing wounds, Can Med Assoc J 128:685, 1983.
21. Gosnell DJ: An assessment tool to identify pressure sores, Nurs Res 22:55-59, 1973.
22. Gosnell DJ: Pressure sore risk assessment, part II: Analysis of risk factors, Decubitus 2:40-43, 1989.
23. Glugla M and Mulder GD: The diabetic foot: medical management of foot ulcers. In Krasner D, editor: Chronic wound care: a clinical source book for healthcare professionals, King of Prussia, Penn, 1990, Health Management Publication, Inc.
24. Haley RW, Culver DH, Morgan WM, et al: Identifying patients at high risk of surgical wound infection, Am J Epidemiol 121:206-215, 1985.
25. Hohn DC: Host resistance to infection: established and emerging concepts. In Hunt TK, editor: Wound healing and wound infection: theory and surgical practice, New York, 1980, Appleton-Century-Crofts.
26. Holden-Lund C: Effects of relaxation with guided imagery on surgical stress and wound healing, Res Nurs Health 11:235-244, 1988.
27. Hughes LE: Wound measurement, Can J Surg 26:210, 1983 [Letter].
28. International Association for Enterostomal Therapy: Standards of care for dermal wounds; pressure ulcers, revised ed, Irvine, Calif, 1991.
29. Knighton DR, Fiegel VD, Ciresi KF, et al: Classification and treatment of chronic nonhealing wounds, Ann Surg 204:322-330, 1986.
30. Kundin JI: A new way to size up a wound, Am J Nurs 89:206-207, 1989.
31. Kundin JI: Designing and developing a new measuring instrument, Perioperative Nurs Q 1:40-45, 1985.
32. Lecomte de Nouy P: Biological time, New York, 1937, The Macmillan Co.
33. Levine ME: The four conservation principles of nursing, Nurs Forum 2:22-35, 1967.
34. Levine ME: Holistic nursing, Nurs Clin North Am 6:253-264, 1971.
35. Levine ME: Introduction to clinical nursing, Philadelphia, 1973, FA Davis.
36. Levine ME: The four conservation principles twenty years later. In Riehl-Sisca JP, editor: Conceptual models for nursing practice, ed 3, Norwalk, Conn, 1989, Appleton & Lange.
37. Lund CC and Browder NC: Estimation of areas of burns, Surg Gynecol Obstet 79:352, 1944.
38. Maibach H and Rovee D, editors: Epidermal wound healing, St. Louis, 1971, Mosby–Year Book, Inc.
39. National Pressure Ulcer Advisory Panel National Consensus Conference, Washington, DC, 1989.
40. Norton D: Calculating the risk: reflections on the Norton scale, Decubitus 2(3):24-31, 1989.
41. Norton D, McLaren R, and Exton-Smith AN: An investigation of geriatric nursing problems in hospital, London, 1962, National Corporation for the Care of Old People.
42. Percoraro RE and Reiber GE: Classification of wounds in diabetic amputees, Wounds 2:65-73, 1990.
43. Pinchofsky-Devin G: Nutritional assessment and intervention. In Krasner D, editor: Chronic wound care, King of Prussia, Penn, 1990, Health Management Publications.
44. Pories WJ, Schear EW, Jordon DR, et al: The measurement of human wound healing, Surgery 59:821-824, 1966.
45. Resch CS, Kerner E, Robson MC, et al: Pressure sore volume measurement, Am J Geriat Soc 36:444-446, 1988.
46. Rodeheaver G: Controversies in topical wound management, Wounds 1(1):19-34, 1989.
47. Shea JD: Pressure sores: classification and management, Clin Orthop 112:89, 1975.

48. Thomas AC and Wysocki AB: The healing wound: a comparison of three clinically useful methods of measurement, Decubitus 3:18-25, 1990.

49. Waltz CF, Strickland OL, and Lenz ER: Measurement in nursing research. Philadelphia, 1986, FA Davis.

50. Wells FC, Newsom SWB, and Rowlands C: Wound infection in cardiothoracic surgery, Lancet 1:1209-1210, 1983.

51. West JM: Wound healing in the surgical patient: influence of the perioperative stress response on perfusion, AACN Clin Issues in Crit Care Nurs 1:595-601, 1990.

52. Whitney JD: The influence of tissue oxygen and perfusion on wound healing, AACN Clin Issues in Crit Care Nurs 1:578-584, 1990.

53. Wilson AP, Treasure T, Sturridge MF, and Grüneberg RN: A scoring method (ASEPSIS) for postoperative wound infections for use in clinical trials of antibiotic prophylaxis, Lancet (8476):311-313, 1986.

54. Winter GD and Scales JT: Effect of air drying and dressings on the surface of a wound, Nature 197:91, 1963.

55. Wood RA, Williams RH, and Hughes LE: Foam elastomer dressing in the management of open granulating wounds: experience with 250 patients, Br J Surg 64:554-557, 1977.

4 Acute Surgical Wounds

DIANE M. COOPER

OBJECTIVES

1. State two factors that make it difficult to apply current wound-healing research to the acute wound-repair process.

2. Describe an acute surgical wound.

3. Discuss the negative impact at least four factors (direct and indirect) have on the acute surgical wound-repair process.

4. Distinguish the relevance of tissue oxygen and arterial oxygen to wound healing.

5. Describe at least 10 nursing interventions that optimize acute surgical wound healing.

6. Describe five parameters of the surgical incision site that should be assessed.

7. Compare and contrast four wound-measurement techniques.

As with other phenomena in the human experience, the ideal exists only in textbooks or in our minds, so too, in reality, the notion of an ideal wound is a myth, if not a contradiction. Examples of the extent to which the general surgery patient might go if the goal of healing was a "perfect" scar are to return to one's infancy during which time scarring is less than in later life, submit to the deep sea environment in order to increase tissue oxygenation and the constant bathing of the wound in physiologic solutions, or undergo plastic surgical procedures for cosmetic modification of the suture line.

The majority of clinicians, however, function at or above sea level and in the real world, where often they are faced with caring for patients experiencing less than ideal healing situations that challenge the clinician's knowledge and creativity. In the midst of all this, the following becomes clear: Healing is an extremely complex process that is triggered by injury, influenced by multiple microenvironmental and macroenvironmental variables, subject to modification, not universally inevitable, and incapable of producing the quality of tissue integrity present in uninjured areas of the body.[2,22] In addition, although a great deal has been learned about tissue repair over the last several decades, much of the information has been acquired from bench research and animal studies. Although vital in the development of knowledge, a great many of these findings continue to demand reformulation and testing on humans before use in everyday clinical practice. Thus what at first appears revolutionary and capable of radically influencing the course of healing for the better remains inaccessible to the clinician in everyday practice.

One example of the difficulty inherent in reformulating information for use by clinicians can be seen in attempts to create a schema by which human wounds can be classified along a continuum from optimal to suboptimal states.[3-5] Accomplishing just this apparently simple translation is no easy task, for in a review of the literature it becomes clear that wounding and healing, even in the abstract sense, are not the generic concepts they were once believed to be. Instead, wound "types" (such as the pressure ulcer and the burn wound) are appreciated increasingly for their uniqueness and diversity.

Writers have categorized wound types in humans variously, pointing out the fact that each possesses distinguishing attributes that may significantly affect the course and quality of healing: A wound acquired as a result of an accident, for example, faces a set of obstacles during repair different from that of the incision resulting from elective surgery, and the full-thickness wound goes through reparative mechanisms in excess of those required of the partial-thickness injury.

Clinicians caring for wounds in the acute care setting are faced with yet another dilemma, the fact being that a great deal of the clinically relevant literature on healing addresses chronic or problematic wounds; less information is synthesized about the relatively "healthy" wound that can be optimized. The acute wound, in particular the uncomplicated surgical wound, is an example of a healthy, potentially "optimizable" wound. If assisted knowledgeably, this wound has been demonstrated to fare better than if left to heal passively.[1,14,43] Healing in this circumstance can be enhanced, and although the results, when one compares unassisted and assisted wounds, may appear similar, there is mounting evidence indicating that in the long run the knowledgeably treated wound will, in fact, do better. This chapter focuses on a description of the acute wound, in particular the surgical wound, with postoperative conditions that optimize or maximize its healing potential being emphasized. Available methods of assessing this wound type are presented also.

DEFINITION OF THE ACUTE SURGICAL WOUND

Other than the classical phases of tissue healing, no universally accepted definition of the acute, non–accident derived wound is used. One author succinctly described acute wounds as those "that heal rapidly and uneventfully" whereas the chronic wound represents "failure of the normal healing process."[13] One expert described acute wounds simply as those that "heal by themselves" whereas chronic wounds "need help to heal."[17a]

For the most part, definitions of chronic wounds revolve around the lack of the wound's adherence to the *time* frames put forth in the classical healing trajectory. Using time as a framework for the definition of the acute surgical wound, one could say that the acute surgical wound is acquired as the result of an operative procedure and progresses in a timely fashion along the healing trajectory, with at least external manifestations of healing apparent early in the postoperative period. By this very definition then, because of protracted healing, surgical wounds left to close by secondary intention would be excluded from this definition, as would dehisced wounds or those classified other than clean or clean-contaminated.[7]

FACTORS AFFECTING HEALING OF THE ACUTE SURGICAL WOUND

Despite the fact that it would be efficient to discuss the acute wound in an isolated fashion, separate from the patient, such an approach is neither acceptable nor theoretically sound. Just as ideal wounds do not exist, neither can wounds be discussed separate from the person in whom they reside. Discussion of healing in a holistic fashion requires that both indirect and direct factors influencing healing be addressed and that the wound never be evaluated apart from the person in whom it resides.

Similarly, just as it is impossible to separate the wound from the patient, so too it is difficult for one to discuss a patient's wound at a single moment in time, ignoring the history. In a very real sense, patients and the wounds they acquire have "lives"; there is the time before, during, and after wounding. Just as the indirect and direct factors affecting healing must be evaluated, so too the preoperative, perioperative, and postoperative periods must be evaluated carefully when one is discussing factors affecting healing in the patient with the acute surgical wound; each of these periods impinges on the outcome. And, although an in-depth discussion of all three phases is beyond the scope of this chapter, some of the factors crucial to quality healing in the postoperative period are emphasized.

Indirect Factors

Of the number of factors indirectly influencing healing in the patient with an acute surgical wound, some are controllable, such as the manner in which a patient's skin is prepped before the incision is made or the type of suture material is selected, whereas other factors, such as length of hospitalization before surgery and the degree of scrupulousness with which health care professionals comply with established protocols are less easily controlled. Specifics about perioperative issues known to reduce the potential for infection and maximize the recovery of operative patients are thoroughly covered elsewhere.[7-9] Suffice it to say, the strongly held belief that most wound infections *begin* in the operating room probably holds true. Where operating room protocols are strictly adhered to and surgeons practice meticulous technique, wound infection rates have been demonstrated to be low. When technique is other than meticulous, patients suffer.[10,12] It is obvious then that whenever overall surgical infection rates rise all personnel coming into contact with patients must be monitored but perhaps none more closely than those who interact with the patient in the operating room. Vigilant attention by all health care professionals to the numerous factors that might ultimately lead to a problem in healing is one of the first ways to ensure that healing of the acute surgical wound is optimized.

Direct Factors

The key factors directly influencing healing are those that impinge on the systemic state of the person and range from the presence of underlying medical conditions or malignancy, to the management of postoperative therapies, including the manner in which the patient's wound is tended. An in-depth discussion of the specific impact of multiple conditions on healing is not the purpose of this chapter; rather the discussion focuses on those physiologic states over which the nurse has some control. Knowledgeable monitoring of factors that directly influence healing will greatly facilitate optimal wound healing in the surgical patient.

Diabetes Mellitus. An increasingly aging population makes up most of those undergoing surgical procedures. One condition affecting a large number of older persons and yet amenable to treatment is diabetes mellitus. Proper monitoring and control of diabetes can assist greatly in optimizing the healing environment. Therefore any clinician evaluating the status of a patient's wounds must, of necessity, evaluate the person's ability to metabolize glucose.

Numerous factors have been suggested as contributing to the potential for infection in patients with diabetes, among them being age, obesity, malnutrition, and reduced inflammation. Although only some of these are controllable, several writers suggest that careful control of the patient's blood glucose level (that is, maintained at less than 200 mg/dL) is perhaps the single most advantageous action clinicians can take to "normalize" healing in these persons.[15,16,33,38]

One of the crucial factors to consider when one is evaluating the surgical patient with diabetes is the effect of stress, in particular the stress of surgery on healing. The diabetic patient, whether diagnosed or undiagnosed, responds to stress by pouring out a series of "stress" hormones (that is, epinephrine, glucagon, cortisol, and growth hormone), the effect of which is to reduce the amount of circulating insulin while increasing the amount of circulating glucose. Two serious consequences of elevated glucose levels are a reduction in the effectiveness of neutrophils as phagocytes and an alteration in the deposition of collagen by fibroblasts, with subsequent reduction in wound strength (that is, tensile strength).

An additional negative outcome of poorly managed diabetes and ongoing hyperglycemia is malnutrition. Because of the lack of insulin, cells become starved for nutrients, and proteins and fats gradually are used as fuel; consequently the patient becomes catabolic. Obviously, fuel is required for the synthesis of new tissue, and catabolism, as reflected most specifically in reduced serum albumin and transferrin levels, is nonsupportive of healing.

Pointing up the fact that the chance of a person with diabetes developing a postoperative wound infection ranges between 6% and 40%, Rosenberg[38] urged nurses "to become actively involved in the ongoing management of diabetes mellitus throughout the perioperative period." She stated that "nurses must not view diabetes as merely a separate 'background' or 'secondary' diagnosis in the surgical patient." The nurse who carefully monitors the surgical patient's glucose level can significantly assist in optimizing healing and often prevent an acute wound from becoming chronic.

Oxygen-to-Volume Requirements. The starving do not heal. Personifying the wound for a moment, neither will a "starving wound" heal; it requires nutrition to exist and grow (that is, repair itself). Oxygen, one of the key nutrients of the wound, is so essential to optimal healing that without it the synthesis of collagen by fibroblasts is impaired leading to decreased wound strength,[34] new vessels formation is compromised,[28] epithelialization is slowed,[37] and the potential for infection is increased greatly.[18]

Translating this theory into therapeutic directives, a growing number of researchers have suggested that oxygen be supplied routinely to postoperative patients (particularly patients undergoing abdominal surgery) during the first few days after surgery, specifically for the purpose of increasing and ensuring greater oxygen delivery to the reparative site.[1,34,35,44] Simply providing supplemental oxygen, however, is not enough; to ensure that oxygen reaches the wound, a well-perfused vascular system is also essential, as are reduction in vasoconstriction, adequate blood supply, and reduction of tissue edema.[34] In one study of patients who had undergone general surgery, approximately 30% had reduced tissue oxygen tension levels ($Ptco_2$) despite adequate urinary output (that is, ≥50 ml/hour) and adequate arterial oxygen levels (Pao_2).[1] Furthermore, tissue oxygen levels could be corrected with infusion of fluids. Thus tissue oxygen and volume are inextricably linked. This underscores the fact that arterial oxygen levels are not reflective of tissue oxygen perfusion. Unfortunately, at present, no clinically appropriate techniques or indices are available to determine adequate tissue perfusion.

Although the average person breathing room air maintains an arterial oxygen above 80 mm Hg and a tissue oxygen pressure greater than 50 mm Hg, the postoperative patient experiencing pain, cold, fear, and at times narcosis is prone to significantly reduced oxygen levels within the wound.[42] The hormones secreted in response to these noxious or stress stimuli, in particular norepinephrine, have been shown to be "elevated for days" after surgery in some patients and to effect vascular changes that result in oxygen reduction.[42] Thus reducing postsurgical patients' pain, rehydrating, and warming them (all traditional nursing therapies used with surgical patients) are not only theory-based actions but also of great significance in the knowledgeable treatment of the postoperative patient whose healing the clinician is attempting to optimize.[17]

Although for centuries people have gone on to heal in the presence of decreased oxygen, this by no means implies that healing in these patients was optimal. Inadequate tissue oxygen levels in some wounds, no doubt, is the reason that the course of healing changes from adequate to problematic. Obviously, when reduced oxygen levels are coupled with other medical conditions, the threat to optimal healing is compounded. Clinicians of today then can ill afford to ignore research indicating that inadequate tissue oxygen may be the cause of poor healing. Among the important clinical messages regarding oxygen and healing in the surgical patient are (1) that a change in tissue oxygen occurs before changes in other parameters such as blood pressure or pulse or urine output[1,24,27,43] and (2) that Pao_2 is a poor indicator of tissue oxygenation.[43] Because few reliable indices of tissue-oxygen status are available, careful and ongoing assessment of the patient's fluid status and pulmonary status, as well as progressive activity can help to ensure improved tissue oxygenation and increase the likelihood of optimal healing.

Nutrition. Over the past decade, awareness of the importance of meeting the nutritional needs of healing patients has increased. Most clinicians base their practice on the premise that without the building blocks of protein (that is, amino acids) and the fuel supplied by glucose and fats, anabolism will be thwarted. Vitamins and trace elements, in particular vitamins A, B, C, and D and zinc, have likewise received attention for the contribution each makes in optimizing the healing environment.[29,40]

Because the focus of this chapter is the healthier patient undergoing surgery, the necessity of rectifying serious malnutrition should not be a concern. If this were the case, however, the chance of problematic healing would increase greatly. Despite this, in addition to meeting all healing patients' ongoing nutritional needs, it is important that clinicians evaluate each patient's dietary pattern immediately before surgery, including those whose dietary intake appears to have been adequate. One study[46] of interest in regard to the apparently well-nourished surgical patient demonstrated that "an adequate recent food intake is able to maintain the wound healing response regardless of the patient's nutritional status. An inadequate food intake over the week before surgery is able to impair the wound healing response [as assessed by hydroxyproline accumulation in Gore-tex implants]. . . ."

Worry, sleeplessness, pain, x-ray examinations, and medications are but a few of the reasons that a person's preoperative dietary intake might be altered. Knowledgeable questioning regarding intake immediately before surgery can serve as data to assist in replacement of nutritional substances before or immediately after surgery. Such attention to the total needs of the patient can assist greatly in optimizing healing.

THE INCISION

Regardless of their origins, all wounds progress through the same phases of the reparative process: inflammation, angiogenesis, fibroplasia and matrix deposition, and epithelialization.[30] In the case of the surgical incision closed by primary intention, however, the dynamics of these processes are less apparent to the naked eye than in wounds closing by secondary or tertiary intention. Because at the external surface the edges of the wound healing by primary intention are approximated, the mechanisms underlying healing must be inferred. One of the most basic standards against which healing can be assessed in this type of wound then is the progress of the process since the *time* of wounding (that is, surgery). In addition, clinicians can and should make several other valuable assessments. For the most part, these concern the incision itself and the way healing is supported in that area. Careful evaluation of the incisional area and support of the healing taking place there are activities reflected in the practice of the skilled clinician. Knowledgeable assessments of the patient's surgical incision site include the following: the primary dressing, epithelial resurfacing, wound closure, healing ridge, and local changes at the wound site.

The Primary Dressing

Initially, the majority of the patient's postoperative wounds are covered with some form of dressing. This first dressing, frequently referred to as the primary dressing, acts to absorb drainage, maintain a sterile environment, and serve as a barrier against further trauma to the delicate incisional surface. Careful selection of nonadherent, absorptive dressings that do not become incorporated within dried incisional drainage serves greatly to reduce the potential for suture-line injury (that is, rewounding) when the time comes for the initial dressing to be removed.

Gauze, a traditional dressing material still in use with many surgical patients, is known to become incorporated within wound fluid as it dries. Removal of the primary dressing in this situation can and often does result in disruption of portions of the intact incision. Although the reopened area may be small, when this occurs, it results in a new wound at that site, as well as a potential new site for infection.

Nurses can play a significant role in optimizing healing by becoming well informed about effective and theoretically sound surgical dressing materials specifically designed to cause "no harm" to incisions. Such materials exist, and although individually they are costlier than traditional dressings, use of these healing supportive materials can in the long run result in reduction in the numbers of far more costly sequelae. Expending effort to ensure that healing-promoting dressing materials are available for use with patients, in particular surgical patients, constitutes a significant healing- and cost-saving activity on the part of clinicians.[6]

Epithelial Resurfacing

Because of the presence of multiple intact epithelial appendages (that is, hair follicles, sebaceous glands, and sweat glands) and the relatively short distance that cells in the interrupted epithelial tissue must "travel" before meeting like cells, resurfacing of the wound closed by primary intention occurs relatively soon after wounding. Most incisions closed by primary intention are resurfaced by 72 hours or within 2 to 3 days after surgery. Granted that the ability of the wound to withstand force (that is, its tensile strength) is limited; still for all intents and purposes the resurfaced wound is closed and, if left uninterrupted, impenetrable to bacteria.

Theoretically, incisional dressings become unnecessary after this time. Despite this fact, many patients prefer that the wound remain covered. As healing evolves, some incisions begin to itch and, if a dressing is present, patients are reminded to approach them with caution. For others, time is needed before they desire to view the surgical scar. The presence of a dressing allows these patients gradually to incorporate changes in body image. Finally, although an incisional dressing is no longer necessary after epithelial cells have resurfaced the wound, once the patient begins to wear street clothes and undergarments a soft dressing placed over the suture line often limits local irritation and provides additional comfort and protection.

Wound Closure

Increasingly and appropriately, over the past decade, surgeons have chosen Steri-Strip tapes as the method by which to approximate the edges of incisional wounds. In areas where drainage is expected to be minimal, these tapes eliminate the microwounds created by suture materials.[23] The very presence of sutures, "foreign bodies" (be they catgut, cotton, silk, synthetic absorbables or multifilament plastics), increases the inflammatory response at the wound edge, as well as the potential for infection. If more sutures are placed than are necessary, or if they are pulled too tight or become taut secondary to tissue edema, the potential for compromised healing at the wound edge only increases. Tissue ischemia, inflammation, and the unsightly pinpoint scarring that can result around sutures left in place too long can be avoided through the use of Steri-Strips.[11,12,23]

When sutures are used in the healthy person, they should not be left in place for extended periods of time; rather, they should be removed within days of the surgery and, if necessary, replaced with Steri-Strip tapes. Monitoring the length of time since surgery and encouraging timely removal of sutures is a positive healing action on the part of the nurse.

Healing Ridge

Deposition of collagen in the wound begins in the inflammatory phase (that is, the moment of wounding to day 4 or to day 6) and peaks during the proliferative, or fibroblastic, phase (that is, day 4 to day 21 after injury). In the healthy person the clinician should be able to detect the accumulation of this new tissue synthesis by palpating what is referred to as a "healing ridge" (that is, an "induration beneath the skin extending to about 1 cm on each side of the wound"[21]) forming directly under the suture line between day 5 and day 9 after surgery. If no ridge is apparent, this circumstance is cause for concern and could be prodromal to wound dehiscence. Hunt[21] pointed out that "almost all dehiscences occur by the fifth to eighth postoperative day in patients who have not yet developed a cutaneous healing ridge and about half are associated with infection." Furthermore, he stated that when a healing ridge is present even retention sutures can be removed, "since the risk of separation has passed."

The knowledgeable nurse can certainly form a theoretically based assessment of healing by carefully palpating the incision to determine the presence or absence of such new tissue synthesis. It is unlikely that a "healing ridge" will be absent in the healthy patient whose healing has been optimized, but if it were, interventions reducing the amount of strain placed on the wound and promoting collagen synthesis would need to be instituted promptly.

Local Changes at the Wound Site

Although most postoperative wounds go on to heal without incident, some manifest changes that bear close observation and institution of a coordinated therapeutic plan. Obviously, the presence of drainage from a previously intact suture line would be an untoward symptom with the need for immediate follow-up assessments. Most frequently, such an occurrence heralds wound dehiscence, or, in extreme cases, fistula formation. If either of these situations were to occur, careful, supportive local wound care treatments should begin, and the wound would go on to heal by secondary intention. Needless to say, the patient and his or her family members would need thoughtful reassurance, explanation, and eventually instruction in how to care for the wound healing in this way.

Changes in skin coloration, induration, increased temperature at the wound site, and unresolved pain after surgery all represent classical signs of infection or hematoma and require immediate consultation with the surgeon. Most nurses are extremely adept at identifying these markers of altered healing and institute appropriate interventions.

Of greater concern in the current era of healthcare delivery is the early discharge of patients from the acute care setting, or "day surgery" procedures. Although the majority of these discharges are nonproblematic, the need for thorough teaching regarding resumption of activities, wound observations, and so forth demand patience and expertise on the part of the clinician. Depending on the type of surgery, instruction in deep-breathing techniques, activity and rest patterns, the need for hydration, and, when appropriate, the use of stool softners to reduce straining the incisional area all need to be addressed. Frequently, this instruction occurs at a time when the patient is fatigued and somewhat overwhelmed by the entire surgical experience. Teaching, in this case, is best reinforced by providing the patient or family member with written guidelines. Research on the best time and method for accomplishing this important aspect of care needs to continue.

WOUND MEASUREMENT

A description of the status of wound measurement and assessment appears elsewhere in this book (see Chapter 3). Four approaches to the assessment of wounds healing by primary intention have been reported; ASEPSIS,[44] Wound Assessment Inventory (WAI),[19] Wells, Newsom, and Rowlands "grading scale,"[41] and a series of observational and palpation assessments described for care of the patient in the home.[37] Of these, only the ASEPSIS and the WAI have undergone any testing for reliability and validity.

ASEPSIS is an acronym for seven wound assessment parameters: four subjective (that is, serous drainage, erythema, purulent exudate, separation of deep tissue) and three objective (that is, additional treatment, isolation of bacteria, stay prolonged over 14 days). ASEPSIS (Table 4-1) was developed to evaluate wound infections in clinical trials of antibiotic regimens. Content validity testing of the items on the scoring method has not been described, though preliminary interrater reliability testing has been reported.[45] Because ASEPSIS was developed specifically for patients with wound infections, it does not appear appropriate for the healthy patient who remains infection free.

Table 4-1   The wound score: ASEPSIS

Criterion	Points
*A*dditional treatments	
Antibiotics	10
Drainage of pus under local anesthesia	5
Débridement of wound (general anesthesia)	10
*S*erous discharge*	daily 0-5
*E*rythema*	daily 0-5
*P*urulent exudate*	daily 0-10
*S*eparation of deep tissues*	daily 9-10
*I*solation of bacteria	10
*S*tay as inpatient prolonged over 14 days	5

From Wilson APR, Treasure T, Sturridge MF, and Grüneberg RN: A scoring method (ASEPSIS) for postoperative wound infections for use in clinical trials of antibiotic prophylaxis, Lancet (8476):311-313, 1986.

*Given scores only on day 5 of first 7 postoperative days.

Category of infection: total score 1 to 10 = satisfactory healing; 11 to 20 = disturbance of healing; 21 to 30 = minor wound infection; 31 to 40 = moderate wound infection; greater than 40 = severe wound infection.

Wound Assessment Inventory (WAI)

The WAI,[19] an instrument designed to "provide a means of quantifying the major signs of inflammation in three-day-old surgical wounds," directs the clinician to assess edema, erythema, and exudate at the incision site. These classical signs of infection are rated on a four-point scale (0 = absent to 3 = marked). Content validity of the items has been reported, as well as interrater reliability scores (0.70 on 12 paired ratings). The potential for subjectivity affecting scoring is great, and the instrument focuses on an outcome that can be affected by multiple, unassessed variables. The merit of this instrument lies in the fact that it begins to log some of the parameters clinicians presently assess in a less than systematic way.

Grading System

Wells, Newsom, and Rowlands[41] interested in monitoring wound infection in patients undergoing cardiothoracic surgery, developed a grading system by which to classify the external incision: "grade 1 = normal incision; grade 2 = inflamed with some exudate; and grade 3 = breaking down with purulent exudate." "A single observer visited the patients . . . and classified wounds." Obviously the range of possibilities between these grades is great, and the system ignores more subtle or covert cues of wound infection. The potential for subjectivity, particularly when clinicians have not been provided with clear objective guidelines for each grade, leaves assessments open to broad interpretation. Validity and reliability data on this approach have not been reported.

Observational and Palpation Assessments

Siddall,[39] citing the difficulty of monitoring the postsurgical patient's wound in the home, suggested a list of assessments the nurse might make to assist in objectifying the process. Validity and reliability of this cluster of assessments nurses frequently make have not been reported.

Certainly generation of research-based tools to evaluate the status of all types of wounds, but particularly wounds closed by primary intention, bears diligent work and concerted effort. This task should, of necessity, involve the active input of clinicians, particularly nurses.

SUMMARY

In 1980,[25] Hunt stated that the goal (in regard to surgical wound healing) was "now clear . . . patients (and surgeons) would no longer need to suffer through failed wounds, leaking anastomoses, and critical wound infections." That phrase has long bothered me, for it seems that the renowned wound-healing researcher inadvertently forgot to include a key member of the healing milieu—the nurse. Levine,[32] a nurse theorist, put it best when she stated that:

The success of the ultimate healing depends in large measure on what happens to the individual during that time. The nurse is the person on the health team who shares the most time with the patient, and thus no worker can influence the success of the healing process more than the nurse. Nursing processes of every kind are dedicated to the promotion of healing.

Only recently have nurses begun to acknowledge their inherent responsibility for wound management.[6] Through research and lively communication, today's nurses will and must assume their role as one of the essential links in continuing to identify and describe activities and states that *optimize* healing. It is no longer good enough to say "the patient healed"; rather the questions astute, knowledgeable clinicians must challenge one another with is: Did we conserve the patient's energy?[32] Did we inflict no further harm by insuring that theory-based therapies were implemented? And, perhaps most important: Did we do everything possible to optimize the healing environment and the healing experience?

SELF-EVALUATION

QUESTIONS AND PROBLEMS

1. State two factors that complicate the application of wound-healing research to the acute wound-repair process.
2. Define three parameters characteristic of an acute surgical wound.
3. True or false: Indirect factors that affect the acute surgical wound are more controllable than direct factors.
4. Which of the following factors contribute to the potential for an infection in a patient with diabetes?
   a. Age and reduced platelet function
   b. Obesity and amount of insulin required
   c. Malnutrition and site of insulin injection
   d. Reduced inflammation and age
5. Negative consequences of elevated glucose levels include:
   a. reduced effectiveness in neutrophil phagocytosis.
   b. enhanced collagen deposition.
   c. overproduction of fibroblasts.
   d. overconsumption of oxygen by tissues.
6. True or false: Blood oxygen levels (Pao_2) is a measure of tissue oxygen levels ($Ptco_2$).
7. State four nursing interventions that support acute wound healing.
8. Describe the significance of the healing ridge in an acute surgical wound.
9. Describe four methods of assessing a wound and their relevance to the acute surgical wound.
10. State four classical signs of an infection at an acute surgical wound site.

SELF-EVALUATION

ANSWERS

1. 1. Research on tissue repair is primarily in the form of animal studies.
   2. Human wounds can vary in status on a continuum of optimal to suboptimal states.
   3. Human wounds are unique and diverse as a consequence of different causes and the presence of different combinations of factors that impinge on the repair process.
   4. Human wounds each possess distinguishing attributes that affect the course and quality of healing. For example, a partial-thickness wound probably goes through a more extensive reparative process than the incision resulting from elective surgery.
2. 1. Results from an operative procedure.
   2. Improves and progresses in a timely fashion.
   3. Wound edges are approximated.
   4. External manifestations of healing are apparent early in the postoperative period.

3. True

4. d

5. a

6. False

7.
   1. Monitor glucose levels closely.
   2. Reduce and control postoperative pain using a variety of modalities (analgesics, repositioning, relaxation techniques, and so on).
   3. Monitor the patient's hydration status and intervene to assure adequate hydration.
   4. Maintain patient's warmth with blankets, slippers, and so on.
   5. Provide information and comfort to allay the patient's anxiety and fears (that is, comments to inform the patient that he is progressing as expected).
   6. Obtain an accurate preoperative (1-week) dietary history.
   7. Encourage ambulation during periods when the postoperative pain is controlled.
   8. Avoid procedures in the area of the wound that potentially constrict blood vessels such as poorly sized antiembolism stockings on the "donor" leg after a coronary artery bypass.

8. The healing ridge can be palpated and forms directly under the suture line between day 5 and day 9 after surgery. Hunt defines the healing ridge as the induration beneath the skin extending to about 1 cm on each side of the wound. The presence of a healing ridge marks the deposition of collagen in the wound.

9.
   1. ASEPSIS: An acronym for seven wound-assessment parameters, which are serous drainage, erythema, purulent exudate, separation of deep tissue, additional treatment, isolation of bacteria, and stay prolonged over 14 days. Application of ASEPSIS to acute infection-free surgical wounds is not appropriate because this tool was developed specifically for patients with wound infections.
   2. Wound Assessment Inventory (WAI): An instrument designed to quantify the major signs of inflammation of 3-day-old surgical wounds. Again the instrument focuses on wound infection versus status of noninfected surgical wounds.
   3. Grading system: A method of classifying the external incision. *Grade 1* = normal incision; *grade 2* = inflamed with some exudate; *grade 3* = breaking down with purulent exudate. Unfortunately, the three parameters are vague and leave room for wide interpretation. No validity or reliability data have been reported for this tool.
   4. Observation and palpation: A list of assessments developed in an attempt to objectify the wound-assessment process. Validity and reliability of this approach have not been reported.

10.
   1. Changes in skin color.
   2. Induration.
   3. Increased temperature at the wound site.
   4. Unresolved incisional pain.

REFERENCES

1. Chang N, Goodson WH, Gottrup F, and Hunt TK: Direct measurement of wound and tissue oxygen tension in postoperative patients, Ann Surg 197:470–478, 1983.
2. Clark RA and Henson PM: The molecular and cellular biology of wound repair, New York, 1988, Plenum Press.
3. Cooper DM: Clinical assessment/measurement of healing: evolution and status, Clinical Materials. (In press.)
4. Cooper DM: Challenge of open wound assessment in the home setting, Progressions 2(3):11-18, 1990.
5. Cooper DM: Human wound assessment: status report and implications for clinicians, AACN Clin Issues in Crit Care Nurs 1:553-563, 1990.
6. Cooper DM: Optimizing wound healing: a practice within nursing's domain, Nurs Clin North Am 25:165-180, 1990.
7. Cruse PJ: Wound infections: epidemiology and clinical characteristics. In Howard RJ and Simmons RL, editors: Surgical infectious diseases, ed 2, East Norwalk, Conn, 1988, Appleton & Lange.
8. Cruse PJ: Incidence of wound infection on the surgical services, Surg Clin North Am 55:1269, 1975.
9. Cruse PJ and Foord R: A five year prospective study of 23,649 surgical wounds, Arch Surg 107:206, 1973.
10. Dykes ER and Anderson R: Atraumatic technic: the sine qua non of operative wound infection prophylaxis, Cleveland Clinic 28:157, 1961.
11. Edlich RF, Rodeheaver G, Golden GT, and Edgerton MT: The biology of infections: sutures, tapes and bacteria. In Hunt TK, editor: Wound healing and wound infection: theory and surgical practice, New York, 1980, Appleton-Century-Crofts.
12. Forrester JC: Sutures and wound repair. In Hunt TK, editor: Wound healing and wound infection: theory and surgical practice, New York, 1980, Appleton-Century-Crofts.
13. Fowler E: Chronic wounds: an overview. In Krasner D, editor: Chronic problem wounds, King of Prussia, Penn, 1990, Health Management Publications Inc.
14. Goodson WH and Hunt TK: Development of a new miniature method for the study of wound healing in human subjects, J Surg Res 33:394-401, 1982.
15. Goodson WH and Hunt TK: Wound healing and the diabetic patient, Surg Gynecol Obstet 149:600, 1979.
16. Goodson WH and Hunt TK: Wound healing in experimental diabetes mellitus: importance of early insulin therapy, Surg Forum 29:95, 1978.
17. Heidenreich T and Guiffre M: Postoperative temperature measurement, Nurs Res 39:153-155, 1990.
17a. Harris, David, MD: Personal communication, April 6, 1991.
18. Hohn DC: Host resistance to infection: established and emerging concepts. In Hunt TK, editor: Wound healing and wound infection: theory and surgical practice, New York, 1980, Appleton-Century-Crofts.
19. Holden-Lund C: Effects of relaxation with guided imagery on surgical stress and wound healing, Res Nurs Health 11:235-244, 1988.
20. Howard RA and Simmons PM: Surgical infectious diseases, East Norwalk, Conn, 1988, Appleton & Lange.
21. Hunt TK: Disorders of repair and their management. In Hunt TK and Dunphy JE, editors: Fundamentals of wound management, New York, 1979, Appleton-Century-Crofts.
22. Hunt TK and Dunphy JE, editors: Fundamentals of wound management, New York, 1979, Appleton-Century-Crofts.
23. Hunt TK and Van Winkle W: Normal repair. In Hunt TK and Dunphy JE, editors: Fundamentals of wound management, New York, 1979, Appleton-Century-Crofts.
24. Hunt TK, Zederfeldt BH, and Goldstick TK: Tissue oxygen tension during controlled hemorrhage, Surg Forum 18:3, 1967.
25. Hunt TK: Wound healing and wound infection, New York, 1980, Appleton-Century-Crofts.

26. Jensen JA, Goodson WH III, Vasconez LO, and Hunt TK: Wound healing and anemia, West J Med 144:465-466, 1986.

27. Jonsson K, Jensen JA, Goodson WH, et al: Assessment of perfusion in postoperative patients using tissue oxygen measurements, Br J Surg 74:263-267, 1987.

28. Knighton DR, Silver IA, and Hunt TK: Regulation of wound-healing angiogenesis: effect of oxygen gradients and inspired oxygen concentration, Surgery 90:262-269, 1981.

29. Krasner D: Chronic wound care, King of Prussia, Penn, 1990, Health Management Publications Inc.

30. LaVan FB and Hunt TK: Oxygen and wound healing, Clin Plast Surg 17:463-484, 1990.

31. Leite JF, Antunes CF, Monteiro JC, and Pereira BR: Value of nutritional parameters in the prediction of postoperative complications in elective gastrointestinal surgery, Br J Surg 74:426-429, 1987.

32. Levine M: Introduction to clinical nursing, ed 2, Philadelphia, 1973, FA Davis.

33. Morain WD and Cohen LB: Wound healing in diabetes mellitus, Clin Plast Surg 17:493-499, 1990.

34. Niinikoski J: The effect of blood and oxygen supply on the biochemistry of repair. In Hunt TK, editor: Wound healing and wound repair: theory and surgical practice, New York, 1980, Appleton-Century-Crofts.

35. Niinikoski J, Heughan C, and Hunt TK: Oxygen tensions in human wounds, J Surg Res 12:77, 1972.

36. Niinikoski J: Effect of oxygen supply on wound healing and formation of experimental granulation tissue, Acta Physiol Scand Suppl 334:4-72, 1969.

37. Pai MP and Hunt TK: Effect of varying oxygen tensions on healing of open wounds, Surg Gynecol Obstet 135:756-758, 1972.

38. Rosenberg CS: Wound healing in the patient with diabetes mellitus, Nurs Clin North Am 25:247-261, 1990.

39. Siddall S: Wound healing: an assessment tool, Home Healthcare Nurse, pp 35-40, 1983.

40. Stotts NA and Washington DF: Nutrition: a critical component of wound healing, AACN Clin Issues in Crit Care Nurs 1:585-592, 1990.

41. Wells FC, Newsom SWB, and Rowlands C: Wound infection in cardiothoracic surgery, Lancet 1(8335):1209-1210, May 28, 1983.

42. West JM: Wound healing in the surgical patient: influence of the perioperative stress response on perfusion, AACN Clin Issues in Crit Care Nurs 1:595-601, 1990.

43. Whitney JD: The influence of tissue oxygen and perfusion on wound healing, AACN Clin Issues in Crit Care Nurs 1:578, 1990.

44. Wilson APR, Treasure T, Sturridge MF, and Grüneberg RN: A scoring method (ASEPSIS) for postoperative wound infections for use in clinical trials of antibiotic prophylaxis, Lancet (8476):311-313, 1986.

45. Wilson AP, Webster A, Grüneberg RN, et al: Repeatability of ASEPSIS wound scoring method, Lancet 1(8491):1208-1209, May 24, 1986.

46. Windsor JA, Knight GS, and Hill GL: Wound healing response in surgical patients: recent food intake is more important than nutritional status, Br J Surg 75(2):135-137, 1988.

5 Pressure Ulcers

RUTH A. BRYANT
MARY L. SHANNON
BARBARA PIEPER
BARBARA J. BRADEN
DONALD J. MORRIS

OBJECTIVES

1. Distinguish between incidence and prevalence.

2. Describe the data reporting the prevalence of pressure ulcers in hospitals and nursing homes and in the elderly and spinal cord injured.

3. Define pressure ulcer.

4. Identify three most common locations for pressure ulcers to develop.

5. Describe the role of subcutaneous tissue and muscle in preventing pressure ulcers.

6. Identify four factors that cause pressure ulcer formation.

7. Differentiate between capillary pressure, capillary closing pressure, and interface pressure.

8. Describe the role of tissue tolerance, intensity of pressure and duration of pressure in the development of pressure ulcers.

9. Describe the impact of the following factors on pressure ulcer development: blood pressure, temperature, smoking, psychosocial status, and age.

10. Describe the phenomena of reactive hyperemia, blanching erythema and nonblanching erythema.

11. Describe the pathophysiologic consequences of pressure damage including the changes that occur at the cellular level and the cone-shaped pressure gradient.

12. Discuss five variables that influence the extent of tissue damage as a consequence of pressure.

13. Differentiate between reliability, validity, specificity, and sensitivity.

14. Describe three pressure-sore risk-assessment scales including the parameters each scale measures.

15. Identify therapeutic features that can be provided by support surfaces.

16. Explain the relevance of capillary closing pressure in selection of support surfaces.

17. Distinguish between the three categories of support surfaces: overlay, replacement mattress, and specialty bed.

18. Identify four criteria for the use of therapeutic foam.

19. Compare and contrast the following in terms of advantages and disadvantages:
    a. Foam overlays
    b. Water overlays
    c. Gel overlays
    d. Static air overlays
    e. Low air loss overlay
    f. Alternating air overlay
    g. Replacement mattresses
    h. Low air loss bed
    i. High air loss bed
    j. Kinetic therapy bed

20. Establish two criteria for use of each of the following:
    a. Pressure-reduction device
    b. Pressure-relief device
    c. Kinetic therapy device

21. Describe the effect of the following on interface pressure: sheepskin, donuts, repositioning.

22. Describe one situation when surgical intervention for a pressure ulcer is preferred and one situation when surgical intervention is not preferred.

23. Identify the major principles underlying all surgical procedures.

24. Distinguish between fasciocutaneous flap and myocutaneous flap.

25. Describe the nursing implications in the care of a patient after a myocutaneous flap with regard to wound drainage, positioning, and activity level.

Pressure ulcers present a significant health care threat to patients with restricted mobility or chronic disease and to older patients. The National Pressure Ulcer Advisory Panel[110] estimates that well over 1 million people in hospitals and nursing homes suffer from pressure ulcers. Hospital-acquired pressure ulcers add to the patient's length of stay, delay the patient's recuperation, and increase the patient's risk for developing complications. Additionally, pressure ulcers often necessitate hospitalization (in certain patient populations such as the elderly and patients with a spinal cord injury) because of sepsis, or the need for débridement or surgical repair. At a time of increasingly scarce health care dollars, pressure ulcers consume intense resources in the form of dressing changes, nursing care, physical therapy, medications, nutritional support, and physician services. A significant mortality is associated with pressure ulcers; approximately 60,000 people are estimated to die from complications related to pressure ulcers every year.[89]

ECONOMIC IMPACT

The financial cost of pressure ulcers to the U.S. health economy is essentially a matter of conjecture. The literature reports quite a range of costs for pressure ulcer management. Cost estimates ranging from $5,000 to $27,000 per ulcer have been cited.[6,77] In 1978, Robinson, Coghlan, and Jackson[126] reported treatment costs for four paraplegic patients as $218,649, an average of $53,729 per patient. Pressure ulcer treatment costs for five paraplegic patients at a California hospital center ranged from $10,564 to $46,341 per patient.[108]

Unfortunately the costs that are reported to be incurred while a pressure ulcer is being managed must be viewed cautiously; the studies are not all comparable. Some studies account for all costs: room, nursing care, supplies, medications, physician fees, and so forth. Other studies examine only direct costs such as the supplies or medications specifically indicated for that particular problem. The result is that there are a great many opinions in the literature and little else.

Alterescu[8] thoughtfully reviewed the difficulties inherent in "costing out" pressure ulcer management. He found that when the patient was admitted for a problem other than the pressure ulcer, the average variable cost of pressure ulcer management per patient was $1300. In contrast, if the patient was admitted specifically for the pressure ulcer, the costs were almost tripled, averaging $3746. If the conservative figure of $1300 is used to calculate the cost of the treatment for the estimated 1 million patients with pressure ulcers in the United States,[110] the annual cost would be 1.3 billion.

SCOPE OF THE PROBLEM

The scope of the pressure ulcer problem in the United States is as unknown as the true costs of managing the pressure ulcer. This may be attributed to two factors: (1) a pressure ulcer is not a reportable condition, and (2) institutions believe that the presence of pressure ulcers is a negative reflection on the quality of care. In fact, the quality assurance guidelines of some state and federal agencies have reinforced the belief that pressure ulcers reflect negatively on quality of care.

Prevalence

Prevalence and incidence are sometimes unfortunately used interchangeably when the pressure ulcer problem is being reported. Box 5-1 outlines the differences between these two measurements.

Reported prevalence varies widely according to country, patient population, and methodology. For example, international studies report a prevalence of 8.85% to 7.19%.[41,67] In general, these studies include all inpatients and outpatients receiving care on one specific day and exclude all maternity patients, ambulatory patients, psychiatric patients, and physically mobile, mentally retarded patients.

It should be noted that these prevalence reports contrast considerably with an earlier prevalence study conducted in Denmark in 1971.[118] This report encompassed 98% of all hospital departments, nursing homes, and visiting nurses and found that 43.1 patients per 100,000 population had pressure ulcers (0.043%).

Nationally, reported pressure ulcer prevalence in the hospital varies from a low of 1.5% to a high of 18.3%.[101,106,128] This wide discrepancy in rates can be attributed to the fact that some studies include intact pressure-damaged skin (stage 1), whereas other studies will

---

Box 5-1   DEFINITION OF INCIDENCE AND PREVALENCE

INCIDENCE
The rate at which new cases develop.
Requires repeated observations (over time).
Observation is one specific population (such as all residents of a state, all males, all patients over 60 years of age).

PREVALENCE
The number of cases at any given point in time.
Requires only one observation.
Observation is of one specific population.

EXAMPLE
A survey is conducted of all the nursing homes in one city. There are 1000 nursing home residents. On May 1, 90 patients are found to have pressure ulcers. Eight weeks later, there are 92 patients with pressure ulcers, and 30 of these have developed since the last survey. The *incidence* is 30 new cases per 8 weeks or 3.75 cases per week or 15 cases per month. Expressed as a percentage, the incidence per week is 3.75 cases per 1000 patients, or 0.375%. The *prevalence* on May 1 was 90 cases per 1000 patients (9.0%); eight weeks later the *prevalence* was 92 cases per 1000 patients (9.2%). Prevalence should remain relatively stable over time unless the frequency of the disease is changing.

---

exclude such lesions. Lower prevalence rates are reported when intact pressure-damaged skin is excluded from the sample.[6,137] However, prevalence can also be overestimated by erroneous inclusion of patients with ordinary hyperemic responses such as pressure-damaged intact skin. Thus it is imperative that data collectors accurately distinguish between stage 1 pressure ulcers and other causes of erythema.

Eckman[50] reported a 23.6% prevalence of pressure ulcers among a unique sample of 1378 subjects in 130 funeral homes. Based on these findings, Eckman extrapolated that dermal ulcers were present in 500,000 of the 2.13 million people who died in the United States in 1987.[50]

Some populations, such as the elderly and the spinal cord injured, are at especially high risk for pressure ulcers.[4,5] Although the spinal cord–injured patients from World War II had a pressure ulcer prevalence of 57% to 85%,[78,144] these rates have fortunately declined to a range of 25% to 40.4% in recent studies.[137,140,158]

Pressure ulcers are also common in the elderly, with a prevalence of 11.6% to 27.5%.[34,136,156,159] The study of Clarke and colleagues[41] underscored the risks of advancing age; among patients less than 70 years of age, only 6% had pressure ulcers, whereas for those 70 years of age and older, the prevalence almost doubled to 11.6%.

Pressure ulcer prevalence also varies with the health care setting. According to the National Pressure Ulcer Advisory Panel (NPUAP),[110] the prevalence of pressure ulcers in acute care settings is 3% to 14% whereas the prevalence range among patients admitted to nursing homes is between 15% and 25%[6,11,14,51,159] Much of this difference occurs because nursing homes have a more concentrated population of patients from high-risk groups.[5] Similar high prevalence rates, 24%, have been reported among patients admitted to a hospital geriatric unit.[113]

Incidence

Determining the incidence of pressure ulcers is inherently difficult because such studies require longitudinal observations. As with prevalence, incidence will vary by setting; among community-dwelling people from 55 to 75 years of age the 10-year incidence of pressure ulcers is 1.85%[64] In contrast, 7.7% of hospitalized patients expected to be confined to bed or chair for at least 1 week may develop a pressure ulcer within 3 weeks.[6] Geriatric and orthopedic units of acute care settings report a higher incidence (24%) of pressure ulcer development during hospitalization periods of approximately 3 weeks.[114,120,125,156] The incidence of pressure ulcers in nursing homes is not easily obtained from the literature; however, over a 6-month period a 26% incidence was reported for one nursing home.[120]

If stage 1 pressure ulcers are included in the study, the reported incidence is higher. Of the patients admitted to a medical intensive care unit, 40% developed a pressure ulcer during a 2-week observation.[26]

SUMMARY

In summary, several factors contribute to the difficulty in accurately determining the size and scope of the pressure ulcer problem. Variations in patient populations and study designs, inappropriate attempts to generalize findings from small population samples,[136] and frequently the expertise of the researchers make data comparisons inaccurate. Other problems include the lack of a uniform classification system (that is, staging or grading), confusion in the use of the terms "prevalence" and "incidence" (see Box 5-1), and inconsistencies in the definition of pressure ulcer; some studies include data on stage 1 pressure ulcers whereas other studies exclude them.

Finally, it should be remembered that many of the large-scale studies were conducted in the 1970s and outside of the United States. Patients now are older and sicker; they are hospitalized for shorter periods of time and are discharged to home or to intermediate or long-term care facilities at a more acute stage of illness. These changes in the patient population can be expected to increase the numbers of people at risk for pressure ulcers, increase the number of high-risk patients in extended care and home care settings, and potentially alter the incidence and prevalence of pressure ulcers in each setting.

TERMINOLOGY

Over the years, several terms have been used to describe pressure ulcers: bedsore, decubitus ulcer, decubiti, and pressure sore. Pressure ulcers is the accepted term because it is more accurate and descriptive.

The origin of the term "bedsore" is not known but predates "decubitus." *Dēcubitus*, a Latin word referring to the reclining position,[56] dates from 1747 when the French used it to mean 'bedsore.'[13] This term, however, is inaccurate because it does not convey the tissue destruction associated with these lesions and because these lesions result from positions other than the lying position (such as sitting). Additionally, although *decubiti* is used as the plural form of *decubitus*, it too is incorrect. *Dēcubitus* is a fourth-declension Latin noun and "fourth declension nouns form their plural with the ending -ūs. . . ."[13] Therefore the plural of *dēcubitus* is *dēcubitūs;* in fact the English plural "decubitus ulcers" would be better.

Several definitions for pressure ulcers have been proposed in the literature;[38,117] all commonly describe impaired blood supply. According to the National Pressure Ulcer Advisory

Panel[110] pressure ulcers are defined as "localized areas of tissue necrosis that tend to develop when soft tissue is compressed between a bony prominence and an external surface for a prolonged period of time."

Pressure ulcers occur most commonly over a bony prominence such as the sacrum, ischial tuberosity, trochanter, and calcaneus; however, they may develop anywhere on the body (as underneath a cast or splint). Approximately 65% of pressure ulcers develop in the area of the pelvis.[3,82,100] Fig. 5-1 demonstrates the typical locations for pressure ulcers and the frequency of ulcer formation at each site.

Bony locations are the areas most prone to pressure ulcer formation because a person's body weight is concentrated on these areas when resting on an unyielding surface. Those who have atrophy of the subcutaneous and muscle tissue layers are at even greater risk for the "mechanical load" of pressure and thus increased soft tissue and capillary compression.

ETIOLOGY

Pressure

Pressure is the major causative factor in pressure ulcer formation. However, several factors play a role in determining whether pressure is sufficient to create an ulcer. The pathologic effect of excessive pressure on soft tissue can be attributed to (1) intensity of pressure, (2) duration of pressure, and (3) tissue tolerance (the ability of both the skin and its supporting structures to endure pressure without adverse sequelae). Two models describe how these factors, in addition to the three major factors that cause pressure ulcers (shear, friction, and nutritional debilitation), contribute to pressure ulcer development (see Fig. 5-2 and pp. 335 and 336).

Intensity of Pressure. To understand the importance of intensity of pressure, it is important to review the terms "capillary pressure" and "capillary closing pressure." Capillary pressure tends to move fluid outward through the capillary membrane.[65] Exact capillary pressure is not known because of the difficulty of obtaining the measurement. Various methods have been used to estimate capillary pressure.

One method used to measure capillary pressure is by direct cannulation of the capillary with a microscopic glass pipet. A manometer is then attached to the pipet and a pressure reading obtained. Capillary pressures have been obtained in animals and in the fingernails of humans using this method. Using such techniques capillary pressures have been reported as follows: 32 mm Hg in the arteriolar limb, 12 mm Hg in the venous limb, and 20 mm Hg in the midcapillary[91] (Fig. 5-3). More commonly, capillary pressures are reported as 30 to 40 mm Hg at the arterial end, 10 to 14 mm Hg at the venous end, and about 25 mm Hg in the middle of the capillary.

Two indirect methods to measure capillary pressure have been reported and result in a pressure termed the "functional" capillary pressure, or the pressure (17 mm Hg) believed necessary to keep the capillary system open and functional.[65] According to Guyton,[65] "indirect measurements are probably nearer to the normal values for capillary pressure than are the micropipet measurements."

The term "capillary closing pressure," or "critical closing pressure," describes the minimal amount of pressure required to collapse a capillary.[36] Tissue anoxia develops when externally applied pressure causes vessels to collapse. It is generally believed that the amount of pressure required to collapse capillaries must exceed capillary pressure. It is

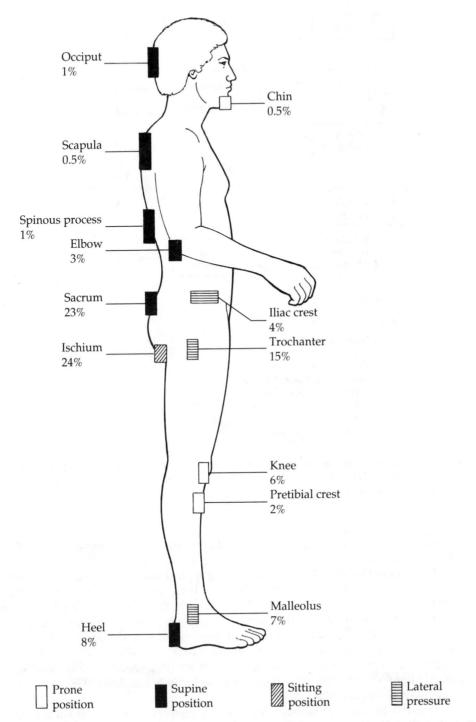

Fig. 5-1   Common sites for pressure ulcers and frequency of ulceration per site. (Data from Agris J and Spira M: Clin Symp 31(5): 2+, 1979.)

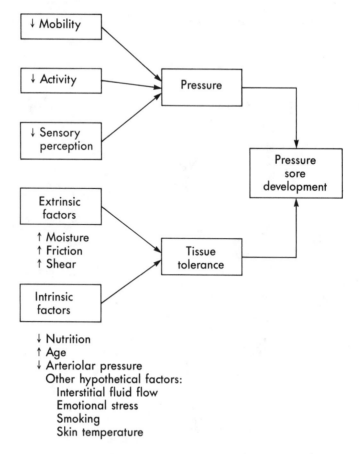

Fig. 5-2 Factors contributing to the development of pressure ulcers. (From Braden B and Bergstrom N: Rehabil Nurs 12(1):8, 1987.) See pp. 335 and 336 for a greater detailed etiologic (causal) model of pressure sore production.

common to use capillary pressures of 12 to 32 mm Hg as the numerical "standard" for capillary closing pressure.

To quantify the intensity of pressure being applied externally to the skin, one measures the interface pressures. Numerous studies have been conducted to measure interface pressures.[79,80,97] Interestingly, these studies have shown that the interface pressures attained while one is in the sitting or supine position commonly exceed capillary pressures.[20]

In 1961, Lindan[97] used an experimental "bed" to calculate the pressure distribution over the skin of a healthy adult male in the supine, prone, side lying, and sitting positions. The range of interface pressures was from 10 to 100 mm Hg. Interface readings as high as 300 mm Hg have been obtained over the ischial tuberosity of healthy able-bodied male subjects when sitting in an unpadded chair.[79]

Fortunately, interface pressures in excess of capillary pressure will not routinely result in ischemia. Healthy people with normal sensation regularly shift their weight in response

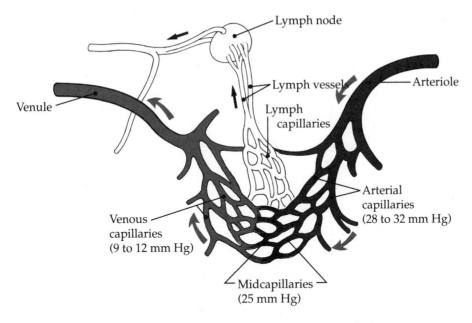

Lymph node

Lymph vessels

Arteriole

Venule

Lymph capillaries

Arterial
capillaries
(28 to 32 mm Hg)

Venous
capillaries
(9 to 12 mm Hg)

Midcapillaries
(25 mm Hg)

Fig. 5-3 Capillary pressures within the capillary bed.

to the discomfort associated with capillary closure and tissue hypoxia. Unfortunately, pathologic processes such as spinal cord injury or sedation impair a person's ability to recognize or respond to this discomfort. Tissue hypoxia can then develop and progress to tissue anoxia and cellular death.

Duration of Pressure. Duration of pressure is an important fact that influences the detrimental effects of pressure and must be considered in tandem with intensity of pressure.[35] An inverse relationship exists between duration and intensity of pressure in creating tissue ischemia.[35,79,149] Specifically, low-intensity pressures over a long period of time can create tissue damage just as high-intensity pressure can over a very short period of time. See Fig. 5-4.

Husain[69] underscored the significance of the relationship between duration and intensity of pressure. Husain found that a 100 mm Hg pressure applied to rat muscle for 2 hours was sufficient to produce only microscopic changes in the muscle; the same pressure applied for 6 hours, however, was sufficient to produce complete muscle degeneration.

Tissue Tolerance. Tissue tolerance is the third fact that determines the pathologic effect of excessive pressure and describes the condition or integrity of the skin and supporting structures that influence the skin's ability to redistribute the applied pressure. Compression of tissue against skeletal structures and the resulting tissue ischemia can be avoided by effective redistribution of pressure.

The concept of tissue tolerance was first discussed in the literature in 1930 by Trumble,[149] who recognized the need to identify how much pressure skin could "tolerate."

Later, Husain[69] introduced the concept of sensitizing the tissue to pressure and consequently to ischemia. Rat muscle was sensitized with a pressure of 100 mm Hg applied for 2

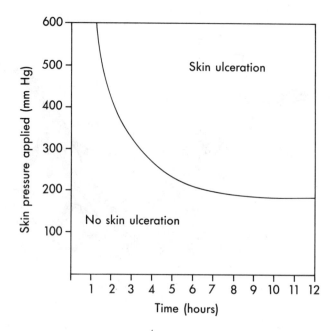

Fig. 5-4   Graph demonstrating relationship between intensity and duration of pressure. (From Kosiak M: Arch Phys Med Rehabil 42:24, 1961.)

hours. Seventy-two hours later, a mere 50 mm Hg pressure applied to the same tissue caused muscle degeneration in only 1 hour. This muscle destruction resulted during the second application of pressure even though the intensity and duration of pressure was lower than the initial intensity and duration.

This finding has significant implications for the patient population at risk for pressure ulcers; it indicates that episodes of deep tissue ischemia can occur without cutaneous manifestations and such episodes can sensitize the patient's skin. Small increments of pressure, even if only slightly above normal capillary pressure ranges, may then result in breakdown.

Tissue tolerance is influenced by the ability of the skin and underlying structures (that is, blood vessels, interstitial fluid, collagen) to "work together as a set of parallel springs that transmit load from the surface of the tissue to the skeleton inside."[81] Several factors can alter the ability of the soft tissue to perform this task, as described in Fig. 5-2.

Shear

Shear was first described in 1958 as a contributing element in pressure ulcers.[123] Shear is caused by the interplay of gravity and friction; it exerts force parallel to the skin and is the result of both gravity pushing down on the body and resistance (friction) between the patient and a surface such as the bed or chair. For example, when the head of the bed is elevated, the effect of gravity on the body is to pull the body down toward the foot of the bed. However, the resistance generated by the bed surface tends to try to hold the body in place. What is actually held in place is the skin, whereas the weight of the skeleton continues to pull the body downward. Fig. 1-8 demonstrates shear force.

Because the skin does not move freely, the primary effect of shear occurs at the deeper fascial level of the tissues overlying the bony prominence. Blood vessels, which are anchored at the point of exit through the fascia, are stretched and angulated when exposed to shear. This force also dissects the tissues "in the plane of greater concentration which is observed clinically as a large area of undermining which extends circumferentially."[123]

Shear causes much of the damage often observed with pressure ulcers. In fact, some lesions are termed "pressure ulcers" that may result solely from shear. According to Bennett and Lee[21] as many as 40% of reported pressure ulcers could be misinterpreted; they could actually be shear injury, rather than pressure injury.

Friction

Friction is a significant factor in pressure ulcer development because it acts in concert with gravity to cause shear. Alone, its ability to cause skin damage is confined to the epidermal and upper dermal layers. In its mildest form, friction abrades the epidermis and dermis similar to that of a mild burn, and such skin damage is often reported as a "sheet burn." This type of damage most frequently develops in patients who are restless.

When friction acts with gravity, however, the effect of the two factors is synergistic, and the outcome is shear. It is not possible to have shear without friction. However, it is possible to have friction without significant shear (such as moving the palm of the hand repeatedly against a bed sheet).

Moisture, specifically incontinence, is frequently cited in the literature as a predisposing factor to pressure ulcer development.[31,145] The mechanism may be that moisture alters the resiliency of the epidermis to external forces.

According to Adams and Hunter[2] both shear and friction are increased in the presence of mild to moderate moisture. However, it appears that shear and friction actually decrease in the presence of profuse moisture. Contrary to earlier beliefs, studies have shown that the high-moisture environment created by urinary incontinence is not a major factor in the production of pressure ulcers.[6,75,137]

Nutritional Debilitation

Although it is undeniable that good nutrition is necessary for wound healing, the role of significant nutritional debilitation in *producing* pressure ulcers is often less appreciated. Numerous studies have indicted poor nutrition as a significant factor in the development of pressure ulcers.[6,71,119,121,156]

Severe protein deficiency renders soft tissue more susceptible to breakdown when exposed to local pressure because hypoproteinemia alters oncotic pressure and causes edema formation.[109] Oxygen diffusion and transport of nutrients in ischemic and edematous tissue is compromised. Additionally, there is a decreased resistance to infection with low protein levels because of the effect on the immune system.[29,111] The stage is set for skin breakdown in the older patient when protein depletion is coupled with the normal aging process.

Certain vitamin deficiencies, particularly vitamins A, C, and E, may also contribute to pressure ulcer development. Vitamin A deficiency delays reepithelialization, collagen synthesis, and cellular cohesion. Vitamin C deficiency compromises collagen production and immune system function and results in capillary fragility. Vitamin E deficiency may decrease cell-mediated immunity and may also increase tissue damage from toxic free radicals.

Other factors that have been identified as important in the development or predisposition to pressure ulcer formation include advanced age, low blood pressure, smoking, and elevated body temperature.

Advanced age. Several changes occur in the skin and its supporting structures with the aging process: (1) loss of lean body mass, (2) decrease in serum albumin levels, (3) diminished inflammatory response, (4) loss of elasticity in the tissue, and (5) reduced cohesion between the epidermis and the dermis.[19,54,74] With these changes, the ability of the soft tissue to distribute the mechanical load without compromising blood flow is impaired.[31,81] These changes combine with many other age-related changes that occur in other body systems to make the skin more vulnerable to pressure, shear, and friction.[24,74] For example, studies have shown that the blood flow in the area of the ischial tuberosity while one is sitting on an unpadded surface is lower in paraplegic and geriatric populations than in normal patients.

Low blood pressure. When Trumble[149] identified the need to study tissue tolerance, he looked at the amount of external pressure needed to create skin "pain" in relationship to the patient's blood pressure, instead of capillary pressure. He postulated that "skin pressure tolerance varies slightly with blood pressure."

In fact, systolic blood pressures below 100 and diastolic pressures below 60 have been associated with pressure ulcer development.[60,107] Hypotension may shunt blood flow away from the skin to more vital organs, thus decreasing the skin tolerance for pressure by allowing capillaries to close at lower levels of interface pressure.

Psychosocial status. Psychosocial issues such as motivation, emotional energy, and emotional stress[10] have been associated with pressure ulcer formation. Cortisol may be the trigger for lowered tissue tolerance when a person is under stress. Cortisol is the primary glucocorticoid secreted when a person is exposed to a stressor and lacks appropriate coping mechanisms to mediate the stress-related hormonal response.[30,81]

There are two mechanisms by which cortisol might decrease the ability of the skin to absorb mechanical load. (1) Cortisol may alter the mechanical properties of the skin by disproportionately increasing the rate of collagen degradation over collagen synthesis.[42,127] In fact, loss of skin collagen has been associated with the development of pressure ulcers among spinal cord–injured patients.[127] (2) It is also possible that glucocorticoids may trigger structural changes in connective tissue and may affect cellular metabolism by interfering with the diffusion of water, salt, and nutrients between the capillary bed and the cells.[132]

Smoking. Evidence that smoking may contribute to pressure ulcer formation is beginning to accumulate. Cigarette smoking has been reported to correlate positively with the presence of pressure ulcers in a group of spinal cord–injured patients.[90] The incidence and extent of existing ulcers was greater in those patients with higher pack-per-year histories.

Elevated body temperature. Elevated body temperature has been associated with pressure ulcer development in several studies.[6,31,60] In elderly subjects, even mild temperature elevations may increase the risk for pressure ulcer development.[24] Although the mechanism of this association between elevated body temperature and pressure ulcer development is not proved, it may be related to increased oxygen demand in already anoxic tissue.

Miscellaneous factors. Other conditions, such as those that create sluggish blood flow, may also be significant intrinsic factors jeopardizing tissue tolerance. For example, greater tissue damage has been associated with increased blood viscosity and high hematocrit.[134] This may explain why dehydration is sometimes mentioned as a contributing factor to pressure ulcer development.

PATHOPHYSIOLOGIC CHANGES

Clinical Presentation

The pathophysiologic tissue changes that occur with pressure ulcer formation are a predictable series of events.[117] Clinical presentation can vary from nonblanching erythema to ecchymosis and then to frank necrosis.

Obstruction of capillary blood flow by externally applied pressure creates tissue ischemia (hypoxia). If the pressure is removed in a short period of time, blood flow returns and the skin can be seen to flush. This phenomenon, known as "reactive hyperemia," is a compensatory mechanism whereby blood vessels in the pressure area dilate in an attempt to overcome the ischemic episode. Reactive hyperemia by definition is transient and may also be described as blanching erythema. Blanching erythema is an area of erythema that becomes white (blanches) when compressed with a finger. The erythema promptly returns when the compression is removed. The site may be painful for the patient with intact sensation. Blanching erythema is an early indication of pressure and will usually resolve without tissue loss if pressure is reduced or eliminated.

When the hyperemia persists, deeper tissue damage should be suspected. Nonblanching erythema is a more serious sign of impaired blood supply and is suggestive that tissue destruction is imminent or has already occurred; it results from damage to blood vessels and extravasation of blood into the tissues. The color of the skin can be an intense bright red to dark red or purple; many people misdiagnose pressure-induced nonblanching erythema as a hematoma or ecchymosis (bruise). When deep tissue damage is also present, the area is often either indurated or boggy when palpated. Nonblanching erythema attributable to ischemia is seldom reversible.

Cellular Response

When pressure occludes capillaries, a complex series of events is set into motion. Surrounding tissues become deprived of oxygen, and nutrients and metabolic wastes begin to accumulate in the tissue. Damaged capillaries become more permeable and leak fluid into the interstitial space to cause edema. Because perfusion through edematous tissue is slowed, tissue hypoxia worsens. Cellular death ensues and more metabolic wastes are released into the surrounding tissue. Tissue inflammation is exacerbated, and more cellular death occurs (Fig. 5-5).

Muscle Response

Muscle damage may occur with pressure ulcers and is more significant than the cutaneous damage. In fact, pressure is highest at the point of contact between the soft tissue (such as muscle or fascia) and the bony prominence.[17,79] This cone-shaped pressure gradient indicates that deep pressure ulcers initially form at the bone–soft tissue interface, not the skin surface, and extend outward to the skin (Fig. 5-6).[138] The skin damage seen in pressure ulcers is often referred to as the "tip of the iceberg" because a larger area of necrosis and ischemia is expected at the tissue-bone interface.

It has been further suggested that muscle damage is more extensive than skin damage because the muscle is more sensitive to the effects of ischemia.[37] An understanding of the structure of the vascular system allows one to form a rationale for this enhanced muscle damage. The vascular circulation can be divided into three sections: segmental, perforator, and cutaneous.[45] The segmental system is composed of the main arterial vessels arising

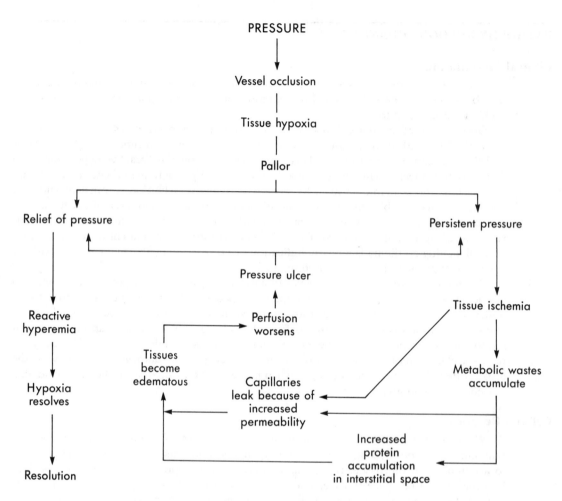

Fig. 5-5 Cellular response to pressure.

from the aorta. The perforator system supplies the muscles but also serves as an interchange supply to the skin. The cutaneous system consists of arteries, capillary beds, and veins draining at different levels of the skin and serves to provide thermoregulation as well as limited nutritional support. This indicates that occlusion of the perforator system may initiate muscle damage and may also create some of the cutaneous ischemia. The significance of the perforator blood flow to skin damage has been demonstrated when musculocutaneous flaps have been elevated surgically.

"Interruption of the blood supply to the muscle can lead to skin necrosis, emphasizing the importance of the relationship of the physiological blood supply to the skin *from* underlying muscle. It is reasonable to suspect that the same type of tissue breakdown or necrosis could result from pressure-induced *muscle* ischemia in bedridden patients, and that in some cases the cutaneous lesions are secondary to the impaired muscle circulation."[45]

Because the skin receives its blood supply from both the perforator and the cutaneous systems, the skin actually receives more blood than necessary to meet metabolic needs.[117] It

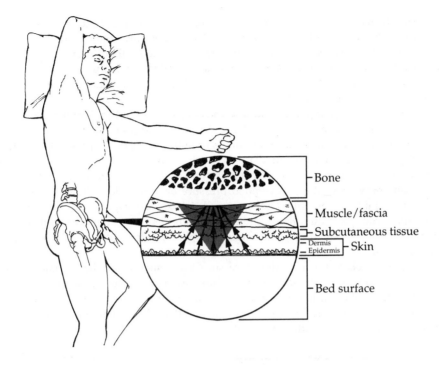

Fig. 5-6   Diagram of extent of tissue damage at muscle and skin level

is possible that the occlusion of "perforators" may be of more significance than occlusion of the cutaneous system and may produce more extensive tissue damage.

Variables Influencing Extent of Tissue Damage

If pressure is not relieved, ischemic changes occur as a consequence of decreased perfusion; however, the occlusion also triggers a cascade of events that further intensifies the extent of tissue ischemia. Hence the tissue damage typically seen with pressure is precipitated by pressure but then worsened by events such as venous thrombus formation, endothelial cell damage, redistribution of blood supply in ischemic tissue, alteration in lymphatic flow, and alterations in interstitial fluid composition.

Externally applied high pressures, even when applied for a short duration, damage the blood vessels directly, which in turn causes tissue ischemia. In 1961, Kosiak[79] described the changes in larger vessels and the formation of venous thrombi impairs the normal reactive hyperemia that should occur once pressure is removed. Thus tissue remains ischemic even after the pressure has been alleviated.

Compression of the capillary wall also damages the endothelium.[39] Once pressure is removed and reperfusion begins, the damaged endothelial cells are shed into the bloodstream and proceed to occlude the blood vessel. As the endothelium is shed, platelets are activated by the underlying collagen and clot formation is triggered. Furthermore, damaged endothelial cells lose their usual anticoagulant characteristics and release thrombogenic substances that exacerbate vessel occlusion and ultimately cause increased tissue ischemia.

The redistribution of the blood supply that occurs in ischemic skin further aggravates pressure-induced tissue hypoxia. Because of the externally applied pressure, blood flow to surface capillaries is reduced, and such reduction renders them more vulnerable and more permeable than before. The extent of ischemia created can be further worsened when neutrophils are present in the tissue because their resting oxygen demands are 30 times greater than resting epithelial cells.[131]

Alteration in the lymphatic flow and the composition of the interstitial fluid also affects pressure-induced ischemia.[124] Lymphatic flow in pressure-damaged skin ceases. Likewise, the normal movement of interstitial fluid is inhibited by both the pressure and the ischemia. Consequently, protein is retained in the interstitial tissues causing increased interstitial oncotic pressure, edema formation, dehydration of the cells, and tissue irritation.

In summary, extensive or extended pressure occludes blood flow, lymphatic flow, and interstitial fluid movement. Tissues are deprived of oxygen and nutrients, and toxic metabolic products accumulate. Interstitial fluids retain proteins that dehydrate cells and irritate tissues. The ensuing tissue acidosis, capillary permeability, and edema contribute to cellular death.[124]

Abruzzese recently stated that "pressure sores should not be a major problem."[1] An essential component in the reduction or elimination of pressure ulcers is the understanding of risk factors. With an in-depth review of the etiology of pressure ulcer formation and the pathophysiologic process involved, those factors that place a patient at risk for developing a pressure ulcer become readily apparent.

PREVENTION OF PRESSURE ULCERS

A formal, comprehensive pressure ulcer prevention program is essential to effectively prevent pressure ulcers. Such a program is best developed and implemented with a multidisciplinary team who can provide a holistic approach. Typically, members of this team should consist of representatives from the following specialties: nursing, medicine, physical therapy, occupational therapy, and nutritional support.

Background

Pressure ulcer prevention programs establish guidelines that allocate resources and describe activities aimed at decreasing the probability that a patient will develop a pressure ulcer. When allocating resources for pressure ulcer prevention, clinicians have three options: (1) assume all patients are at risk and use preventive resources on all patients, (2) depend on their clinical judgment and intuitive sense to identify those patients at risk, or (3) use a risk assessment tool to identify patients who are at risk.

The assumption that all patients are at risk and thus preventive measures should be universally applied is difficult to defend in the majority of settings; this blanket rule likely represents an extremely inefficient use of resources. The following serves as an example of this problem. In one hospital setting, 84% of the patients in a general medical surgical unit and 58% of the patients admitted to an intensive care unit (ICU) stepdown unit were judged "not at risk" and did not go on to develop pressure ulcers. In the ICU, 45% of patients admitted were judged "not at risk"; 15% went on to develop a pressure ulcer.[25] Cumulatively, these data demonstrate that 65% of the patients studied were judged not at risk, and this judgment was correct in 97.6% of the cases. To treat all patients in such settings as being at risk would be a tremendously wasteful approach to care. However, such an approach is probably acceptable practice in neurologic centers, especially spinal cord rehabilitation, where the degree of immobility is so profound that all patients should be considered at risk.

The accuracy of clinical judgment and intuitive sense in identifying those at risk has not been studied extensively, but Bergstrom, Demuth, and Braden found that using a risk-assessment tool more accurately identified those patients who would develop a pressure ulcer than the nurse's "best guess."[25] Furthermore, clinical judgment is likely to be much less reliable (consistent) than risk scales because it will be based on highly variable individual experience and knowledge. Risk scales should be both more reliable and more accurate than clinical judgment; they may also enhance the judgment of the novice clinician and focus the attention of the expert clinician.

The most cost-efficient method of implementing a pressure ulcer prevention program is to use a risk-assessment scale so that those patients who are most in need of preventive care can be targeted. Therefore risk assessment becomes an essential ingredient in a pressure-ulcer prevention program. Such a program should provide guidelines that (1) identify patients at risk for developing pressure ulcers and (2) minimize the negative effects of identified risk factors. From these guidelines, policies or standards of care can be established.

Identify Patients at Risk

Screening tests or risk-assessment tools are the backbone of any pressure-prevention program. Screening tests facilitate prevention primarily by distinguishing those who are at risk for developing pressure ulcers from those who are not, thus allowing for judicious allocation of resources. The second function of this type of assessment is to identify the extent to which a person exhibits specific risk factor, thus prompting the nurse to initiate individualized preventive interventions.

Features of Risk-Assessment Tools. Screening tests vary in terms of cost, invasiveness, utility (ease of use, time required), reliability, and predictive validity. Although the cost-benefit ratio of a screening tool can be a particularly difficult determination, it should be considered. How high a cost can be tolerated for detection on a per case basis? What kind of costs are either incurred or avoided based on the outcome of the test? How often would a test have to be repeated to effectively identify those at highest risk?

The selection of screening tests require practical and ethical considerations. For example, interface pressure might be an excellent predictor of pressure ulcer risk yet be impractical for routine screening. Although serum albumin might be moderately predictive of pressure ulcer risk, it may be more invasive and expensive than could be justified in certain settings, such as nursing homes and home care.

Rating scales are the most common screening tool used by nurses to identify patients at risk for pressure ulcer development. Although rating scales have the advantage of being low cost and noninvasive, a critical evaluation of their performance is necessary. Specifically, information concerning reliability and validity is crucial. Does the tool accurately (validly) predict the development of a pressure ulcer? Do different uses consistently (reliably) assign the same rating to the same patient? Additionally, several related questions should be considered. Does the educational background (RN, LPN, NA) of the rater or the shift during which the rater worked affect reliability? Is the scale consistent in predicting pressure-ulcer development regardless of age? Does patient population (such as nursing home, acute care, or critical care) affect the predictive ability of the scale? Finally, does the timing of the assessment influence the predictive validity?

Common measures of predictive validity are sensitivity, specificity, predictive power of positive results, and predictive power of negative results (Table 5-1).[92,95] Sensitivity and specificity are the two measures that best reflect predictive validity; these measures are less likely to be influenced by the pressure ulcer prevalence of different patient populations.[152] Sensitivity addresses the question, Of the patients who developed pressure ulcers, what percentage were identified by the screening tool as being at risk (true positives)? Specificity addresses the question, Of the patients who did not develop a pressure ulcer, what percentage were identified by the screening tool as being at no risk (true negatives)?

Rating scales can also create false-positive and false-negative results. Patients who were predicted to develop a pressure ulcer but do not are referred to as false positives, whereas patients who are predicted to remain pressure ulcer free and do not are referred to as false negatives. Both sensitivity and the predictive value of negative results are influenced by the number of false negatives; the number of false positives influences specificity and the predictive value of positive results.

The ideal screening test would be 100% sensitive and 100% specific, but this is rarely achieved, even by tests intended for diagnosis rather than screening. This ideal is still less likely to be achieved when one is attempting to predict a condition that is preventable. Nevertheless, these measures of predictive validity are invaluable, when one compares the results of various instruments for screening (Table 5-2).

Several instruments designed to predict the risk of pressure ulcers have been reported in the literature.[24,61,118] These instruments use summative rating scales based on contributing factors and specify critical scores for identifying patients are risk. An example of the Gosnell scale, Braden scale, and Norton scale can be found in Appendix A.

Table 5-1 Definitions of measures of validity for screening tools to predict development of pressure sores (PS+/PS−)

		PS+	PS−
Positive test:		TP (true positive)	FP (false positive)
Negative test:		FN (false negative)	TN (true negative)

Sensitivity. Of those who became PS+, the percentage who had a positive test	$\dfrac{TP}{TP + FN} \times 100$
Specificity. Of those who remained PS−, the percentage who had a negative test	$\dfrac{TN}{TN + FP} \times 100$
Predictive value of positive results. Of those who had a positive test, the percentage who became PS+	$\dfrac{TP}{TP + FP} \times 100$
Predictive value of negative results. Of those who had a negative test, the percentage who remained PS−	$\dfrac{TN}{FN + TN} \times 100$

Table 5-2 Reliability and validity data on selected risk-assessment tools

	Reliability studies with interrater reliability		Validity studies						
	% agreement	Raters	Setting	n	Range	Age	Standard deviation	% sensitive	% specific
Norton scale									
Roberts and Goldstone (1979)	NR	RNs	Orthopedic wards	59	NR	(Over age 60)		92	57
Goldstone and Goldstone (1982)	NR	NR	Orthopedic wards	40	NR	(Over age 60)		89	36
Lincoln et al. (1986)	39.7	RNs	Acute Med-surg	50	65-89	72.2	15.8	0	94
Gosnell scale									
Gosnell (1973)	NA	—	Extended care	30	65-91	78.8	NR	50	73
Gosnell (1988)	90	RNs							
Braden scale									
Bergstrom et al. (1987)[26]	88	RNs	Med-surg	99	18-92	57.2	16.8	100	90
Bergstrom et al. (1987)[26]	15	LPN, NA	Stepdown	100	14-102	50.5	24.0	100	64
DeMuth (1987)	NA	—	Adult ICU	60	21-84	58.5	14.5	83	64

NR, Not reported; *NA*, not applicable.
Differences in outcome criteria and timing of assessment exist between studies and interfere with comparisons. Some adjustments were made for these differences when reporting was adequate.

Norton scale. The Norton scale has been studied extensively,[58,59,96,125] and consists of five parameters: physical condiction, mental state, activity mobility, and incontinence. Each parameter is rated on a scale of 1 to 4, with one- or two-word descriptors for each rating. The sum of the ratings for all five parameters yields a score that can range from 5 to 20, with lower scores indicating increased risk. Norton found an almost linear relationship between the scores of the elderly patients and the incidence of pressure ulcers, with a score of 14 indicating the "onset of risk" and a score of 12 or below indicating a high risk for pressure ulcer formation.

A summary of reliability and validity data from three studies can be found in Table 5-2.[58,96,125] Only one study reported interrater reliability, which was a low-percentage agreement among RN raters. This study also reported disagreement among experts concerning face validity.

Gosnell Scale. In 1973, Gosnell[60] adapted the Norton scale by adding nutrition and deleting physical condition. The Gosnell scale consists of five parameters (mental status, continence, mobility, activity, and nutrition), which were further clarified by descriptors. Additionally, two- or three-sentence descriptive statements were added for each rating on each parameter. Gosnell also studied several additional variables, such as body temperature, blood pressure, skin tone and sensation, medication, and medical diagnoses. However, these variables were given no weight in the score.

The range of possible scores for the Gosnell scale is 5 to 20. Although early studies[60] reported that lower scores denoted higher risk (16 was the critical cutoff score), a later revision[61] shows the scoring to be reversed (high scores denote high risk). Testing to determine the cutoff score is in progress. Since all ratings have historically been done by the investigator, early reports did not address interrater reliability. Most recent testing demonstrates a percent agreement of 90% when used by RNs.[62] A review of the reliability and validity of the Gosnell scale is summarized in Table 5-2.

Braden scale. A third instrument, the Braden scale[25,26,32] is composed of six subscales that conceptually reflect degrees of sensory perception, skin moisture, physical activity, nutritional intake, friction and shear, and ability to change and control body position. All subscales are rated from 1 to 4, except for the friction and shear subscale, which is rated from 1 to 3. Each rating is accompanied by a brief description of criteria for assigning the rating. Potential scores range from 4 to 23, and an adult hospitalized patient with a score of 16 or below is considered at risk.[25] In older populations, a score of 17 or 18 may be a more efficient predictor of pressure ulcer formation.[26]

This instrument has undergone testing in three settings (critical care, acute care, and extended care) and validity has been established by expert opinion. Raters have been registered nurses, licensed practical nurses, and nurse aides. Data demonstrate the Braden scale is highly reliable when used by registered nurses, as shown in Table 5-2.[25,26,32]

Implementing Risk Assessment

When implementing the risk-assessment component of a pressure-ulcer prevention program, one must make several decisions. First, it must be determined what caregiver can perform the assessment. Since only registered nurses have been found to reliably use any of these scales, it seems wise to specify that assessments be performed by registered nurses whenever possible. The one test of interrater reliability, in which raters were practical nurses and nurse aides, tested personnel untrained in use of the tool and found an unacceptably low percent agreement. Therefore, in settings where practical nurses or nurse aides are the predominant bedside caregivers, the registered nurse must "train" these personnel in the correct use of the tool. Furthermore, their assessment should be validated until there is consistently no more than one point difference in the total score assigned to any patient.

Another decision involves the timing of risk assessment. The prevailing practice has been to assess the patient only on admission. Although admission assessment is important because it allows the nurse to identify those at highest risk, the nurse is rarely able to learn enough during the admission assessment to accurately identify lesser degrees of risk. For this reason, as well as the propensity for this patient's condition to change, risk assessment should be repeated 24 to 48 hours after admission and repeated when the patient's condition changes. In establishing a protocol, it is wise to specify an interval for reassessment that reflects how quickly the patient's condition changes in that setting. For example, one might set the interval at daily in the ICU, every 48 hours on medical-surgical floors, weekly in skilled nursing facilities, and monthly in intermediate care facilities. None of these tools requires more than 30 seconds to complete when the nurse is familiar with the patient, and so frequent assessment should not be burdensome.

In summary, risk assessment involves more than simply determining the patient's score on an assessment tool. It involves synthesizing risk factors identified through use of an assessment tool with knowledge of additional contributing factors as well as nursing judgment based on experience. The nurse should be aware that a risk score on an assessment tool is an important piece of data but that knowledge of the score without recognition of the specific deficits contributing to that score is insufficient for determining a program of prevention.

Minimize the Negative Effects of Risk Factors

Identification of factors (intrinsic and extrinsic) that place the patient at risk for developing a pressure ulcer is, in itself, insufficient to prevent pressure ulcers. Risk assessment must serve as a basis to identify measures that will alleviate, reduce, or minimize the negative effects of identified risk factors.

Assessment. The nurse must first determine which risk factors are present for an individual patient. Because pressure is the causative factor of pressure ulcers, reduction or elimination of the interface pressure is essential. Positions that may result in pressure ulcer formation, such as supine, sitting, or an operative position, must be determined. For example, patients who spend much of their time sitting in a chair are prone to pressure-ulcer formation over the ischial tuberosities. For these patients pressure relief or reduction in the bed will not be beneficial; pressure reduction in the chair is imperative.

Coexisting factors predisposing to pressure-ulcer formation must also be assessed. Reduction of pressure alone will not be sufficient if the patient is subjected to shear, friction, or fungal infection, for example. Interventions appropriate for prevention of these types of skin damage are discussed in detail in Chapter 1.

During the assessment process, it is also important to ascertain the effectiveness of the current plan such as the turning frequency or the support surface. For example, an every 2-hour turning schedule for a hemodynamically unstable patient is not appropriate. Likewise, although the support surface may be appropriate, it may be performing suboptimally because of improper inflation.

Interventions: Positioning. For years frequent repositioning of the patient has been recommended to prevent capillary occlusion, tissue ischemia, and pressure ulceration.[78,133,149] Although repositioning does not reduce intensity of pressure, it does reduce the more critical element of pressure-ulcer formation, duration. In 1961, Kosiak recommended the frequency of repositioning to be hourly to every 2 hours[79] based on the interface pressure readings from healthy able-bodied subjects. Currently, the Agency of Health Care Policy and Research (AHCPR)[23] recommends repositioning at least every 2 hours.

Unfortunately, because capillary closing pressures vary among persons and pressure points, the frequency of repositioning required to prevent ischemia is variable and unknown. Furthermore, there are many other factors that impinge on the frequency of repositioning (such as pain, hemodynamic instability, staffing). Therefore frequent repositioning alone may not be sufficient to prevent tissue ischemia.[70]

Additionally, one should avoid the side-lying position when repositioning,[23,134] because this position exerts such intense pressure directly over the trochanter. Instead, the 30-degree lateral position as described by Seiler and Stahelin should be used alternately with the supine position (Fig. 5-7).[135]

Heels can be protected from pressure when they are kept off the bed with a pillow under the lower leg or by use of specially designed heel protectors. Because support surfaces vary in their ability to reduce interface pressure under the heels, these additional interventions may be indicated in combination with the support surface.

Interventions: Outdated. Many devices used to prevent pressure in the past are now known to be deleterious. For example, foam or rubber rings (that is, donuts) are never indicated to relieve pressure because they actually concentrate the intensity of the pressure to

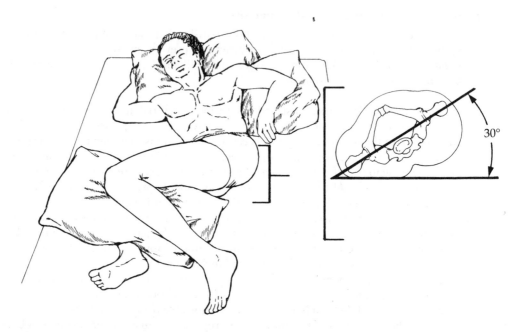

Fig. 5-7   Thirty-degree lateral position at which pressure points are avoided.

the surrounding tissue.[3] Furthermore, sheepskin has no effect on pressure and so is inappropriate for pressure prevention.[9]

Support Surfaces

A cornerstone in the reduction or elimination of interface pressures is the use of support surfaces. These products reduce tissue-interface pressures over the bony prominences by maximizing contact and redistributing weight over a large area.[86,133,153]

Support surfaces are available in a variety of sizes and shapes that are appropriate for beds, chairs, examining tables, and operating room tables. The construction of the support surface and the process for selecting a support surface for an individual is similar regardless of the size or shape needed. Unfortunately, the use of support surfaces for the chair or operating room are frequently overlooked.

In addition to pressure reduction or relief, many support surfaces also provide shear and friction reduction, moisture control, or kinetic therapy.[68] To use support surfaces efficiently and effectively, the nurse must be knowledgeable of their indications, contraindications, advantages, and disadvantages.

Once a plan for reducing or eliminating pressure is developed and the plan is implemented, the effectiveness of the intervention (turning, support surface, and so on) should be evaluated. Within 24 hours a decrease in the dimensions of blanching erythema should be evident. Furthermore, no progression or new development of ischemic tissue should appear or a reevaluation of interventions is warranted.

Tissue Interface Pressure. The capillary closing pressure (12 to 32 mm Hg) is used as a measure of the effectiveness of support surfaces. It is implied that as the skin–resting surface interface pressure nears capillary closing pressures, the support surface is more effective and less likely to interrupt or occlude capillary blood flow. However, this overreliance on capillary pressure values as absolutes when making determinations about pressure prevention equipment is under scrutiny for several reasons.[85] First, capillary closing pressure was measured in the fingertips of young healthy males. Second, lower capillary pressures have been reported in older patients. Third, it is an assumption that skin–resting interface pressures actually reflect pressure at the bone-tissue interface. Skin–resting pressures do not necessarily assure that blood flow through the capillaries is unimpeded.

Because skin–resting surface interface pressure is the method currently used to evaluate support surfaces and their ability to reduce pressure, it is important to understand how interface pressure is calculated. Interface pressure is a measurement obtained by placement of a sensor between the skin and the resting surface and can be measured using several methods.

A one-time interface pressure measurement can be obtained with an electropneumatic pressure sensor that is connected to an inflation system and an aneroid gauge. Even with widely different transducer dimensions (31 and 100 mm), good agreement has been reported between the electropneumatic sensors and internal tissue compression.[40] Thus they are considered to be a meaningful measurement tool.

A SCP (subcapillary pressure) monitor attached to a electropneumatic pressure sensor allows continuous readings. Pressure duration and magnitude can then be reported.[40]

The Texas Interface Pressure Evaluator System (TIPE) is another tool used to measure tissue interface pressure and consists of a display unit, interconnected cable, and an extralarge plastic sensor pad. The sensor pad is composed of a matrix of 144 pneumatically activated switches. Each switch is connected to a light-emitting diode (LED) readout in the display unit. The pad is placed between the patient and the surface being evaluated. The TIPE is used to locate the points of maximum pressure, the pressure gradient, and the body area being "loaded."[143]

Because instrumentation used to measure interface pressures (that is, the size, shape, and positioning of the pressure sensor) affects the absolute value of the pressure readings, interface pressures collected from different instruments and different investigators are not comparable.[85] Krouskop and Garber propose that comparisons are best made when interface pressures are stated as a percentage against a standard surface, such as a standard hospital mattress. For example, mean interface pressures on a standard hospital mattress have been reported as follows: sacrum, 36 to 48 mm Hg; trochanter, 62 to 97 mm Hg; and heel 98 mm Hg.[73,87,104] Therefore, if a company reports an interface pressure for a bony prominence of 23 mm Hg on their surface and a pressure of 68 mm Hg for the same area on a standard bed, the percentage of the standard surface would be 33.8.

The standard deviation associated with the mean peak pressures should also be made available.[85] A small standard deviation implies that most measured pressures were close to the reported mean value. By definition, 95% of measurements lie within 2 standard deviations of the mean. Thus a larger standard deviation implies less reproduceability in pressure measurements and a wider range of pressure values.

When one is interpreting the significance of reported pressure readings, it is important to consider a number of issues. (1) Both the range of pressure readings obtained per site and the number of readings conducted per site should be reported instead of one single pressure reading per site. (2) The procedure used to acquire the pressure reading should be described. (3) The population tested should be described (that is, healthy subjects versus patients). (4) Researchers should state how often equipment was recalibrated because the sensors are fragile and may malfunction. (5) Finally, factors known to affect the results of interface pressure measurements should be disclosed.[122] These factors include the transducer size and shape, the load shape and its interaction with the support material, the method of equilibrium detection, and the uniformity of the measurement technique.[122]

The importance of the shape of the load is exemplified by the fact that a healthy person with normal muscle mass will support and distribute weight more effectively than a debilitated person. As a result, the healthy subject will usually demonstrate lower pressure readings than the debilitated subject. Uniformity of the measurement technique is necessary because the skill of the person taking the readings may make a difference.[122,154]

As noted earlier, in addition to reducing tissue interface pressure, many support surfaces also reduce shear, friction, and moisture. Products that have a slick surface (such as low air-loss beds) are believed to decrease friction and shear. Surfaces with porous cover material through which air flows help to reduce moisture between the body and support surface, thus preventing maceration.

Categories of support surfaces. Support surfaces can be categorized many ways (see Box 5-2). First they can be described as a pressure-reducing or pressure-relieving device. In the *Standards of Care: Dermal Wounds: Pressure Sores*, pressure-relieving devices are defined as those that consistently reduce pressure below capillary closing pressure.[70] The indications for use are (1) to prevent skin breakdown in people who cannot be turned, (2) to prevent further skin breakdown, and (3) to promote healing in the patient who already has skin breakdown involving multiple surfaces.

Box 5-2   CATEGORIES OF SUPPORT SURFACES

I. Management of pressure
  • Pressure reduction
  • Pressure relief
II. Air or fluid support
  • Dynamic
  • Static

III. Type of device
  • Overlay
  • Replacement mattress
  • Specialty bed

Pressure-reducing devices are those that lower pressure as compared to a standard hospital mattress or chair surface but do not consistently reduce pressure to less than capillary closing pressure. Pressure-reducing devices therefore must be used with a turning schedule that is tailored for the individual patient. The turning schedule is determined by evaluation of the status of the skin after progressive lengthening of the interval between position changes. A turning schedule should include not only major position changes but also the often neglected minor weight shifts.

Second, support surfaces can be categorized according to whether support is dynamic or static.[55,154] Dynamic systems typically use electricity to alter inflation and deflation and thus decrease tissue interface pressure (such as alternating pressure pad). Static devices reduce pressure by spreading the load over a larger area. A constant inflation is maintained by use of a material that molds to the body surface (such as foam, gel, water, and some air-filled overlays).

Third, support surfaces can be categorized as overlays, replacement mattresses, and specialty beds. Overlays are products that are applied on top of the hospital mattress and utilize foam, air, water, or gel to distribute the load and reduce pressure. Replacement mattresses are complete hospital mattresses designed to reduce pressure as compared to the standard hospital mattress. Specialty beds are entire units that are used in place of the hospital bed. This category includes low air-loss, high air-loss, and kinetic therapy beds. Kinetic therapy is continuous passive motion designed to counteract the negative effects of immobility.

Overlay Mattresses. Overlay mattresses are devices that are applied over the surface of the hospital mattress; most overlays provide pressure reduction. Overlay mattresses require a one-time charge, a setup fee, a daily rental fee, or a combination (such as one-time charge of mattress and daily rental of pump). Because overlay mattresses are applied over an existing hospital mattress, the height of the bed is increased, and such an increase may complicate patient transfers in and out of bed and alter the fit of linens.

Overlays may be static (foam, gel, water, air filled, low air loss) or dynamic (alternating air). Most overlay mattresses are single patient use items that present environmental issues relative to disposal of the product. Gel, water, and some air-filled overlays are reusable (multiple patient use). Because moisture entrapment against the skin is a problem with certain patient populations, some air-filled, low air-loss and alternating air-filled overlays provide air movement designed to reduce moisture buildup.

Static overlays

FOAM. Foam overlays have been used for many years and are probably the most universally used overlay. Foam is a static system and provides pressure reduction. Several characteristics of foam are important for effective pressure reduction: base height, density, indentation load deflection (ILD), and contours.[84,86,88] Base height refers to the height of the foam from the base to where the convolutions *begin* (not to the peak of the convolution). Density is the weight per cubic foot, is a measurement of the amount of foam in the product, and reflects the foam's ability to support the person's weight. ILD is a measurement of the firmness of the foam and is determined by the number of pounds required to indent a sample of foam with a circular plate to a depth of 25% of the thickness of the foam. For example, because 25% of a 4-inch foam is 1 inch, the 25% ILD would measure the number of pounds required to make a 1-inch indentation in the 4-inch foam. If this takes a 30-pound weight, the ILD would be stated as 25% ILD of 30 pounds. Likewise, 60% ILD of a 4-inch foam measures the number of pounds required to make a 2.4-inch depression in the foam (60% of 4 inches is 2.4 inches). ILD describes the foam's compressibility and conformability and indicates the ability of the foam to distribute the mechanical load. A low ILD is desirable. A relationship of 60% ILD to 25% ILD is an important characteristic in a therapeutic foam because it reflects the relationship between support and conformability. This ratio is recommended to be 2.5 or greater. Practically speaking, because the desired 25% ILD is 30 pounds, the 60% ILD should be at least 75 pounds (2.5 × 30). This indicates that 30 pounds would make a 1-inch depression in the 4-inch foam, whereas at least 75 pounds would be needed to make a 2.4-inch depression in the same foam.

Contours describe the surface of the foam pad, that is, egg crate, slashed, smooth, and so on. Benefits of one surface over another are largely subjective currently.

The base height of foam overlays varies widely. A foam overlay with a 2-inch base does not significantly reduce pressure when compared with a standard hospital mattress.[88] Therefore it is appropriately used only as a comfort device for persons at low risk for skin breakdown. However, Berjian and colleagues reported that two 2-inch foam overlays reduced pressure more than a standard hospital mattress.[27] A convoluted foam overlay with a 4-inch base significantly reduced pressure under the scapula ($p = .005$) and sacrococcygeal area ($p = .005$). The mean trochanter pressure remained high at approximately 52 mm Hg; however, these pressure readings still represent a significant reduction when compared to a standard mattress.

In summary, the following features in a therapeutic foam overlay are recommended:[83,84]
- Base height of 3 to 4 inches
- Density of 1.3 to 1.6 pounds per cubic foot
- 25% ILD of about 30 pounds
- Ratio of 60% ILD to 25% ILD of 2.5 or greater

The manufacturer's guidelines will state the amount of body weight the foam product will support and its length of use. When used for long-term pressure reduction, the staff or family must examine the product at intervals and replace the foam when effectiveness appears reduced. Advantages and disadvantages of foam overlays are listed in Box 5-3.

WATER. Water-filled overlays and water beds have long been used to reduce interface pressure.[139] Several studies have demonstrated that the water bed provides significantly lower interface pressure than a hospital mattress does.[94,141,153] According to Berecek, pressure points are eliminated because the function of the water bed is based on Pascal's law: "the weight of a body floating on a fluid system is evenly distributed over the entire support-

---

Box 5-3 FOAM OVERLAYS: ADVANTAGES AND DISADVANTAGES

ADVANTAGES	DISADVANTAGES
One-time charge	May be hot and trap perspiration
No setup fee	Washing removes flame-retardance
Light weight	coating
Cannot be punctured by needle or metal	Foam has a limited life
traction	Plastic protective sheet necessary for
Available in many sizes (bed, operating	protection from incontinent episodes
tables, chairs)	
Requires no maintenance	

---

ing system."[22] Unfortunately, the water bed presents three considerable concerns: leaks, maintenance of bed warmth, and appropriate filling. Although water-filled devices are quite popular for the home, their many disadvantages make them inappropriate for acute care or long-term care settings. Advantages and disadvantages are listed in Box 5-4.

GEL. Gel-flotation pads are constructed of Silastic (silicone elastomer), silicone, or polyvinyl chloride.[22] These surfaces provide flotation with pressure reduction, may be single-patient or multipatient use, require minimal maintenance, are available in a variety of sizes and shapes, and have a surface that is easy to clean. These features make them attractive for use in long-term care settings and operating rooms. However, gel-filled overlays tend to be expensive and heavy and lack air flow for moisture control.[9] Friction control is variable depending on the surface of the gel. Gel-filled pads are particularly useful in wheelchairs.

Gels may be combined with foam to create a mattress. Foam sections are removed and the gel pad is inserted where the pressure-reducing effect of the gel is desired. A list of advantages and disadvantages of gel-filled overlays is listed in Box 5-5.

Box 5-4 WATER OVERLAYS: ADVANTAGES AND DISADVANTAGES

ADVANTAGES	Patient transfers may be difficult
Readily available in community	Inadvertent needle punctures will create
Baffle system available to control motion	leaks
effects	Water leaks can create safety hazards
Easy to clean	Maintenance is needed to prevent
	microorganism growth
DISADVANTAGES	Heavy
Requires water heater to maintain	Cannot raise head of bed unless mattress
comfortable water temperature	has compartments
Fluid motion makes procedures difficult	Can be overfilled or underfilled
(that is, positioning or cardiopulmonary	
resuscitation)	

Box 5-5   GEL-FILLED OVERLAYS: ADVANTAGES AND DISADVANTAGES

ADVANTAGES	DISADVANTAGES
Low maintenance	Heavy
Easy to clean	Expensive
Multipatient use	Limited research on effectiveness
Impermeable to punctures with needles	

AIR FILLED. Static air-filled overlays consist of interconnected bulbous cells that are inflated with an air blower to an appropriate pressure level. These overlays are available in a chair size and a bed size and as operating room pads. Static air-filled overlays are considered pressure reducing and should be used for patients who can reposition themselves.

Makelbust and colleagues[102,103] tested one single-patient-use static air-filled overlay (Gaymar Sof-Care, Orchard Park, New York) on healthy volunteers and reported the following mean interface pressures: 12 to 16 mm Hg for the sacrum, 17 to 25 mm Hg for the trochanteric area, and 52 to 77 mm Hg for the calcaneous area.

Another unique static air-filled overlay (RoHo, St. Louis, Missouri) is a reusable, multiple-patient-use device that consists of many flexible air cells attached to a common manifold. With proper individualized inflation, this type of static air-filled device provides low surface tension, the ability to conform to any shape, and a suspension force that is uniform and independent of immersion depth. The following mean interface pressures have been reported for this type of device: less than 25 mm Hg for the sacrococcygeal and scapula areas and less than 50 mm Hg for the trochanter.[88] All pressures were significantly ($p = .005$) less than a standard hospital mattress. Advantages and disadvantages of static air-filled overlays are listed in Box 5-6.

LOW AIR-LOSS OVERLAY. Recently, low air-loss overlays have been introduced. These static overlays, however, are attached to motorized pumps that maintain a constant inflation and provide slight air movement against the skin to prevent moisture buildup. The fabric covering for these overlays is air permeable, bacteria impermeable, and waterproof and reduces shear and friction. Advantages and disadvantages of low air-loss overlays are listed in Box 5-7.

Dynamic Overlays

ALTERNATING AIR-FILLED OVERLAY. The objectives for use of an alternating air-pressure overlay are to prevent constant pressure against the skin and to enhance blood flow by cre-

---

Box 5-6   STATIC AIR-FILLED OVERLAYS: ADVANTAGES AND DISADVANTAGES

ADVANTAGES	DISADVANTAGES
Easy to clean	Can be damaged by sharp objects
Multipatient use products available	Requires regular monitoring to determine
Low maintenance	proper inflation
Repair of some products is possible	
Durable	

Box 5-7 LOW AIR-LOSS OVERLAYS: ADVANTAGES AND DISADVANTAGES

ADVANTAGES	DISADVANTAGES
Easy to clean	Can be damaged by sharp objects
Maintains a constant inflation	Noisy
Deflates to facilitate transfers, cardiopulmonary resuscitation, and so on	
Setup provided by company	
Moisture control	

---

ating high-pressure and low-pressure areas. These pressure-reducing, dynamic systems consist of a configuration of chambers through which air is pumped at regular intervals to provide inflation and deflation. Typically, interface pressures are lower than capillary closing pressure when the cylinders are deflated; interface pressures are then higher than capillary closing pressure when the cylinders are inflated. Interface pressures in the trochanter area commonly remain high during both phases; however, because interface pressures are significantly less than a standard hospital bed for the sacrum, scapula, and trochanter, pressure reduction in these areas is attained.[88] Advantages and disadvantages for this overlay are listed in Box 5-8.

Replacement Mattress. Recently, replacement mattresses that are designed to reduce interface pressures and replace the standard hospital mattress have been introduced. Replacement mattresses vary in design; most are made of foam and gel combinations or layers of different foam densities (that is, very firm, high-density foam for the periphery or bottom layer and low-density, more comfortable foam for the upper layer).[12,73,88] Some replacement mattresses have removable foam shapes, and some have a replaceable foam core. Still other replacement mattresses are a series of air-filled chambers covered with a foam structure. All replacement mattresses are covered with a conformable bacteriostatic cover that can be maintained with standard terminal cleaning.

Maintenance of replacement mattresses will vary with their type of design. Although some mattresses have to be turned (or flipped) regularly to maintain efficacy, others cannot be turned because of their design. This feature is significant to the institution because it

---

Box 5-8 ALTERNATING AIR-FILLED OVERLAY: ADVANTAGES AND DISADVANTAGES

ADVANTAGES	DISADVANTAGES
Easy to clean	Assembly required
Pump is reusable	Sensation of inflation and deflation may bother patient
Quick deflation for emergencies	Requires electricity
	Motor may be noisy

may reduce the employee's risk of low back injuries resulting from such activities. Another feature of some replacement mattresses is air flow to reduce moisture buildup against the skin.

Although many companies are developing replacement mattresses, few published research studies are available to document effectiveness and efficacy.[73,88,12] From these few studies, interface pressures are reported as being lower than a standard hospital mattress. Even though Andrews and Balai[12] found a decrease in healing time of sacral ulcers when patients were placed on a replacement mattress, there was no significant difference in the incidence of pressure ulcers after admission.

Purchase of these mattresses entails a significant initial expense and are probably most justifiable in settings with a large number of high-risk patients or whenever large numbers of overlays are used. Because some third-party payers limit reimbursement for overlays (particularly Medicaid and Medicare), institutions with a large percentage of Medicare and Medicaid patients who are at high risk for pressure ulcer development may find that replacement mattresses are a more cost-effective alternative. However, the use of specialty beds may not be reduced by use of replacement mattresses.[12] Advantages and disadvantages are listed in Box 5-9.

Specialty Beds. High and low air-loss beds were developed to allow deformation of the bed surface to the body contours, thereby reducing tissue-interface pressure below capillary closure. In addition to providing pressure *relief,* these specialty beds also eliminate shear and friction and decrease moisture.[44,93] Specialty beds replace hospital beds and are the most costly of all support surfaces. Electricity (or a battery pack) is required for a specialty bed to function.

Investigators have examined the pressure-relief capacity of both types of air-loss beds. With proper adjustment, the pressure relief and redistribution characteristics of high air-loss and low air-loss specialty beds do not differ.[87]

High air-loss beds. High air-loss beds, initially developed to treat persons with burns, consist of a bed frame containing silicone-coated beads and incorporating both air and fluid support.[112] Fluidization of the beads occurs when air is pumped through the beads making them behave like a liquid.[66,147] The person "floats" on a sheet with one third of the

---

Box 5-9   REPLACEMENT MATTRESSES: ADVANTAGES AND DISADVANTAGES

ADVANTAGES	DISADVANTAGES
Reduce use of overlay mattresses	Initial expense high
Reduce staff time	Some mattresses have removable sections, which may be misplaced
Do not add height to mattress	
Provides certain level of pressure reduction automatically	May not control moisture
	Potential for excessive delay in using other support surface
Multiple patient use	
Easy to clean	No objective method for determining when or if product loses effectiveness
Uses standard hospital linens	
Low maintenance	

body above the surface and the rest of the body immersed in the warm, dry fluidized beads.[151] High air-loss beds have bactericidal properties because of their temperature, alkalinity (pH 10), and entrapment of the microorganisms by the beads.[147]

Ryan[130] reported in his randomized study of men undergoing elective aorta-femoral grafts assigned to a conventional bed at 22° C or a high air-loss bed at 32° C that urinary nitrogen loss was significantly less in the patients placed in the high air-loss bed. It is postulated that the high air-loss bed's warm environment (30° to 32° C) may reduce the body's catabolic activity in the seriously ill person; this, however, needs further study. When the high air-loss bed is turned off, it quickly becomes firm enough for cardiopulmonary resuscitation or for repositioning the patient for dressing changes.

Although some evidence indicates that high air-loss beds enhance pressure-ulcer healing rates,[116] occipital and calcaneous skin–resting surface interface pressures may remain sufficient to occlude capillary perfusion. Occipital and calcaneous ulcers have been reported to develop in patients while on the high air-loss surface.[116]

High air-loss beds have also been compared to the standard hospital mattress in wound-healing studies.[7,18,63,72] Researchers generally agree that ulcers decrease significantly in size, and fewer ulcers develop in the patients placed on a high air-loss bed.

High air-loss beds are recommended for patients with burns or multiple stage III or IV pressure ulcers. They may be used to rewarm a person with hypothermia, since they can quickly narrow the gap between the core and peripheral temperatures, thus reducing vasoconstriction and improving peripheral circulation.[150] This may reduce shivering and the subsequent increased oxygen demand. Patients with severe debilitating pain are often more comfortable on this bed because of the "cocooning" effect and decreased need to be turned.[142] Furthermore, appetite is reported to improve with high air-loss therapy; this effect may correlate with the pain control provided by the bed.[46,47,72,76] High air-loss beds are not recommended for patients with pulmonary disease, or with unstable spines, or patients who are ambulatory. Advantages and disadvantages are listed in Box 5-10.

Low air-loss beds. A low air-loss bed consists of a bed frame with a series of connected air-filled pillows. The amount of pressure in each pillow is controlled and can be calibrated to provide maximum pressure reduction for the individual patient. The low air-loss bed deflates quickly for cardiopulmonary resuscitation.

As with the high air-loss beds, low air-loss beds are also indicated for patients who need pressure relief (that is, patients who cannot be frequently repositioned or who have skin breakdown on more than one surface).[70] These beds have the added features of a regular hospital bed frame. Low air-loss beds are contraindicated for patients with an unstable spine. Some low air-loss beds include pulsation therapy, and although this is believed to enhance cutaneous blood flow and to reduce edema, further research is needed. Advantages and disadvantages are listed in Box 5-11.

Kinetic therapy. Some specialty beds provide kinetic therapy. These beds are designed to counteract the effects of immobility by continuous passive motion or oscillation therapy. Some beds are a combination of oscillation therapy and low air loss. Oscillation therapy is believed to (1) provide mobilization of respiratory secretion, thus decreasing the incidence of atelectasis and pneumonia and improving oxygenation of blood; (2) prevent urinary stasis, thus reducing the risk of urinary tract infection, and (3) reduce venous stasis and risk of deep vein thrombosis and pulmonary emboli. Thus kinetic therapy may have a significant positive effect on multiple body systems.

Box 5-10   HIGH AIR-LOSS SPECIALTY BEDS: ADVANTAGES AND DISADVANTAGES

ADVANTAGES
Less frequent repositioning required
Improved patient comfort
Traction can be applied
Procedures can be facilitated by turning the bed off
Quickly become firm for cardiopulmonary resuscitation and procedures
Reduce shear, friction, and edema to site
May facilitate management of copious wound drainage or incontinence
Sales force can provide setup, monitoring, and on-call services

DISADVANTAGES
Continuous circulation of warm, dry air may dehydrate patient
Bed may be hot or make room hot
Additional wound care measures are necessary to prevent wound desiccation
Coughing is less effective in mobilizing secretions

Leakage of beads (microspheres) may irritate the eyes and respiratory tract and make floor slippery
Width of bed may preclude care to obese patients or patients with a contracture
Height of bed makes some nursing care difficult, and a step is needed to facilitate care
Transfer of patient out of bed is difficult
Bed is heavy and not easily transferrable
Some patients become disoriented or complain of feeling weightless
Dependent drainage of catheters may be compromised because the patient is immersed in the bed
The head of the bed cannot be raised; semi-Fowler's position is achieved by use of a series of foam wedges
Size may be too large for most homes

Kinetic therapy is available with a low air-loss surface or with a firm, slightly padded surface. A kinetic treatment table has a firm, slightly padded surface. By rotating slowly side to side, the treatment table alternates pressure points; it does not reduce shear or moisture. Access to body parts is possible by opening special hatches without affecting body alignment. This device is primarily indicated to stabilize the spine or for victims of major trauma requiring traction. It is not used if a patient is hemodynamically unstable or for the patient with severe claustrophobia.

Kinetic therapy with low air-loss support is indicated for patients who need pressure relief and will also benefit from kinetic therapy. This type of specialty bed is contraindicated for patients in cervical or skeletal traction.

Selecting support surfaces for institution or agency. Selecting a pressure-relief or pressure-reduction device for a specific patient and for the institution or agency presents many challenges. Generally, one product alone is not sufficient for an institution, and a range of products is more appropriate. Several factors should be considered when one is determining what support surfaces to have available in an institution or agency.

1. What are the common needs for the patient population typically served? For example, an institution that has many high-risk patients for pressure ulcer development may find replacement mattresses to be effective at reducing their number of overlays. An institution with a wide variety of acutely ill patients will have different patient needs and may need a

---

Box 5-11   LOW AIR-LOSS SPECIALTY BED: ADVANTAGES AND DISADVANTAGES

ADVANTAGES

Head and foot of bed can be raised and
   lowered
Transfers in and out of bed easily
   accomplished
Portable motor available to maintain inflation
   during bed transfers
Less frequent turning schedules required
Sales force provides setup, monitoring, and
   on-call services

DISADVANTAGES

Portable motors are quite noisy
Bed surface material is quite slippery, and
   caution must be used so that patients do not
   slide down or out of bed when being
   transferred

---

range of products such as an overlay mattress, a specialty bed, and a kinetic therapy product. Rehabilitation centers or nursing homes, on the other hand, will need access to mattress overlays, replacement mattresses, or a select combination of both, as well as wheelchair overlays. Settings where many grafts or flaps are performed will need access to specialty beds and appropriate "stepdown" support surfaces.

Additionally, the type of surgical procedures performed within the institution should be assessed. Duration and type of surgical procedures is becoming increasingly recognized as factors contributing to pressure ulcer formation. This association was demonstrated in a study of 125 surgical patients at a large metropolitan teaching hospital where patients who were elderly or undergoing procedures requiring extracorporeal circulation were at higher risk for this type of injury.[77] Other researchers have found that patients undergoing orthopedic procedures, particularly for fractured femurs, are at a higher risk.[125,156]

2. The costs of the support surface should be considered. Some devices are available on a rental basis, whereas others have a one-time fee. The cost of the device should be considered in conjunction with the length of time the product will be used, goals for use, and length of product efficacy.

Indirect costs associated with the use of support surfaces, such as the time commitment of the staff to utilize the product, must also be considered. How long does it take the staff to set up the device? Will the staff need to provide some degree of maintenance or frequent checks to assure effective inflation? The ease with which the product can be used and maintained are important features to minimize staff time required by the device. A device that requires daily maintenance is probably not appropriate in a low staffing situation.

3. Company performance and service should also be assessed. Services such as setup, maintenance, storage, and disposal may be provided. The company should be examined for its shipping and delivery policy and guarantee. Some companies provide in-service programs for the staff. A trial of the product may be possible. Talking with other nurses who have used the product may help identify the advantages and disadvantages of a company and the product.

Product disposal is becoming a critical environmental issue. If it is costly for the hospital to dispose of trash, a rented, reusable overlay may be more cost effective than a disposable overlay. Storage of the standard hospital bed while a specialty bed is in use is also a concern in some facilities where space is limited.

4. Do effectiveness studies exist for this particular product? There should be available independently written literature that describes the range and standard deviation of interface pressures for the product. The method of recording interface pressures, the age and health of the study sample, and size of sample need to be considered. The size of the sensor measuring the pressure is important, since a small sensor may be misplaced and not even obtain the highest reading. Test data should be published in a reputable scientific journal, not literature produced by the manufacturer's marketing department.

It would be less than ideal to select a support surface without efficacy studies or based on the results of one study (especially if the study used a limited sample). For example, many studies regarding interface pressures are done on healthy, young adults; generalizability of these measurements to an older person and ill population is not known. A small sample size may increase the risk of saying a product makes a significant difference when it does not. Sample sizes need to be large enough to account for the type of statistical analysis performed and ability to predict a significant effect. When limited research on products of interest is available, the nurse would be well advised to design and conduct a test to evaluate the product's effectiveness.[22]

Selecting support surface for individual patient. Once a decision is made as to what products to have available in the agency or institution, attention must turn to educating the staff as to appropriate use of the products. Guidelines for selecting a support surface for a specific patient are necessary to enable appropriate staff decision making and proper utilization.[49,155] Although no specific decision tree exists, several factors should guide the selection process.

1. Does the patient need pressure reduction or relief? The patient who cannot be repositioned or who has breakdown involving multiple surfaces requires pressure relief.

2. Is this support system needed on a short-term or a long-term basis? For example, an acutely ill patient may need pressure relief during an illness crisis but by discharge may not require any support surface. A patient in a nursing home or with a chronic disease may require long-term pressure reduction. Surgical patients may need pressure relief during the surgery and only mild pressure reduction or no pressure reduction postoperatively. Some patients confined to a chair need no pressure relief in bed but need pressure reduction while in the chair.

3. Is the patient, staff, or family compliant with repositioning? Because most overlays or replacement mattresses do not eliminate the need for a turn schedule, they may be inappropriate for patients who are hemodynamically unstable. Likewise, the patient has to cooperate and stay repositioned. The family of a bed-bound patient has to be able to turn the patient at appropriate intervals, understand the importance of repositioning, and provide consistency and followthrough.

4. Will the support surface interfere with the patient's independent functioning? For example, the height an overlay can add to a mattress may complicate a rehabilitation patient's ability to transfer. Certainly, a high air-loss bed would not be indicated for a patient who is getting in and out of bed.

5. What is financially feasible? Institutions cannot afford to have all support systems available. Many institutions establish contractual relationships with companies to control

costs and to provide access to a specific range of products. Reimbursement for products in the home or nursing home setting is quite limited and should be explored before a decision is made.

6. What mechanism is needed to ensure appropriate functioning of the support surface? Air- or water-filled overlays must be checked on a regular basis to ascertain appropriate flotation. Many of the low air-loss overlays and specialty beds have service people to monitor this; however, staff or family still require some degree of familiarity with features and functions.

7. The patient's surrounding environment needs to be examined. Are there adequate outlets for electrical equipment in the patient's room or would an overlay that does not use electricity be a better choice? How noisy is the product and can the patient tolerate this additional noise? Some products generate heat, which may also be poorly tolerated by some patients.

8. Are there other therapeutic effects needed in addition to pressure reduction or relief? For example, a closed head-injury patient may need a support surface that reduces pressure but also controls moisture.

Once a product is selected its effectiveness for that particular patient needs to be reevaluated at regular intervals. As the patient recuperates, a less aggressive support surface may be warranted. Conversely, if the patient is deteriorating, a more aggressive support surface or a product with more features may be indicated.

Summary. Selecting the most appropriate support surface involves many considerations. The primary goal for use of a support surface is to prevent and manage skin breakdown; thus products are examined in terms of their therapeutic effects.

Unfortunately, the state of the art for determining therapeutic effectiveness of support surfaces is in its infancy. First, there is a lack of consensus as to what constitutes capillary closing pressure. Second, there is a dearth of reliable tools and methods for accurate measurement of tissue-interface pressures. And third, there is an assumption that skin–resting surface interface pressures reflect the more important muscle-bone interface pressures.

The process of selecting support surfaces will continue to be refined as new products are developed and as more is learned about measuring effectiveness. The nurse should keep abreast of these changes so that products can be used in an effective, efficient fashion.

MANAGEMENT OF PRESSURE ULCERS

Doughty[48] states that "effective wound management is predicated on scientific principles that form the basis for nursing intervention." Chapter 3 details a holistic approach to effective wound management based on principles of wound care: relieve or eliminate the source, optimize the microenvironment, support the host, and provide education. Although optimizing the microenvironment through topical wound care and supporting the host with nutritional interventions are important components of pressure ulcer management, effective elimination or reduction of skin–resting interface pressure is imperative and cannot be overemphasized. Optimizing the wound environment and supporting the host can be marginally successful, if at all, in the presence of continued pressure. Interventions for interface pressure management and wound care have been discussed; this section highlights nuances of wound care that are specific to ulcers precipitated by pressure.

Optimize the Microenvironment

Historically, pressure ulcers have been managed with a vast array of poorly researched or scientifically unsubstantiated treatment modalities. The heat lamp, antacids, honey, insulin, and maggots are just a few therapies that need to be put to rest. Likewise, the practice of massaging pressure points, which for many years was believed to stimulate circulation to areas injured by pressure, should be critically evaluated.[52] Recent studies demonstrate that the effects on local skin blood flow varies between individuals, within individuals, and between normal skin and injured skin. Furthermore, some researchers suggest that massage, especially extended massage, may further injure ischemic, fragile capillaries.[115] Several articles provide a very interesting review of old wound treatment and their perceived mode of action.[15,22,33,43,129]

Before selecting topical therapy, the pressure ulcer should be carefully examined for undermining or tunneling. Because of the shear force that often contributes to pressure ulcer formation, undermining of the ulcer edges is common. This is particularly true in the sacrococcygeal area. A cotton-tipped applicator can be used to ascertain the extent of undermining or the presence of tunnels. The topical therapy selected must include a method of filling this "dead space" created by undermining or tunneling.

As with all wounds, careful accurate wound assessment and documentation of wound status at regular intervals is critical for evaluation of the progress of wound repair. Regular reevaluation of topical therapy based on these assessments is also essential to ensure appropriateness of interventions. Appropriate topical therapy means using dressings that are best indicated for the ulcer, therapy that is manageable by those providing the care, and therapy that is consistent with the patient's health status, prognosis, and care objectives. For example, the patient who is being managed with twice-daily dressing changes requires a reevaluation before being discharged to home care; the goal is to develop a care plan that can be effectively implemented by the caregivers or home care nurses. It is important to remember that topical wound care is not static; it must be reevaluated and changed as the wound changes and as the patient's needs change.

When measurable improvement in the wound has not been observed for a significant period of time (such as 2 to 4 weeks), the patient should be reevaluated for the presence of factors that would prevent healing (such as pressure, shear, malnourishment). Extrinsic factors must be corrected; if intrinsic factors are uncorrectable, the goals for the ulcer healing must be reconsidered.

Support the Host

Once the pressure has been eliminated attention must be given to the patient's nutritional status. As discussed in Chapter 9, protein, calories, vitamins, and minerals are essential to support the wound-repair process and prevent extension of the ulcer. Nutritional support may be in the form of snacks, oral supplements, adjunctive tube feedings, or parenteral nutrition. The method selected is guided by the extent of the patient's nutritional needs.

Local or systemic infection must be controlled or eliminated. Because necrotic tissue harbors bacteria, aggressive débridement of necrotic wounds that appear clinically infected is indicated. Systemic antibiotics are commonly used to control the release of toxins during and immediately after débridement.

Osteomyelitis must also be considered in infected pressure ulcers. A radiologic exam and its interpretation by an expert are indicated to rule out osteomyelitis.

Provide Education

Pressure ulcer care and prevention is not a passive process for the patient or caregivers. The patient or the primary caregivers must understand the cause of pressure ulcer formation, the significance of factors contributing to pressure injury, preventive measures, the significance of nutrition in wound repair, and the indicators of wound healing.[16] All health care personnel providing care to the patient need to appreciate the role they *must* play in preventing pressure ulcers.

Formal patient education programs are common for patients with a spinal cord injury in rehabilitation centers.[53] These could serve as a model for similar educational programs for patients with any chronic disease that limits mobility as the disease progresses and increases risk for pressure injury (that is, multiple sclerosis, terminal cancer). Family members should be included in such programs.[16] Likewise, high-risk patient populations should be routinely assessed specifically for indications of pressure damage. Education of the patient, staff, caregivers, and family members is the key to effective prevention of pressure ulcers and to successful management of existing pressure ulcers.

SURGICAL INTERVENTIONS FOR PRESSURE ULCERS

Before any planned surgical treatment for pressure ulcers the general condition of the patient must be optimized. A team approach, including an internist, rehabilitation specialist, nursing staff, surgeon, ET (enterostomal therapy) nurse, nutritionist, orthopedist, and physical therapist, must be utilized to obtain good results.

Optimize Patient

Along with fine tuning of the basic functional processes, there are specific requirements before operative intervention. All spasticity must be controlled, either pharmacologically or surgically. Infection at the site of the ulcer or elsewhere must be overcome by intravenously administered antibiotics and appropriate débridement. The cause of the ulcer must be identified (whether secondary to repeated shear forces, immobility, or trauma) and corrected. Most importantly, the patient must be nutritionally sound because protein malnutrition is a leading cause of flap failure. Serum albumin is a readily available test that can act as a rough guide to the patient's condition. With rare exception, flap closure of a pressure ulcer should not be done with serum albumin less than 3.0 g/dl.

Evaluate Tissue Damage

Coincident with optimization of the patient's general condition, the ulcer itself should be evaluated and staged as per the National Pressure Ulcer Advisory Panel:[98]

Stage I: Nonblanchable erythema of intact skin

Stage II: Partial-thickness skin loss

Stage III: Full-thickness skin loss and involvement of underlying subcutaneous tissue, superficial to deep fascia

Stage IV: Full-thickness skin loss with destruction of tissues deep to the deep fascia (muscle, bone, ligament, tendon, and so forth)

Surgical therapy is based upon ulcer staging:

Stage I. These lesions should be considered as a warning. They will heal spontaneously, without operative intervention, provided that the cause of the lesion is understood and measures are taken to correct the patient's poor positioning, hygiene, or susceptibility to shear forces.

Stage II. These lesions appear similar to partial-thickness burns with loss of epidermis and exposed, injured dermis. Careful evaluation of the wound is needed because these lesions may herald a larger, deeper stage III lesion. The true stage II lesion, with only partial-thickness skin loss, should also heal with local therapy if one assumes that there is correction of the cause. These lesions heal by reepithelialization from remaining epidermal structures (hair follicles, sweat glands, and so forth). In the true stage II lesion there is little or no role for surgical intervention because viable dermis still exists.

Stage III. These larger lesions show full-thickness skin loss with injury to underlying tissue layers. On presentation, many often contain a large amount of necrotic material and show significant associated cellulitis. Systemic toxicity is not uncommon. Necrotic tissue must be removed and infection controlled; such steps are usually best accomplished by intravenous antibiotics and immediate surgical débridement. Débridement may be done at the bedside; however, a more thorough job can be done in the operating room.

Most of these patients show clear physical and biochemical signs of protein malnutrition. Intervention in this regard is at least as crucial as operative intervention. Because of the significant protein loss from the wound, these patients require an unusually high caloric intake with protein supplementation. If the patient is unable to maintain adequate protein intake, nasogastric tube feedings or parenteral hyperalimentation, or both, are warranted.

Once débridement of any grossly necrotic tissue is complete, appropriate topical therapy is then begun. Standard gauze dressings moistened with saline solution are frequently used and are an appropriate choice to support wound débridement. The gauze should be loosely placed into the depths of the wound and not packed; vigorous packing prevents the naturally helpful process of wound contraction from occurring. With adequate nutritional support and proper positioning, the wound will clean up rapidly. Healthy, red granulation tissue at the wound base and new epithelialization at the wound margin are sure signs that the wound is ready for surgical closure. Indeed, if there is a paucity of granulation tissue present or if no new epidermis is present at the wound edge, surgical closure should be delayed. The patient should be further evaluated for the presence of factors affecting wound healing (such as nutritional status, uncorrected causes, infection), which may need to be corrected before surgical closure.

Most stage III ulcers will heal on their own; however, spontaneous closure may take months and may result in an unstable scar that is predisposed to recurrence. For this reason, it is frequently preferable to manage these lesions with surgical excision and closure, barring contraindications.

Stage IV. These deepest of lesions are handled in a fashion similar to the stage III lesion. Débridement is often more radical because there is bony involvement. Localized osteomyelitis is the rule. Deeper extension into the pelvis and fistulas (such as urethroperineal) must be ruled out.

Surgical Options

There are a variety of surgical procedures that may be used to close chronic wounds. The most common are skin grafts and tissue flaps.[28]

Skin grafts. Skin grafts may be either split thickness or full thickness; the most commonly used are split thickness. These grafts involve transfer of the epidermis and a measured portion of the dermis from a donor site to a shallow well-vascularized wound.[146] Skin grafts provide superficial coverage but do not replace deeper tissue layers such as subcutaneous tissue and muscle; thus they are unable to provide the padding needed to protect bony prominences from recurrent breakdown.[28] They are rarely, if ever, used in the surgical management of pressure ulcers; they may, however, be used to close donor sites after layer flap procedures.[146]

Survival of skin grafts is dependent on revascularization of the grafted skin; this is accomplished by ingrowth of capillaries from the vascularized surface into the graft.[146] The two factors most commonly associated with graft failure are (1) failure to adequately immobilize the graft, which is critical to revascularizaton, and (2) infection.[146]

The donor site for the skin graft is a partial-thickness wound, which heals by reepithelialization.[146]

Tissue flaps. Tissue flaps are the procedures most commonly used for surgical management of pressure ulcers.[28] They involve the transfer of skin and underlying structures (such as subcutaneous tissue, fascia, and muscle) to fill a defect. Tissue flaps may be further classified according to tissue layers involved and surgical method used to transfer the tissue into the defect. All flaps involve partial detachment of the tissue from its original site; the base remains attached and provides circulatory support to the flap.[146]

Flaps may be classified as fasciocutaneous (also sometimes called "skin flaps") and myocutaneous. Fasciocutaneous flaps involve elevation and rotation of the epidermis, dermis, and subcutaneous tissue; these flaps provide padding and superficial coverage. These flaps may be further divided into "random" flaps and "axial" flaps. Random flaps are dependent on the dermal and subdermal vessels for their blood supply; since these vessels are rather small, the blood supply to these flaps is somewhat tenuous.[28] Axial flaps are those designed to include a major cutaneous artery; this design increases vascularity and the chances for flap survival.[146]

Myocutaneous flaps involve rotation of all tissue layers, that is, skin, subcutaneous tissue, fascia, and muscle. These flaps provide optional coverage for a bony prominence and are therefore frequently used in surgical reconstruction of pressure ulcers. Myocutaneous flaps are well-vascularized flaps containing major vessels that originate from the base of the flap; these vessels nourish the flap until new capillary systems are established between the flap and the wound bed.[146]

Flaps can also be classified according to surgical technique: common flaps include the advancement flap, the rotation flap, and the transposition flap.[146]

Advancement flaps involve elevation of the tissue to be transferred, undermining of the wound edges, and "advancement" of the tissue into the defect. Advancement flaps are useful in areas where there is significant stretch of the skin.[146]

Rotation flaps are used to fill defects adjacent to the donor tissue; a flap is outlined on three sides, the tissue is elevated, and the flap is "rotated" into the defect. The donor site may be closed surgically or may require a split-thickness skin graft in closure. (Skin-graft closure is adequate, since the tissue is rotated from a site adjacent to but not overlying a bony prominence.)[146]

Transposition flaps are rotation flaps that are moved across normal skin to fill a defect (as opposed to being directly adjacent to the defect).

One other flap that should be mentioned is the "free flap"; this flap is performed less commonly because it requires microvascular surgery techniques. In this approach, the donor tissue is completely removed from the donor site and transferred to the graft site; the vessels are anastomosed by microvascular techniques to vessels in the wound bed.[146]

Tissue Expansion An additional surgical option for pressure ulcer closure is tissue expansion. This option may be utilized when there is not enough tissue adjacent to an ulcer to provide flap coverage. Silastic "expanders" or hollow pouches are placed surgically into the subcutaneous or submuscular tissue layer in an area adjacent to the defect. Sterile fluid is injected into the expander at routine intervals until the pouch is fully expanded; this process induces expansion of the overlying tissue layers. When there is sufficient tissue to provide coverage of the defect, the expander is removed and the ulcer is closed.[146]

Pressure Ulcer Closure

Principles. Although many different techniques and flaps have been described, all follow basic principles:

1. The patient is positioned in the operating room to mimic the position of maximal tension on the flap. This prevents wound dehiscence secondary to tension upon patient positioning postoperatively.
2. Perioperative prophylactic antibiotic therapy specific to wound culture is in order. Forty-eight hours of intravenous therapy is required. Although some authors have found quantitative cultures helpful, most have not found them necessary. Even in patients with a radiologic diagnosis of osteomyelitis additional antibiotic therapy is not needed because all involved bone should be excised at the time of closure.
3. Ostectomy of bony prominence is necessary in order to increase the surface area upon which the patient rests. Total ischiectomy is no longer favored because the weight redistribution results in ulcers on the opposite side or on the perineum.
4. The entire ulcer is excised in "pseudotumor" fashion leaving only healthy, unscarred tissue. This also removes the contaminated granulation tissue, thereby decreasing postoperative infection rates.
5. Incisions are planned to allow for possible recurrences in the same or a different location. Since recurrences are common, the surgeon must be sure that planned incisions do not violate potential future flaps.
6. Incisions are planned to avoid suture lines over bony prominences. Scar tissue directly over a bony prominence predisposes the patient to future pressure ulceration.
7. The defect resulting from excision is filled with healthy, unscarred, well-vascularized tissue. This filling in prevents seroma formation and allows for rapid wound healing.
8. A closed drainage system is used to prevent seroma formation. Drainage can be significant in the early postoperative period. Drainage systems can be discontinued when drainage is minimal (usually 5 to 7 days).
9. Postoperatively the patient is placed in a prone position or on a specialty bed, which provides pressure relief and eliminates shear (such as an air-fluidized bed).[117] Three weeks prone or in a specialty bed is a minimum requirement.
10. Mobility is gradually increased beginning week 3 postoperatively with careful monitoring of skin and suture lines.
11. Skin grafts are not used to close pressure ulcers because they are usually not durable enough in the long term.

Adherence to these basic principles will decrease overall perioperative complications regardless of the site of the ulcer. The ischial ulcer is the most common in the chair-bound

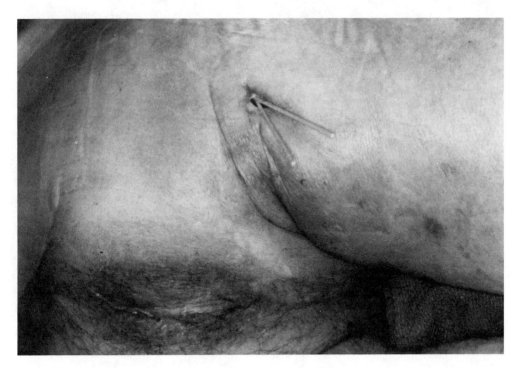

Fig. 5-8   Typical ischial ulcer with small skin defect and large cavity.

spinal cord–injured patient, whereas sacral and trochanteric sores are more common in patients confined to bed.

Ischial Ulcer. Ischial ulcers occur secondary to prolonged sitting without change in position. There is rarely a large skin defect present. The underlying cavity however is frequently very large (Fig. 5-8). The ischial tuberosity is the pressure point and is always involved. As part of the ulcer excision, ischial ostectomy should be carried out to create a smooth, broad surface in order to theoretically distribute weight over a greater surface area. See Fig. 5-9.

The gluteus maximus muscle flap offers a large amount of well-vascularized tissue with which to fill the defect.[105] Even in the spinal cord–injured patient, significant muscle exists. Skin closure of the donor site can be obtained by linear closure in some cases or by a separate inferiorly based fasciocutaneous rotation flap.

The hamstring V-Y myocutaneous flap may be used for patients with recurrent ulcerations in extremely large defects, or when the gluteus is nonusable. See Fig. 5-10 and 5-11. This flap is particularly valuable for layer defects because thorough dissection yields 10 to 12 cm of advancement. It is called a "V-Y flap" because the flap is raised with V-shaped incisions and then closed as a Y.[148] This flap is well vascularized by segmental perforators from the hamstrings originating from the profunda femoris artery.[148] Because the origins and insertions of the muscles are severed, however, this flap cannot be used in an ambulatory patient.

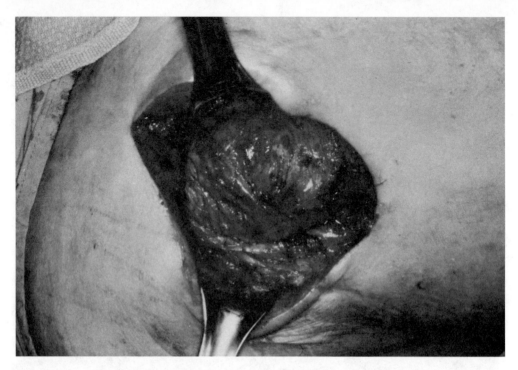

Fig. 5-9   Resultant large defect after excision and ostectomy.

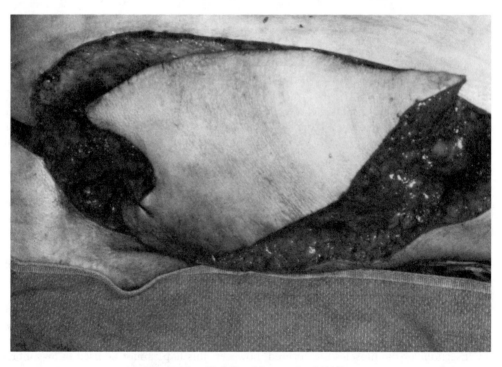

Fig. 5-10   Mobilized hamstring V-Y flap.

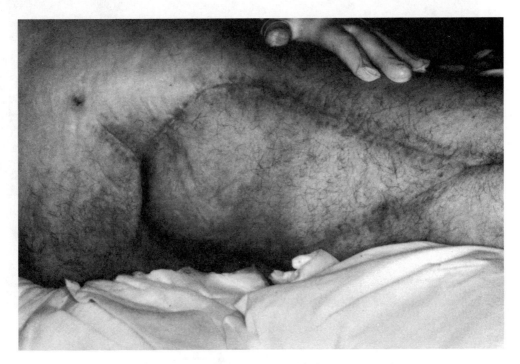

Fig. 5-11 Well-healed flap.

Additional myocutaneous flaps for ischial ulcer closure include the tensor fasciae latae flap, the rectus abdominis flap, and the gracilis flap.

Sacral Ulcer. Unlike ischial ulcers, large skin defects in the sacral area are not uncommon and can be associated with even larger areas of undermining. Fortunately, these ulcers are rarely deep. Ostectomy of the sacral prominence is still mandatory. Coverage is most commonly obtained with a very large fasciocutaneous buttock rotation flap (Figs. 5-12 and 5-13). Other useful flaps include the rhomboid (a diamond-shaped flap) and a simple Z-plasty (a double transposition flap designed to lengthen in one direction and shorten in the other)[146] (Figs. 5-14 and 5-15). Gluteus maximus musculocutaneous V-Y flaps have been advocated but are extensive procedures that are usually more than is needed for these ulcers.[105]

Greater Trochanteric Ulcers. The tensor fasciae latae (TFL) Myocutaneous flap is the workhorse of this region.[99] It is most commonly designed as a transposition flap with a large resultant dog-ear (Figs. 5-16 to 5-18). V-Y advancement and rotation of the TFL flap often gives an excellent functional and better esthetic result (Figs. 5-19 and 5-20).

Other flaps include the rectus femoris myocutaneous flap and random bipedicle or unipedicle fasciocutaneous flaps.

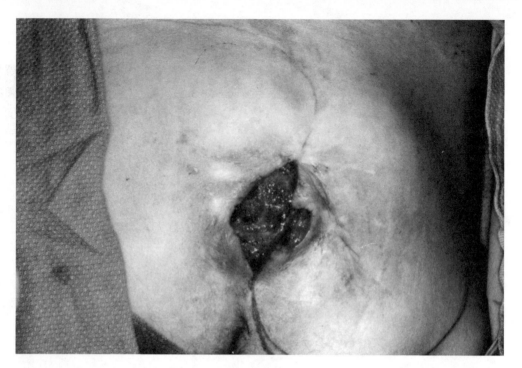

Fig. 5-12   Recurrent sacral ulcer. Notice scar from prior inferiorly based rotation flap.

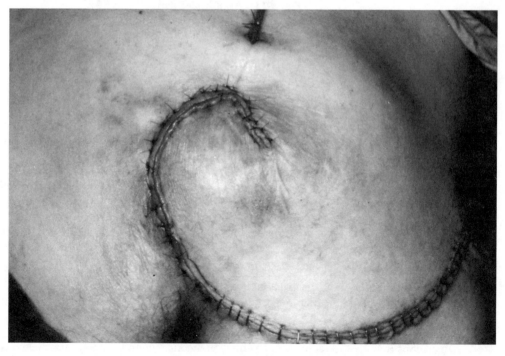

Fig. 5-13   Closure with superiorly based buttock rotation flap.

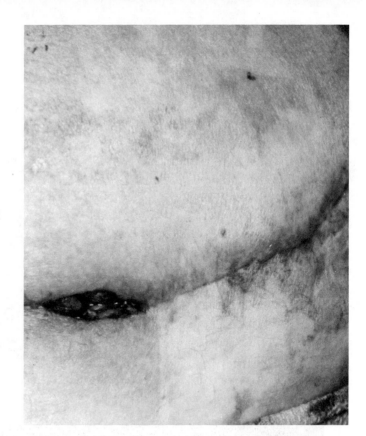

Fig. 5-14 Recurrent sacrococcygeal ulcer at distal end of prior buttock rotation flap.

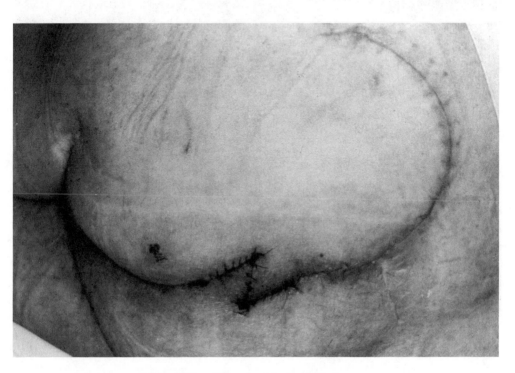

Fig. 5-15 Closure with simple Z-plasty.

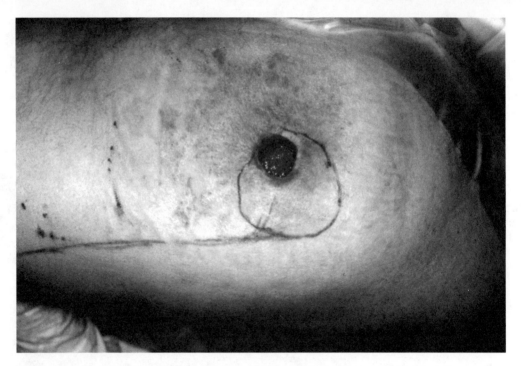

Fig. 5-16 Greater tochanteric ulcer. Markings demonstrate large area of undermining and tensor fasciae latae (TFL) flap design.

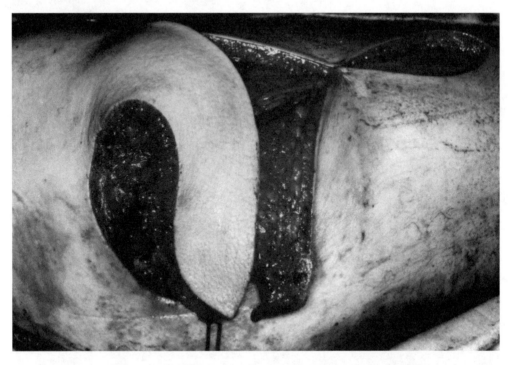

Fig. 5-17 Flap transposed.

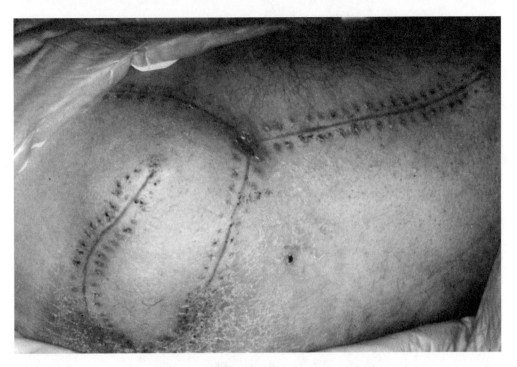

Fig. 5-18 Well healed with large dog-ear.

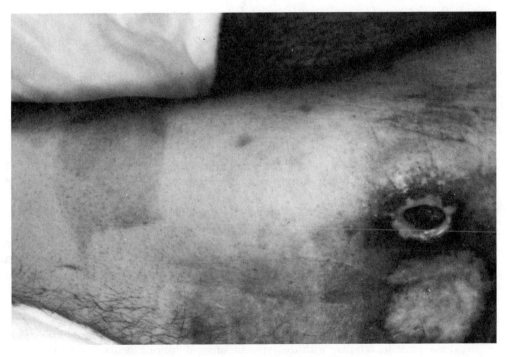

Fig. 5-19 Recurrent greater trochanteric ulcer.

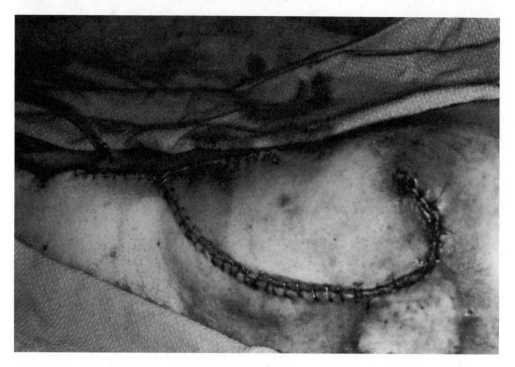

Fig. 5-20   Completed tensor fasciae latae flap. V-Y rotation-advancement flap closure.

Other sites. The olecranon, malleolar, and heel areas are particularly susceptible to pressure injury. Repair of these ulcers follows the same principles outlined above; local and regional fasciocutaneous flaps are most commonly employed.

SUMMARY

Pressure ulcers are a national health concern because, for the most part, they are a preventable costly complication. Pressure ulcers develop as a consequence of the occlusion of capillaries because of unrelieved pressure. The extent of tissue damage is influenced by numerous variables.

Prevention of pressure is a critical element in managing pressure ulcers and requires judicious use of interventions such as support surfaces. Regardless of the presence or absence of tissue damage, interface pressure must be reduced. Appropriate topical therapy must be initiated to enhance the wound repair. When the nurse is familiar with the pathologic process of tissue destruction caused by unrelieved pressure, appropriate interventions can be derived.

Successful surgical treatment of pressure ulcers is based on optimizing the patient's physiologic needs, a team approach, accurate staging, and fundamental surgical principles. Preventive strategies must then be employed to avoid a recurrence of these problem ulcers. The nurse must be familiar with the types of surgical options available for pressure ulcer management and their indications and contraindications to effectively care for these patients.

SELF-EVALUATION
QUESTIONS AND PROBLEMS

1. Define prevalence and incidence.
2. Why are the data describing the prevalence of pressure ulcer formation in hospitals, nursing homes, and high-risk populations so varied?
3. Define pressure ulcer.
4. What is the role of muscle in preventing pressure ulcers?
   a. Muscle redistributes pressure load.
   b. Muscle provides the blood supply to the skin.
   c. Muscle enables blood vessels to resist shear injury.
   d. Muscle concentrates pressure over the bony prominence.
5. State the three factors that play a role in determining the negative effects of pressure.
6. What is the range of pressures measured in the capillary bed?
   a. 5–15 mm Hg
   b. 11-32 mm Hg
   c. 10-20 mm Hg
   d. 15-35 mm Hg
7. Capillary closing pressure is the:
   a. pressure required to keep a capillary patent.
   b. difference in pressures between the arteriolar end of the capillary and the venous end.
   c. pressure needed to occlude the capillary blood flow.
   d. mean capillary pressure.
8. Explain why it is difficult to accurately assign a numerical value to capillary closing pressure.
9. Tissue interface pressures is believed to be an indirect measure of:
   a. capillary closing pressure.
   b. mean capillary pressure.
   c. pressure being exerted on a capillary.
   d. pressure required to keep a capillary patent.
10. Explain the relationship between tissue interface pressure and capillary closing pressure.
11. Describe how intensity of pressure and duration of pressure affect tissue ischemia.
12. Which of the following are major factors that contribute to pressure ulcer development?
    a. Shear, smoking, friction
    b. Age, smoking, blood pressure
    c. Nutrition, moisture, shear
    d. Shear, friction, nutritional debilitation
13. Which of the following statements about blanching erythema is *false?*
    a. It resolves once pressure is removed.
    b. It indicates deep tissue damage.
    c. It is an area of erythema that turns white when compressed.
    d. It implies pressure is not adequately relieved or reduced.
14. State four variables that influence the extent of tissue damage associated with pressure.

15. State at least two variables that contribute to cellular death in a pressure-damaged area.
16. Describe the pressure gradient in pressure ulcer formation.
17. The undermining that is commonly observed with pressure ulcers may be the result of which process?
    a. Shear
    b. Friction
    c. Maceration
    d. Advanced age
18. Differentiate between specificity and sensitivity.
19. Identify at least two differences among the three pressure-sore risk-assessment scales.
20. List therapeutic features that are provided by various support surfaces.
21. Tissue interface pressures are frequently used as indicators of support surface effectiveness. Identify at least three factors that may affect the accuracy of tissue interface readings.
22. Define the following terms:
    a. Overlay
    b. Replacement mattress
    c. Specialty bed
23. List the criteria for a therapeutic foam overlay.
24. Explain why water overlays are more appropriate for long-term and home care use than for acute care settings.
25. Compare and contrast static and dynamic air overlays.
26. Which of the following are considered to be pressure-relieving devices?
    a. Low air-loss beds
    b. Therapeutic foam overlays
    c. Alternating pressure pads and water mattresses
    d. Replacement mattresses
27. Explain the rationale for selection of a pressure-relief versus a pressure-reducing device.
28. List factors to be considered in selecting an appropriate support surface for an individual patient.
29. Describe four conditions that must be controlled before surgical intervention for the patient with pressure ulceration.
30. Briefly describe 11 principles underlying successful surgical management for the patient with pressure ulcers.
31. Myocutaneous flaps such as the gluteus maximus flap are frequently the procedure of choice in pressure-ulcer closure because:
    a. they provide well-vascularized tissue to fill the defect.
    b. they are almost always successful, even in the malnourished patient.
    c. postoperative healing time is half that required for fasciocutaneous flaps and skin grafts.
    d. they are 25% more resistant to repeat breakdown than normal tissue.
32. Which of the following flaps should *not* be used in an ambulatory patient?
    a. Gluteus maximus myocutaneous flap
    b. Tensor fasciae latae flap

     c. Large fasciocutaneous flap

     d. Hamstring V-Y flap

33. Patients undergoing flap closure of pressure ulcers are best managed postoperatively on:

     a. a pressure-reduction device with frequent position changes.

     b. a kinetic therapy device with air-support surface.

     c. a water-flotation device.

     d. a pressure-relief device with nonshear surface.

34. Which of the following patients should be referred to plastic surgery:

     a. A 32-year-old male spinal cord–injured patient with multiple state 2 lesions secondary to friction

     b. A 90-year-old woman with late-stage Alzheimer's and stage IV sacral ulcer

     c. A 45-year-old woman with a state 3 venous hypertension ulcer that is granulating

     d. A 26-year-old paraplegic with a stage IV ischial ulcer

---

SELF-EVALUATION

ANSWERS

1. *Prevalence* reflects the number of observations on a given day or at a specific time. *Incidence* reflects the ratio of the number of patients with a problem out of a specific population over a specified period of time.

2. Differences in the range within similar settings and between settings exist because (1) the data collector's ability to recognize damaged skin varies; (2) a standardized classification system is lacking (that is, some studies define pressure ulcers as always having breaks in the skin, thus overlooking the potential for pressure damage with intact skin); (3) some institutions have a concentrated population of patients shown to be at increased risk for pressure development; and (4) studies vary in population, design, and expertise of researchers. According to the NPUAP, the prevalence of pressure ulcers in acute care hospitals is 3% to 14% and in nursing homes is 15% to 25%. The literature reports a prevalence range of 25% to 40.4% for spinal cord–injured patients and 11.6% to 27.7% in the elderly.

3. A localized area of tissue necrosis that develops when soft tissue is compressed between a bony prominence and an external surface for a period of time.

4. a

5. Intensity of pressure, duration of pressure, and tissue tolerance

6. b

7. c

8. It is difficult to accurately assign a numerical value to capillary closing pressure because:

     • capillary blood pressure is influenced by values such as arterial blood pressure and venous pressure, which vary from individual to individual, from one bony prominence to another, and from time to time.

     • capillary closing pressure, which is commonly reported as 25 to 31 mm Hg, is based on studies in healthy adult males whereas recent studies report capillary closing pressures as low as 12 mm Hg in the elderly.

9. c

10. When tissue interface pressures exceed capillary pressures, capillaries close and tissue hypoxia ensues; tissue hypoxia is tolerable for short periods of time but prolonged ischemia results in tissue necrosis.

11. Amount and duration share an inverse relationship in producing tissue ischemia. It takes a long time for low pressure to create ischemia whereas it takes a short time for high pressure to cause tissue ischemia.

12. d

13. b

14. **a.** Venous thrombus formation
   b. Endothelial cell damage
   c. Redistribution of blood supply in ischemic tissue
   d. Altered lymphatic fluid flow in the area of pressure

15. **a.** Occlusion of capillaries
   b. Impaired perfusion through edematous tissue
   c. Accumulation of metabolic wastes

16. Pressure is highest at the point of contact between soft tissue and bone; thus tissue necrosis initially occurs at the bone–soft tissue interface. Once a pressure ulcer manifests itself cutaneously, deeper tissue damage has already occurred.

17. a

18. *Specificity* measures "true negatives," the percentage of patients who did *not* develop pressure sores and were *not* identified as being "at risk."
   Sensitivity measures "true positives," the percentage of patients who *did* develop pressure sores and *were* identified as being "at risk."

19. Norton scale:
   a. Five parameters
   b. Scale for parameters is from 1 to 4
   c. One- and two-word descriptors are given per rating of parameter
   d. Lower scores indicate increased risk
   Gosnell scale:
   a. Five parameters
   b. Two- and three-sentence descriptive statements for each rating of parameter
   c. High scores denote increased risk
   Braden scale:
   a. Six parameters
   b. Scale for parameters is from 1 to 4 (except for friction or shear category)
   c. Brief descriptions accompany each parameter
   d. Lower scores denote increased risk

20. Pressure reduction
   Pressure relief
   Relief of shear and friction
   Control of moisture and maceration
   Kinetic therapy

21. Transducer size and shape
   Load shape and its interaction with the support material
   Method of equilibrium detection
   Uniformity of measurement technique
   Skill of person doing the testing

22. *Overlay:* Device that is placed on top of a standard hospital mattress.

Replacement mattress: Mattress that is used in place of the standard hospital mattress and provides pressure reduction as well as the features of a standard mattress (long-term use, terminal cleaning).

Specialty bed: Bed used in place of standard hospital bed to provide pressure relief, relief of shear and friction, or kinetic therapy, or all three.

23. Thickness of 3 to 4 inches

Density of 1.3 to 1.6 lb/ft^3

Indentation load deflection (ILD): 25% ILD of about 30 lb; ratio of 60% ILD to 25% ILD of 2.5 or greater

24. Water overlays effectively reduce interface pressure by flotation therapy. However, water overlays have several disadvantages that make them less appropriate for acute-care settings: potential for water leaks, which can create safety hazards; weight; requirement for personnel to set up and maintain overlay; potential for water displacement resulting in higher pressures in heel area; limitations on patient positioning; difficulties with temperature regulation; potential for underfilling or overfilling; difficulty performing procedures (such as CPR) because of fluid motion.

25. Air overlays provide high-level pressure reduction, and some may provide pressure relief. Air overlays can be classified as either static or dynamic.

- Static devices are composed of interconnecting air cells that are inflated before patient use. They are called "static devices" because they reduce interface pressure by maintaining a constant inflation. Many static devices require daily monitoring for loss of air, with reinflation provided as needed; these are most effective in settings with adequate staff. Some static devices (low air-loss overlays) are connected to pumps to maintain constant inflation and provide air flow to control moisture.
- Dynamic devices use electrical currents to create alternating currents of air for weight redistribution; in addition to weight redistribution, this change of air is believed to enhance blood flow by creating high and low pressure areas. Some dynamic devices also provide low levels of air flow to reduce maceration.

26. a

27. *Pressure relief* is indicated for patients who are unable to turn or be turned and for patients who have breakdown involving multiple skin surfaces. The rationale is that these patients need a surface that maintains continuous blood flow to the tissues.

Pressure reduction is indicated for patients who can turn or be turned and whose breakdown (if present) is limited to one turning surface. The rationale is that these patients have at least two turning surfaces and can thus be maintained effectively with pressure reduction and a turning schedule.

28. Therapeutic considerations: need for pressure relief versus pressure reduction, relief of shear and friction, moisture control, or kinetic therapy (in determining need for pressure relief versus pressure reduction, one must consider caregiver compliance with turning)

Duration of therapy

Independence issues, that is, support surface should be selected so that it does not compromise patient's mobility and independence

Setup and maintenance required, and availability of such surfaces

Environmental issues, such as requirement for electricity in home setting

Financial feasibility

29. **a.** Spasticity must be controlled, either surgically or pharmacologically.

   b. Infection must be eliminated.

   c. The cause of the lesion must be identified and corrected.

   d. Nutritional status must be optimized; in general, flap closure should not be done if the patient's serum albumin is less than 3.0 g/dl.

30. **a.** Intraoperative positioning should provide maximal "stretch" on the flap; this reduces the risk of postoperative dehiscence resulting from tension on the flap.

   b. Perioperative antibiotic coverage should be provided based on culture results.

   c. The bony prominence should be partially excised to remove any infected bone and to increase the surface area upon which the patient rests.

   d. The entire ulcer and any granulation tissue should be excised so that only healthy unscarred tissue is left as a wound base.

   e. Incisions should be made with possible recurrences in mind.

   f. Incisions should be made so as to avoid suture lines over bony prominences.

   g. The defect should be filled with healthy, unscarred, well-vascularized tissue.

   h. Gradually increase mobility postoperatively and observe skin and suture lines.

   i. Skin grafts are not indicated because they lack durability.

31. a

32. d

33. d

34. d

REFERENCES

1. Abruzzese RS: Early assessment and prevention of pressure sores. In Lee BY, editor: Chronic ulcers of the skin, St. Louis, 1985, McGraw-Hill Book Co, Inc.
2. Adams T and Hunter WS: Modification of skin mechanical properties by eccrine sweat gland activity, J Appl Physiol 26:417, 1969.
3. Agris J and Spira M: Pressure ulcers: prevalence and treatment, Clin Symp 31(5):2+, 1979.
4. Allman RM: Pressure ulcers among the elderly, N Engl J Med 320:850, 1989.
5. Allman RM: Epidemiology of pressure sores in different populations, Decubitus 2(2):30+, 1989.
6. Allman RM, Laprade CA, Noel, LB, et al: Pressure sores among hospitalized patients, Ann Intern Med 105:337+, 1986.
7. Allman RM, Walker JM, Hart MK, et al: Air-fluidized beds or conventional therapy for pressure sores, Ann Intern Med 107:641, 1987.
8. Alterescu V: The financial costs of inpatient pressure ulcers to an acute care facility, Decubitus 2:14+, 1989.
9. Alterescu V and Alterescu K: Etiology and treatment of pressure ulcers, Decubitus 1(1):28, 1988.
10. Anderson TP and Andberg MM: Psychosocial factors associated with pressure sores, Arch Phys Med Rehabil 60(8):341+, 1979.
11. Anderson KE and Kvorning SA: Medical aspects of decubitus ulcer, Int J Dermatol 21:265+, 1982.
12. Andrews J and Balai R: The prevention and treatment of pressure sores by use of pressure distributing mattress, Decubitus 1(4):14, 1988.
13. Arnold HL: Decubitus: the word. In Parish LC, Witkowski JA, and Crissey JT: The decubitus ulcer, New York, 1983, Masson Publishing, USA.
14. Barbenel JC, Jordan MM, Nicol SM, and Clark MO: Incidence of pressure sores in the greater Glasgow Health Board area, Lancet 2:548+, 1977.
15. Barnes SH: Myths and misconceptions of pressure sore management, J Enterostom Ther 12(1):29+, 1985.

16. Barnes SH: Patient and family education for the patient with a pressure necrosis, Nurs Clin North Am 22(2):463, 1987.
17. Barth P et al: Pressure profiles in deep tissues, Proc 37th Annual Conference on Engineering in Medicine and Biology, Los Angeles, Sept 15-19, 1984.
18. Beaver MJ: Mediscus low air-loss beds and the prevention of decubitus ulcer, Crit Care Nurse 6:32, 1986.
19. Bennett G: Ageing skin and pressure sores, Practitioner 231:834, 1987.
20. Bennett L, Kavner D, Lee BY, et al: Skin stress and blood flow in sitting paraplegic patients, Arch Phys Med Rehabil 65:186+, 1984.
21. Bennett LM and Lee BY: Vertical shear existence in animal pressure threshold experiments, Decubitus 1:18, 1988.
22. Berecek KH: Treatment of decubitus ulcers, Nurs Clin North Am 10:171+, 1975.
23. Bergstrom B: AHCPR guidelines for the prediction, prevention and early treatment of pressure sores, Lecture presented at the Prediction Prevention and Early Treatment of Pressure Ulcers in Adults: A Conference to Review Guidelines Developed by the Agency for Health Care Policy and Research, Arlington, Va, March 6-8, 1991.
24. Bergstrom N and Braden B: The influence of diminished tissue tolerance on pressure sore development in the elderly, 40th Annual Scientific Meeting of the Gerontological Society, Washington, DC, Nov 1987; abstract in The Gerontologist 27 (special issue).
25. Bergstrom N, Demuth PJ, and Braden B: A clinical trial of the Braden Scale for predicting pressure sore risk, Nurs Clin North Am 22(2):417+, 1987.
26. Bergstrom N, Braden B, Laguzza A, and Holman A: The Braden Scale for predicting pressure sore risk, Nurs Res 36(4):205+, 1987.
27. Berjian RA, Bouglass HO, Holyoke ED, et al: Skin pressure measurements on various mattress surfaces in cancer patients, Am J Phys Med 62:217, 1983.
28. Black J and Black S: Surgical management of pressure ulcers, Nurs Clin North Am 22(2):429+, 1987.
29. Bobel LM: Nutritional implication in the patient with pressure sores, Nurs Clin North Am 22(2):379, 1987.
30. Braden BJ: Emotional stress and pressure sore formation among the elderly recently relocated to a nursing home: key aspects of recovery: improving mobility, rest, and nutrition, New York, 1990, Springer Publishing.
31. Braden B and Bergstrom N: A conceptual schema for the study of the etiology of pressure sores, Rehabil Nurs 12(1):8+, 1987.
32. Braden BJ and Bergstrom N: Clinical utility of the Braden Scale for predicting pressure sore risk, Decubitus 2(3):44+, 1989.
33. Braden BJ and Bryant R: Innovations to prevent and treat pressure ulcers, Geriatr Nurs 11(4):182-186, 1990.
34. Brandeis GH et al: Correlates of pressure sores in the nursing home, Decubitus 2:60, 1989.
35. Brooks B and Duncan W: Effects of pressure on tissues, Arch Surg 40:696, 1940.
36. Burton AC and Yamada S: Relation between blood pressure and flow in the human forearm, J Appl Physiol 4:329+, 1951.
37. Cherry GW et al: Functional microcirculatory changes after flap elevation: possible factor in flap failure, Plast Surg Forum 3:206+, 1980.
38. Cherry GW and Ryan TJ: Pathophysiology. In Parish LC, Witkowski JA, and Crissey JT: The decubitus ulcer, New York, 1983, Masson Publishing, USA.
39. Cherry GW, Ryan TJ, and Ellis J: Decreased fibrinolysis in reperfused ischemic tissue, Thromb Diathesis Haemorrhag 32:659, 1974.
40. Clark M: Measuring the pressure, Nurs Times 84(25):72, 1988.
41. Clark MO, Barbanel JC, Jordan MM, and Nicol SM: Pressure sores, Nursing Times 74(9):363-366, 1978.
42. Cohen IK, Diegelmann RF, and Johnson MJ: Effect of corticosteroids on collagen synthesis, Surgery 82(1):15+, 1977.
43. Constantian MB and Jackson HS: Biology and care of the pressure ulcer wound. In Constantian

MB, editor: Pressure ulcers: principles and techniques of management, Boston, 1980, Little, Brown & Co.

44. Counsell C, Seymour S, Guin B, and Hudson A: Interface skin pressures on four pressure-relieving devices, J Enterostom Ther 17(4):150, 1990.

45. Daniel RK and Kerrigan CL: Skin flaps: an anatomical and hemodynamic approach, Clin Plast Surg 6:181, 1979.

46. Davies P and Ryan DW: Stevens-Johnson syndrome managed in the Clinitron bed, Intensive Care Med 9:87, 1983.

47. Dolezal R, Cohen M, and Schultz RC: The use of Clinitron therapy unit in the immediate postoperative care of pressure ulcers, Ann Plast Surg 14:33, 1985.

48. Doughty D: Management of pressure sores, J Enterostom Ther 15(1):39+, 1988.

49. Doughty D, Fairchild P, and Stogis S: Your patient: Which therapy? J Enterostom Ther 17:154, 1990.

50. Eckman KL: The prevalence of dermal ulcers among persons in the U.S. who have died, Decubitus 2:36, 1989.

51. Ek AC and Boman GA: A descriptive study of pressure sores: the prevalence of pressure sores and characteristics of patients, Adv Nurs 7:51+, 1982.

52. Ek AC, Gustavsson G, and Lewis DH: The local skin blood flow in areas at risk for pressure sores treated with massage, Scand J Rehabil Med 17(2):81-86, 1985.

53. Ferguson-Pell MW: Establishing a pressure sore prevention service. In Lee BY, editor: Chronic ulcers of the skin, St. Louis, 1985, McGraw-Hill Book Co.

54. Forbes GB and Reina JC: Adult lean body mass declines with age: some longitudinal observations, Metabolism 19:653+, 1970.

55. Fowler EM: Equipment and products used in management and treatment of pressure ulcers, Nurse Clin North Am 22:449, 1987.

56. Fox J and Bradley R: A new medical dictionary, London, 1803, Darton & Harvey.

57. Garmar Industries: British society for tissue viability holds conference, Pressure Ulcer Forum 4:1, 1989 (Newsletter).

58. Goldstone LA and Goldstone J: The Norton score: an early warning of pressure sores? J Adv Nurs 1:419+, 1982.

59. Goldstone LA and Roberts BV: A preliminary discriminant function analysis of elderly orthopaedic patients who will or will not contract a pressure sore, Int J Nurs Stud 17(5):17+, 1980.

60. Gosnell DJ: An assessment tool to identify pressure sores, Nurs Res 22(1):55+, 1973.

61. Gosnell D: Assessing client risk for pressure sores. In Waltz CF and Strickland OL, editors: Measuring client outcomes, New York, 1988, Springer Publishing Co.

62. Gosnell D: Pressure sore risk assessment: a critique, Decubitus 2(3):32+, 1989.

63. Greer DM, Morris J, Walsh NE, et al: Cost effectiveness and efficacy of air-fluidized therapy in the treatment of pressure ulcers, J Enterostom Ther 15:247, 1988.

64. Guralnik JM, Harris RB, White LR, and Cornoni-Huntley JC: Occurrence and predictors of pressure sores in the national health and nutrition examination survey followup, J Am Geriatr Soc 36:807+, 1988.

65. Guyton AC: Textbook of medical physiology, Philadelphia, 1986, WB Saunders Co.

66. Hargest TS and Artz CP: A new concept in patient care: the air-fluidized bed, AORN J 10:50, 1969.

67. Hawthorne MH, Jefferson JW, and Paduano DJ: The prevalence of dermal wounds, Decubitus 2:64, 1989.

68. Holley LK, Long J, Stewart J, and Jones RF: A new pressure measuring system for cushions and beds—with a review of the literature, Paraplegia 17(4):461-474, 1979.

69. Husain T: An experimental study of some pressure effects on tissues, with reference to the bedsore problem, J Pathol Bacteriol 66:347+, 1953.

70. International Association for Enterostomal Therapy: Standards of care: dermal wounds: pressure sores, Irvine, Calif, 1987.

71. Iverson-Carpenter MS: Impaired skin integrity, J Gerontol Nurs 14(3):25+, 1988.

72. Jackson BS, Chargares R, Nee N, and Freeman K: The effects of a therapeutic bed on pressure ulcers: an experimental study, J Enterostom Ther 15:220, 1988.
73. Jester J and Weaver V: A report of clinical investigation of various tissue support surfaces used for the prevention, early intervention and management of pressure ulcers, Ostomy/Wound Management 26:39, 1990.
74. Jones PL and Millman A: Wound healing and the aged patient, Nurs Clin North Am 25:263+, 1990.
75. Jordan MA and Clark MO: Report on the incidence of pressure sores in the patient community of the Greater Glasgow Health Board, Glasgow, 1977. In Clark MA et al: Pressure sores, Nurs Times 74:363+, 1978.
76. Kalaja E: Clinical results of treatment of patients in the air-fluidized bed (Clinitron) during a one-year period, Scand J Plast Reconstr Surg 18:513, 1984.
77. Kemp MG, Keithley JK, Smith DW, and Morreale B: Factors that contribute to pressure sores in surgical patients, Res Nurs Health 13:293+, 1990.
78. Kosiak M: Etiology and pathology of ischemic ulcers, Arch Phys Med Rehabil 40:62, 1959.
79. Kosiak M: Etiology of decubitus ulcers, Arch Phys Med Rehabil 42:19+, 1961.
80. Kosiak M et al: Evaluation of pressure as a factor in the production of ischial ulcers, Arch Phys Med Rehabil 39:623, 1958.
81. Krouskop TA: A synthesis of the factors that contribute to pressure sore formation, Med Hypotheses 11(2):255+, 1983.
82. Krouskop T: Lecture presented at the 1988 Wound Care Symposium, San Francisco, Calif, April 1988.
83. Krouskop T: Scientific aspects of pressure relief, Lecture presented at the 1989 International Association for Enterostomal Therapy annual conference, Washington, DC, June 8, 1989.
84. Krouskop TA and Garber SL: The role of technology in the prevention of pressure sores, Ostomy/Wound Management 16:45, 1987.
85. Krouskop TA and Barber SL: Interface pressure confusion, Decubitus 2:8, 1989.
86. Krouskop TA, Noble PS, Brown J, and Marburger R: Factors affecting the pressure-distributing properties of foam mattress overlays, J Rehabil Res 23(3):33+, 1986.
87. Krouskop TA, Williams R, and Krebs M: The effectiveness of air flotation beds in lowering the pressures under the recumbent body, CARE, Sci Pract 4(2):9-12, 1984.
88. Krouskop TA, Williams R, Krebs et al: Effectiveness of mattress overlays in reducing interface pressure during recumbency, J Rehabil Res 22:7, 1985.
89. Kynes P: A new perspective on pressure sore prevention, J Enterostom Ther 13(2):42+, 1986.
90. Lamid S and El Ghatit AZ: Smoking, spasticity and pressure sores in spinal cord injured patients, Am J Phys Med 62(6):300-306, 1983.
91. Landis EM: Micro-injection studies of capillary blood pressure in human skin, Heart 15:209, 1930.
92. Larson E: Evaluating validity of screening tests, Nurs Res 35(3):186+, 1986.
93. LeKander BJ and Hoyman K: Improved care of critically ill patients: contributions of therapeutic beds and mattress, Perspect Crit Care 2:49, 1988.
94. Lilla JA, Friedrichs RR, and Vistnes LM: Flotation mattresses for preventing and treating tissue breakdown, Geriatrics 30(9):71-75, 1975.
95. Lillienfeld AM and Lillienfeld DE: Foundations of epidemiology, ed 2, New York, 1980, Oxford University Press.
96. Lincoln R, Roberts R, Maddox A, et al: Use of the Norton pressure sore risk assessment scoring system with elderly patients in acute care, J Enterostom Ther 13:17+, 1986.
97. Lindan O: Etiology of decubitus ulcers: an experimental study, Arch Phys Med Rehabil 42:774, 1961.
98. Linder RM and Morris DM: The surgical management of pressure ulcers: a systematic approach based on staging, Decubitus 3(2):32, 1990.
99. Nahai F: The tensor fasciae latae flap, Clin Plast Surg 7:51, 1980. ["Nahai" is correct.]
100. Maklebust J: Pressure ulcers: etiology and prevention, Nurs Clin North Am 22:359, 1987.

101. Maklebust J: Hospitalwide pressure ulcer audit, Decubitus 2:64, 1989.
102. Maklebust JA, Brunckhorst L, Cracchiolo-Caraway A, et al: Pressure ulcer incidence in high-risk patients managed on a special three-layer air cushion, Decubitus 1(4):30, 1988.
103. Maklebust J, Mondoux L, and Sieggreen: Pressure relief characteristics of various support surfaces used in prevention and treatment of pressure ulcers, J Enterostom Ther 13(3):85, 1986.
104. Maklebust JA, Sieggreen MY, and Mondoux L: Pressure relief capabilities of the Sof-Care bed and the Clinitron bed, Ostomy/Wound Management 21:36, 1988.
105. McCraw J and Arnold P: Gluteus maximus. In McCraw J and Arnold P, editors: Atlas of muscle and musculocutaneous flaps, Norfolk, Va, 1986, Houston Press.
106. Meehan M: Multisite pressure ulcer prevalence survey, Decubitus 3:14, 1990.
107. Moolten SE: Bedsores in the chronically ill patient, Arch Phys Med Rehabil 53:430+, 1972.
108. Motloch WM: Analysis of medical costs associated with healing of pressure sores in adolescent paraplegic, University of San Francisco, Feb 28, 1978. (Unpublished paper.)
109. Mulholland J et al: Protein metabolism and bed sores, Ann Surg 118:1015, 1943.
110. National Pressure Ulcer Advisory Panel: Pressure ulcers prevalence, cost and risk assessment: consensus development conference statement, Decubitus 2(2):24+, 1989.
111. Natow AB: Nutrition in prevention and treatment of decubitus ulcers, Top Clin Nurs 2:39, 1983.
112. Normolle E and Storm H: Five years experience with air-fluidized bed in the care of burned patients, Scand J Plast Reconstr Surg Hand Surg 18:149, 1984.
113. Norton D, McLaren R, and Exton-Smith AN: An investigation of geriatric nursing problems in hospital, London, 1962, National Corporation for the Care of Old People.
114. Norton D, McClaren R, and Exton-Smith AN: An investigation of geriatric nursing problems in hospital, Edinburgh, 1975, Churchill Livingstone.
115. Olson B: Effects of massage for prevention of pressure ulcers, Decubitus 2(4):32+, 1989.
116. Parish LC and Witkowski JA: Clinitron therapy and the decubitus ulcer: preliminary dermatologic studies, Dermatology 19:517, 1980.
117. Parish LC, Witkowski JA, and Crissey JT: The decubitus ulcer, New York, 1983, Masson Publishing, USA.
118. Petersen NC and Bittman S: The epidemiology of pressure sores, Scand J Plast Reconstr Surg Hand Surg 5:62, 1971.
119. Pinchocofsky-Devin GD and Kaminski MV: Correlation of pressure sore and nutritional status, J Am Geriatr Soc 34(6):435+, 1986.
120. Reed JW: Pressure ulcers in the elderly: prevention and treatment utilizing the team approach, Md State Med J 30:45+, 1981.
121. Reed BR and Clark RAF: Cutaneous tissue repair: practical implications of current knowledge, II, J Am Acad Dermatol 13:919+, 1985.
122. Reger SI, McGovern TF, Chung KC, and Stewart TP: Correlation of transducer systems for monitoring tissue interface pressures, J Clin Engineering 13(5):365, 1988.
123. Reichel SM: Shearing force as a factor in decubitus ulcers in paraplegics, JAMA 166:762, 1958.
124. Reuler JB and Cooney TG: The pressure sore: pathophysiology and principles of management, Ann Intern Med 94(5):661+, 1981.
125. Roberts BV and Goldstone LA: A survey of pressure sores in the over sixties on two orthopaedic wards. Int J Nurs Stud 16:355+, 1979.
126. Robinson CE, Coghlan JK, and Jackson G: Decubitus ulcers in paraplegics: financial implications, Can J Public Health 69:199, 1978.
127. Rodriquez G, Claus-Walker J, Kent MC, and Garza HM: Collagen metabolite excretion as a predictor of bone and skin-related complications in spinal cord injury, Arch Phys Med Rehabil 70(6):442+, 1989.
128. Rubin CF, Dietz RR, and Abruzzese RS: Auditing the decubitus ulcer problem, Am J Nurs 74:1820, 1974.
129. Rudolph R: Wound treatments, nostrums and hokums. In Rudolph R and Noe JM, editors: Chronic problem wounds, Boston, 1983, Little, Brown & Co.
130. Ryan DW: The influence of environmental temperature (32° C) on catabolism using Clinitron fluidized bed, Intensive Care Med 9:279, 1983.

131. Ryan TJ: Microvascularization in psoriasis, blood vessels, lymphatics and tissue fluid, Pharmacol Ther 10:27, 1980.
132. Saarni H and Hopsu-Javu VK: The decrease of hyaluronate synthesis by antiinflammatory steroids in vitro, Br J Dermatol 98:445+, 1978.
133. Scales JT: Pressure on the patient. In Kenedi RM and Cowden JM, editors: Bedsore biomechanics, London, 1976, University Park Press.
134. Schmid-Schönbein H, Rieger H, and Fischer T: Blood fluidity as a consequence of red cell fluidity: flow properties of blood and flow behavior of blood in vascular diseases, Angiology 31:301+, 1980.
135. Seiler WO and Stahelin HB: Decubitus ulcers: preventive techniques for the elderly patient, Geriatrics 40(7):53+, 1985.
136. Shannon M: Pressure sores. In Norris C, editor: Concept clarification in nursing, Rockville, Md, 1982, Aspen Publishers.
137. Shannon ML and Skorga P: Pressure ulcer prevalence in two general hospitals, Decubitus 2:38, 1989.
138. Shea JD: Pressure sores: classification and management, Clin Orthopaed Rel Res (112):89+, 1975.
139. Siegel RJ, Vistness LM, and Laub DR: Use of water bed for prevention of pressure sores, Plast Reconstr Surg 51:81, 1973.
140. Silver JR: Management of complications, Mod Geriatrics 5:6, 1975.
141. Sloan DR, Brown RD, and Larson DL: Evaluation of a simplified water mattress in the prevention and treatment of pressure sores, Plast Reconstr Surg 60(4):596+, 1977.
142. Smoot EC: Clinitron bed therapy hazards, Plast Reconstr Surg 77:165, 1986.
143. Solis I, Krouskop T, Trainer N, and Marburger R: Supine interface pressure in children, Arch Phys Med Rehabil 69:524, 1988.
144. Spence WR, Burk RD, and Rae JW: Gel support for prevention of decubitus ulcers, Arch Phys Med Rehabil 48:283, 1967.
145. Stotts NA and Paul S: Pressure ulcer development in surgical patients, Decubitus 1(3):24+, 1988.
146. Stueber K and Goldberg N: Wound coverage: grafts and flaps. In Dagher FJ, editor: Cutaneous wounds, Mt. Kisco, NY, 1985, Futura Publishing Co.
147. Thomson CW, Ryan DW, Dunkin LJ, et al: Fluidized-bead bed in the intensive-therapy unit, Lancet 1:568, 1980.
148. Tobin GR et al: The biceps femoris myocutaneous advancement flap: a useful modification for ischial pressure ulcer reconstruction, Ann Plast Surg 6(5):396, 1981.
149. Trumble HC: The skin tolerance for pressure and pressure sores, Med J Aust 2:724+, 1930.
150. Turnock H: Benefits of a bead bed, Nurs Mirror 156:32, 1983.
151. Viner C: Floating on a bed of beads, Nurs Times 82:62, 1986.
152. Wasson JH, Sox HC, Neff RK, and Goldman L: Clinical prediction rules: applications and methodological standards, N Engl J Med 313:793+, 1985.
153. Wells P and Geden E: Paraplegic body-support pressure on convoluted foam, waterbed, and standard mattresses, Res Nurs Health 7:127, 1984.
154. Whitney J, Fellows BJ, and Larson E: Do mattresses make a difference? J Gerontol Nurse 10(9):20+, 1984.
155. Willey T: High-tech beds and mattress overlays: a decision guide, Am J Nurs 89:1142, 1989.
156. Williams A: A study of factors contributing to skin breakdown, Nurs Res 21:238+, 1972.
157. Wornom IL III: Surgical intervention: grafts and flaps. In Krasner D, editor: Chronic wound care, King of Prussia, Penn, 1990, Health Management Publications.
158. Young JS et al: Spinal cord injury statistics: experience of the regional spinal cord injury systems, Phoenix, 1982, Good Samaritan Medical Center. (Unpublished.)
159. Young L: Pressure ulcer prevalence associated patient characteristics in one long term facility, Decubitus 2(2):52+, 1989.

6 Lower Extremity Ulcers

MARY ZINK
PAUL ROUSSEAU
G. ALLEN HOLLOWAY, Jr.

OBJECTIVES

1. Differentiate ischemic, neuropathic, and venous ulcers in terms of causative factors, pathophysiology, usual location and appearance, and principles of management.

2. Define the following terms: arteriosclerosis, atherosclerosis, plaque.

3. Identify four major risk factors for peripheral vascular disease.

4. Relate the signs and symptoms of arterial insufficiency to the underlying pathophysiologic processes.

5. Describe the three types of neuropathy that may occur in the diabetic in terms of risk for ulcer formation.

6. Identify critical factors to be included in the history and physical examination of the patient with an ischemic ulcer.

7. Briefly describe the following diagnostic tests: segmental pressures, toe pressures, ultrasonic Doppler waveform, pulse volume recorder, transcutaneous oxygen tension, angiography, digital subtraction angiography, plethysmography, and photoplethysmography.

8. Identify indications for culture of an ischemic ulcer.

9. Identify surgical, pharmacologic, and nursing measures to maximize blood flow to the lower extremity.

10. Identify the factors other than topical therapy that impinge on healing of an ischemic ulcer.

11. Explain why débridement may be contraindicated in the management of an ischemic ulcer.

12. Identify appropriate topical therapy options for an ischemic ulcer based on ulcer assessment.

13. Identify patients who require referral for vascular assessment, nutritional assessment, orthotics, or diabetes management.

14. Identify key components of a patient education program for the patient with PVD (peripheral vascular disease) or diabetes, or both, to include routine care and precautions.

15. Identify four states that predispose the patient to develop venous ulcers.

16. Describe the relationship between trauma and lower extremity ulcers.

17. Describe three methods of managing edema in venous ulcerations.

18. Identify the role of surgery in venous ulcer management.

Many chronic, nonhealing ulcers occur on the lower legs and feet, particularly those of vascular origin. Management of lower extremity ulcers is complex and resource intensive. It is essential that a holistic, collaborative approach be provided by a multidisciplinary team who can diligently monitor the patient's health status, since many pathologic conditions are typically associated with ulcerations on the lower extremities[113] (Box 6-1). Diagnostic studies, often invasive, must be conducted to identify the cause of the wound; surgical procedures may be warranted to improve tissue perfusion; and medical management is needed to monitor and manage concurrent diseases such as diabetes mellitus. Finally, consistent, conscientious care must be provided to encourage and support the patient to alter life-style or health habits known to worsen vascular status and hence the wound. This chapter is a discussion of vascular ulcers (arterial and venous) and neuropathic (diabetic) ulcers.

ARTERIAL ULCERS

Arterial ulcers are caused by insufficient arterial perfusion to an extremity or location and are also termed "ischemic ulcers." The term "ischemic ulcer" denotes a skin lesion with

---

Box 6-1   CAUSES OF LOWER EXTREMITY ULCERS

Venous hypertension
Arterial disease
Bacterial, fungal, and syphilitic infections
Diabetes mellitus
Pressure
Malignancy:
   Squamous cell
   Kaposi's sarcoma
   Melanoma
   Lymphoma

Sickle cell anemia
Connective tissue disorders:
   Rheumatoid arthritis
   Lupus erythematosus
   Scleroderma
Trauma
Insect bites
Factitial

tissue loss related to arterial disease and is not used to describe the actual perfusion state of the ulcer. Although arterial insufficiency may affect any area of the body, it usually involves the lower extremities (Fig. 6-1).

Arterial ulcers are not so common as venous ulcers; however, they are often more complex to manage because of coexisting diseases and complications. The difficulty in healing these ulcers of the lower extremity lies in the lack of adequate arterial perfusion to the affected tissue. Of the conservatively estimated 7.5 million people in the United States who have diabetes, 30% have peripheral vascular disease (PVD), and 15% of these people develop ulcers of the lower extremity, especially the feet.[61]

Pathophysiology of Peripheral Vascular Disease

Peripheral vascular disease (PVD) is commonly associated with arterial insufficiency. PVD involves the arteries, veins, and lymph vessels and results in chronic, systemic health

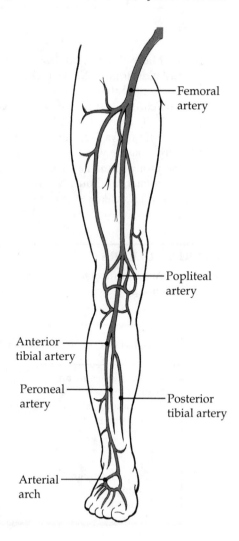

Femoral artery

Popliteal artery

Anterior tibial artery

Peroneal artery

Posterior tibial artery

Arterial arch

Fig. 6-1   Arterial system in leg.

problems. Although symptoms can be palliated (as by revascularization surgery), there is no cure for PVD.

The pathogenesis is arteriosclerosis, a thickening and decreased elasticity of the arterial walls. Atherosclerosis, a form of arteriosclerosis, develops as a result of the accumulation of plaque, lipids, fibrin, platelets, and other cellular debris into and along the wall of the artery.

Current theory postulates that monocytes adhere to the intimal lining of the artery. Macrophages follow and release growth factors, which stimulate growth and migration of vascular smooth muscle cells. Platelets may then adhere to the injury site resulting in a plaque that narrows or blocks the lumen of the artery.[92] In patients with diabetes, this process is accelerated and these patients are 1.2 to 6 times more likely to have PVD, coronary artery, or cerebrovascular disease.[17] In addition, increased platelet adhesiveness and aggregation are believed to be critical in the genesis of atherosclerosis and microthrombi, particularly with diabetes.[17]

The dynamics of blood flow are affected by atherosclerotic plaque. When resting, a person can tolerate up to 70% occlusion of the artery. However, with exercise the increased demands for blood flow cannot be met and muscle ischemia occurs, causing crampy leg pain; 90% or greater occlusion will reduce flow resulting in pain even at rest.[109] Although the exact initiating mechanism of atherosclerosis is unknown,[92] the aging process, life-style habits, and disease can combine to affect both large and small arteries.

Distinctions Between Diabetics and Nondiabetics. Important differences exist between PVD in patients with and that in patients without diabetes, as summarized in Table 6-1. Atherosclerosis is much more common with diabetes, occurs in those at a

Table 6-1.   Differences in diabetic and nondiabetic peripheral vascular disease

	Diabetic	Nondiabetic
Clinical	More common Younger patient More rapid	Less common Older patient Less rapid
Male/female ratio	2:1	30:1
Occlusion	Multisegmental	Single segment
Vessels adjacent to occlusion	Involved	Not involved
Collateral vessels	Involved	Usually normal
Lower extremities	Both	Unilateral
Vessels involved	Tibial artery Peroneal artery Small vessels Arterioles	Aortic artery Iliac artery Femoral artery
Gangrene	Patchy areas of foot and toes	Extensive
In-hospital mortality with amputation	Approximately 3%	Significantly less

From Levin ME and O'Neal LW: The diabetic foot, ed 4, St. Louis, 1988, Mosby–Year Book, Inc.

younger age, more rapidly advances, and is nearly as common in women as in men. In non-diabetic patients, the male-to-female ratio is 30:1. Of particular relevance to lower extremity ulcers are the following:

1. Bilateral lower extremities are usually involved in the patient with diabetes, whereas nondiabetic patients more commonly have unilateral involvement.
2. Vessels affected in the patient with diabetes are most frequently below the knee (tibial and peroneal arteries and smaller distal branches), whereas the femoral, iliac, and aortic vessels are sites in the general population.
3. Occlusion is multisegmental in diabetes, whereas the involvement is singular with a normal, adjacent arterial system in the nondiabetic patient.
4. Gangrene manifests as patchy areas on feet and toes in the patient with diabetes, whereas gangrene is extensive in nondiabetics, since larger vessels are generally occluded proximally.

Contributing Factors In PVD

Several factors, both genetic and environmental, contribute to PVD and are considered risk factors. Most genetic factors are difficult to modulate and may not be amenable to medical management; environmental factors can be altered but require behavioral changes. Major risk factors include smoking, diabetes mellitus, hyperlipidemia, hypertension, and males, whereas obesity, stress, and a sedentary life-style are lesser contributors.[91]

Smoking. It is well known that the physiologic effect of smoking on blood flow is a decrease in both blood flow to the extremities and in skin temperature to the fingers and toes. In addition to this, smoking promotes atherosclerosis, and numerous other adverse effects have been noted.[19] Although the pathogenesis is unknown, atherosclerosis may be related to (1) carboxyhemoglobin, which can injure vessel walls, (2) altered platelet function with resultant thrombus formation, and (3) a decrease in prostacyclin, a prostaglandin that prevents platelet aggregation and promotes vasodilatation.[61]

Diabetes Mellitus. The longer a person has diabetes mellitus, the more likely he is to develop PVD.[61] Therefore a juvenile onset diabetic (type I) may acquire PVD at a younger age.

Patients with diabetes who smoke are severely jeopardizing arterial perfusion because of diabetes-associated PVD. In addition, Klemp and Staberg[50] report that the peripheral vasoconstriction effects of nicotine reduces absorption of insulin from subcutaneous tissue.

Diabetes mellitus is known to trigger an increase in the incidence of atherosclerosis though the exact initiating mechanism is not understood.[91] Good control of blood glucose levels may prevent, stabilize, or improve the microangiopathies (retinopathy, nephropathy, and neuropathy) but, according to several studies so far, preventing hyperglycemia does not seem to affect macrovascular atherosclerosis.[61]

Hyperlipidemia. Hyperlipidemia (hypercholesterolemia and hypertriglyceridemia) significantly affects atherogenesis. A serum cholesterol level greater than 220 mg per 100 ml is considered a sign of hyperlipidemia. Elevated triglyceride levels (over 180 mg/dl) should be evaluated and may also be indicative of hyperlipidemia. Furthermore, the ratio of total cholesterol to high-density lipoprotein (HDL) should be a ratio from 2.5 to 4.8.[56] Patients with hyperlipidemia require dietary restrictions of both fat and sugar. A dietician can advise a dietary regimen in concert with medical evaluation so that the patient's entire health history can be considered. Obesity and a sedentary life-style often coexist in the patient with hyperlipidemia. Maintaining ideal body weight through a combination of diet and regular exercise is known to modify cholesterol levels. The problem with diet therapy is, of course, patient acceptance and compliance. Although we are a nation that espouses healthy dietary habits, we eat "fat." The long-term effects of aggressive dietary programs on atherosclerosis and on survival of the disease itself needs evaluation.[21] Drug therapy may be used when dietary measures fail. Bile acid sequestrants and nicotinic acid have been used. All have side effects that must be managed and may limit compliance.[21]

Hypertension. Hypertension accelerates atherogenesis and increases the incidence of coronary heart disease and cerebrovascular disease. The pathogenesis is not clear but believed to be caused by (1) renin and other hypertensive agents inducing cellular changes in the arteries that contribute to atherosclerosis and (2) increased hemodynamic pressures resulting in injury to arteries, expecially at bifurcations.[91] Dietary, pharmacologic, and biofeedback therapies are current interventional measures.[104]

Summary. From an epidemiologic perspective genetic and environmental risk factors are associated with an increased incidence of atherosclerosis. The individual patient's condition, however, may vary from the group. Furthermore, there is no basis for comparison between risk factors and the severity or extent of atherosclerotic plaques.[91]

Signs and Symptoms of Peripheral Arterial Insufficiency

Peripheral arterial insufficiency of the lower extremity has distinct characteristics that are often sufficient to enable the nurse to distinguish arterial ulcers from venous or neuropathic ulcers based on noninvasive subjective and objective assessments. These characteristics are listed in Box 6-2.

Pain is the most common complaint of the patient with peripheral arterial insufficiency. The situations that produce pain—with exercise, at night, or while one is resting—are a guide to the severity of the patient's PVD.

Box 6-2   SIGNS AND SYMPTOMS OF ISCHEMIC LOWER EXTREMITY DISEASE

PAIN	Pallor on elevation
Exercise (intermittent claudication)	Dependent rubor
Nocturnal	
Rest	**ISCHEMIC SKIN CHANGES**
	Color
IMPAIRED CIRCULATION	Atrophy of subcutaneous tissue
Decreased pulses	Shiny, taut epidermis
Skin-temperature changes	Loss of hair
Delayed capillary and venous	
filling	**GANGRENE**

Intermittent pain or claudication (limping or lameness) is brought on by exercise and is promptly relieved when the exercise is stopped. Cramping, burning, and aching are descriptors used to qualify the sensations. Pain occurs when blood flow to the exercising muscles is unable to meet the increased metabolic demands. The location of the pain is important, since the restriction in blood flow is proximal to the painful area, and pain may occur in the thigh but most often involves the calf or foot (cramping). Pulses distal to the obstruction may be palpated if collateral circulation is developed. Since the muscle mass in the foot is small, the patient may not experience pain.

Most patients with intermittent claudication can be medically managed by cessation of smoking and a regular exercise program to promote development of collateral circulation. Surgical revascularization is reserved for those whose livelihood depends on maintaining activity.[47]

Nocturnal pain may also accompany PVD. As the patient sleeps, blood tends to perfuse the body's core rather than the extremities. Blood pressure drops, and the pressure head that fills the collateral circulation during the awake state is now reduced. Ischemic neuritis often awakens the patient. The patient finds that dangling his feet over the bed may perfuse the vessels by gravity or that getting up and moving around may elevate his blood pressure. The patient may end up sleeping in a chair or recliner to relieve pain only to induce edema secondary to a prolonged, dependent position. Edema further compromises tissue perfusion. Nocturnal pain usually precedes rest pain.[61]

Rest pain is an ominous sign because it indicates a reduction in blood flow below that required for normal tissue metabolism. Elevation, heat, and activity aggravate the pain because these activities increase metabolic demand. This patient is severely incapacitated and usually seeks medical assistance. If the patient with rest pain is not surgically treated, tissue necrosis, ulceration, and gangrene invariably occur.[47] When ischemia coexists with neuropathy, nocturnal and rest pain may not be experienced.

Impaired circulation can often be observed with a change in the quality of pulse. Therefore palpation of lower extremity pulses is a part of routine circulatory assessment. The four lower extremity pulses are usually palpable (femoral, popliteal, posterior tibial, and dorsalis pedis) and can be graded subjectively, according to the system shown in Box 6-3, or more simply as either present or absent.

The popliteal pulse is notoriously difficult to find because it lies deep in the popliteal space. To facilitate palpation the patient should lie down with slightly flexed knees; the

---

Box 6-3   GRADING OF PULSES AND EDEMA

Pulses		Edema		
0	Absent	0 to 1/4 inch	**1+**	(mild)
1+	Barely palpable	1/4 to 1/2	**2+**	(moderate)
2+	Palpable but diminished	1/2 to 1	**3+**	(severe)
3+	Normal			
4+	Prominent, suggestive of aneurysm			

From Hallett JW, Brewster DC, and Darling RC: Manual of patient care in vascular surgery, Boston, 1982, Little, Brown & Co, and Potter DA and Rose MB, editors: Cardiovascular system. In Assessment, Springhouse, Penn, 1983 Intermed Communications, Inc.

examiner then places his or her thumb on the patient's knee and reaches behind it with the first two fingers to feel the pulse.

The dorsalis pedis pulse is on the middorsum of the foot, between the first and second metarsals. Dorsiflexing the foot to 90 degrees will prevent traction on the artery, making this superficial pulse easier to feel.[88] The posterior tibial pulse is found in the groove behind the medial malleolus. A Doppler sensor is helpful in locating or amplifying a weak pulse.

Skin temperature should be evaluated when pulses are palpated by use of the back of the hand and fingers, since these locations are generally more sensitive.

Color (pallor) of the feet on elevation with delayed capillary and venous filling times also indicates ischemia. Ischemia can be evaluated by use of the following technique: with the patient in a supine position, raise the feet to a 45-degree angle until one or both feet blanch. The patient is then instructed to sit up and dangle his legs. The time necessary for the return of color to the extremities is measured and interpreted according to Box 6-4.[61] The extent of ischemia is then interpreted in relation to capillary filling times. Dependent rubor is the observed bluish red color, which is evidence of maximal arteriolar dilatation in the presence of perfusion.[28] A more cyanotic hue can ensue with advancing disease.

Ischemic skin changes can also be present in addition to the color changes cited above. There are several classic skin changes caused by arterial insufficiency. The epidermis is shiny, smooth, and thin and appears tautly stretched over atrophied subcutaneous tissue as exemplified in Plate 19. Atrophy occurs as a result of chronic malnourishment to tissues and muscle. Patients with diabetes may have yellowing of the toenails and fungal infections, which should be aggressively treated.[36] Loss of hair on the lower extremities and feet is another hallmark of arterial insufficiency, but this may occur with old age as well.

Gangrene can develop with tissue hypoxia or anoxia. "Dry gangrene" is the term used to describe black or brown necrotic tissue that eventually contracts into a withered hard mass.[18] This dead tissue may separate and autodebride. Infected necrotic tissue will become soft and boggy, and pus may appear or be palpated.[18] The patient may complain of exquisite tenderness or pain in the proximal, adjacent tissue.

Gangrene is frequently the unfortunate result of inadvertent trauma. Although borderline perfusion to the lower extremity may be sufficient to maintain normal metabolism, injury presents increased blood flow and oxygen demands that cannot be met. Thus trauma may result in gangrene in a previously viable limb. Imminent gangrene and gangrene are strong indicators for vascular surgery or possibly amputation. Referral to the vascular surgeon and, in the case of the patient with diabetes, to the diabetologist is urgent.

Assessment Parameters

The patient with an ischemic ulcer of the lower extremity needs careful evaluation so that appropriate management can be prescribed. Assessment involves the patient's history,

---

Box 6-4 CAPILLARY FILLING TIME ON DEPENDENCY			
Normal:	10-15 seconds	Severe ischemia:	25-40 seconds
Moderate ischemia:	15-25 seconds	Very severe ischemia:	40+ seconds

From Levin ME: The diabetic foot, pathophysiology, evaluation and treatment. In Levin ME and O'Neal LW, editors: The diabetic foot, ed, 4, St. Louis, 1988, Mosby–Year Book, Inc.

physical examination, and diagnostic tests, which may be invasive or noninvasive. Although the patient may have an acute, arterial, ischemic episode with its classic five *P* 's (pain, paresthesias, paralysis, pallor, and pulselessness[34]), the presence of an ulcer is suggestive of a chronic condition.

History. A guided interview is essential to obtain the history most pertinent to the pathogenesis of the ulcer. The patient may be able to accurately relate important symptoms. However, because living with a chronic disease often blunts the patient's discriminatory abilities, a guided interview will assist the patient to recall events or describe symptoms pertinent to arterial insufficiency (Box 6-2).

An accurate history relevant to assessment of the arterial ulcer should address several items as follows:
1. Length of time present ulcer has existed
2. Type of traumatic event initiating ulcer formation
3. Type of topical therapy used
4. History of diabetes, vascular examinations, or surgery
5. History of smoking
6. Presence of coexisting systemic conditions, such as anemia, sickle cell disease, arthritis, or venous insufficiency

The initial encounter with the patient is critical to establishing a positive, therapeutic relationship. Since ischemic ulcers can take months to heal, establishing trust is instrumental for successful patient outcomes.

Physical Examination. Physical examination involves a thorough inspection, palpation, and auscultation of both lower extremities. Ischemic changes of the lower extremity that can be inspected and palpated have been reviewed. Pulses should be assessed by palpation or, if necessary, auscultation with a Doppler unit. Auscultation of the lower extremity arteries is most informative in the femoral area where bruits or arteriovenous fistulas may be suspected.[34]

Ulcer characteristics of ischemic or arterial ulcers are quite distinct as described in Table 6-2. These ulcers are generally painful and may be accompanied by rest pain.

The *location* of arterial ulcers is most typically on the ankle area and feet, which are typical sites distal to the occlusive process. They may also be seen in areas subject to trauma (that is, dorsum of foot, shin, or toes).

The *size* and *depth* of an arterial ulcer are quite variable from the more common, small "punched-out"–appearing lesion to a larger, flatter size. Ischemic ulcer damage may be deep (stage III or IV), especially since there is very little subcutaneous tissue in the distal extremity. The presence of tendon, ligament, and bone should be carefully evaluated.

The *wound bed* in arterial ulcers is usually nonviable, gray yellow, and desiccated, though necrotic eschar is not uncommon. If the wound is clean, the wound bed may be pale pink because of a diminished blood supply.

As with all wounds, it is important to palpate and probe the wound bed and the walls of the wound to determine the presence of tunnels and sinus tracts. Spontaneous drainage of pus and cellular debris can result from a thorough exam. In addition, foreign objects (such as nails or tacks) may be present in the patient with diabetes mellitus. A sterile cotton-tipped applicator can be used to probe and expose these findings as shown in Plate 15.

Table 6-2 Arterial, Venous, and Neuropathic Ulcers of the Lower Extremities: a Comparison

	Arterial	Neuropathic (Diabetic)	Venous
Predisposing factors	Peripheral vascular disease (PVD) Diabetes Advanced age	Diabetic with peripheral neuropathy	Valve incompetence in perforating veins History of deep vein thrombophlebitis and thrombosis Previous history of ulcer Advanced age Obesity
Assessment	Thin, shiny, dry skin Loss of hair on ankle and foot Thickened toenails Pallor on elevation and dependent rubor Cyanosis Decreased temperature Absent or diminished pulses	Diminished or no sensation in foot Foot deformities Palpable pulses Warm foot If patient has coexisting PVD, same assessments as arterial	Firm ("brawny") edema Dilated superficial veins Dry, thin skin Evidence of healed ulcers Lipodermatosclerosis present
Location	Between toes or tips of toes Over phalangeal heads Around lateral malleolus Where subjected to trauma or rubbing of footwear	Plantar aspect of foot Over metatarsal heads Under heel	Medial aspect of lower leg and ankle May extend into malleolar area
Characteristics	Even wound margins Gangrene or necrosis Deep, pale wound bed Painful Cellulitis	Painless Even wound margins Deep Cellulitis or underlying osteomyelitis Granular tissue present unless coexisting PVD	Irregular wound margins Superficial (into dermis) Ruddy, granular tissue Usually painless Exudate usually present
Conservative treatment	Bedrest as feasible Treat any cellulitis Topical care (see Table 6-4) Patient education and support	Treat cellulitis Rule out osteomyelitis Metabolic diabetic control No weight bearing Contact casting Topical care (see Table 6-4) Orthotics Patient education and support	Elevate extremity as feasible Therapeutic vascular compression Topical care: absorption dressings and débridement, as indicated Patient education and support
Surgical treatment	Revascularization Angioplasty	Aggressive débridement Revascularization if coexisting PVD indicates it	Skin grafting

Palpation of the necrotic wound bed with a gloved finger or cotton-tipped applicator can provide information about the condition of the tissue beneath the necrotic tissue. When spongy or boggy tissue is palpated in the wound bed, liquefaction of necrotic tissue and infection should be suspected, and surgical débridement is advised.

Drainage from an arterial ulcer is minimal; some serous exudate may be present even though arterial ulcers bleed very little. If infection is present, pus may be expressed.

Surrounding epidermis must be carefully assessed with arterial ulcers. Normally, blood supply around a wound is increased with the inflammatory phase of wound healing. Generally, the tissues surrounding an arterial ulcer, however, show signs of ischemic disease: cool to the touch and a surrounding band of pale, blanched skin. Slight erythema and warmth may be present if the patient has the circulation necessary to mount an inflammatory response. The patient with diabetes, however, responds to inflammation in areas of marginal perfusion by developing vascular thrombosis and necrosis.[68]

Induration around the wound may be present, particularly in the presence of inflammation. Edema may or may not be present and should be evaluated as described in Box 6-3.

Diagnostic Tests. Although a good history and physical examination will usually provide an accurate indication of the state of vascular perfusion to the lower extremity, it is helpful to determine this in quantitative terms whenever possible. This is done both to corroborate the clinical impression and to provide a base-line value for future reference as to progression or improvement of the disease process. *Noninvasive* tests are the basic studies used and provide the clinical diagnostic information necessary to understand the patient's problem and to identify therapeutic options. *Invasive* tests should generally not be used for diagnosis and should be reserved for use by the vascular surgeon to determine anatomic landmarks and abnormalities once the decision to perform surgical intervention has been made.

Noninvasive Tests. *Segmental pressures* is a basic study done to assess arterial perfusion to both lower and upper extremities. It consists in taking the blood pressure at different levels in the arm or leg, or both. Because the Korotkov sounds heard when a stethoscope is used to determine blood pressure in the arm are not heard at most of these locations, an ultrasonic Doppler instrument is used to determine the systolic pressure over each of several arteries. The diastolic pressure cannot be determined with the Doppler probe.

A standard blood-pressure cuff is placed at the ankle just above the malleoli, and a Doppler signal is detected over the dorsalis pedis artery (Fig. 6-2 shows a typical setup for this test). The cuff is then inflated to a suprasystolic level and, as in any blood pressure measurement, slowly deflated until the return of the Doppler signal is detected. This is the systolic pressure. This procedure is repeated with the Doppler probe placed over the posterior tibial artery. Cuffs can also be placed at more proximal levels on the calf and thigh and pressures taken at these locations to help determine at what levels narrowing or occlusion is present. Pressure readings are repeated three times to ensure accuracy. The higher of the two pressures taken at the ankle is usually interpreted as the "ankle pressure."

Systolic pressures in the leg are normally about 10% higher than the brachial pressure. Pressures may be significantly higher in the thigh if the width of the cuff is too narrow; appropriate cuff width is at least 20% greater than the diameter of the extremity at that location. Special cuffs are available for the larger thigh. A pressure drop of 25 mm Hg between measurement levels is usually considered significant and indicates the presence of a narrowing of physiologic importance.

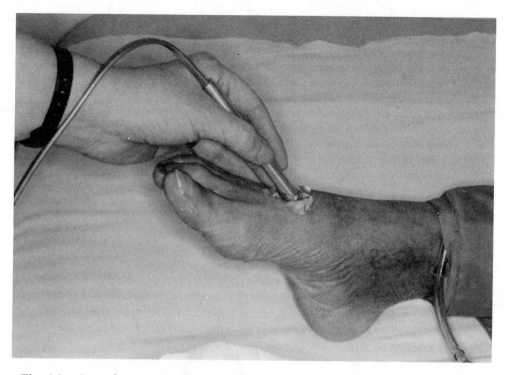

Fig. 6-2   Setup for measurement of ankle pressures. Cuff is placed around ankle above malleoli, with Doppler probe over dorsalis pedis artery in this instance.

Pressures are also commonly compared to pressures in the brachial arteries, which are used as a reference and are assumed to be normal. An "ankle/arm" or "ankle/brachial" index of 1.0 to 1.1 is considered normal, whereas levels below 0.9 indicate the presence of occlusive disease. Intermittent claudication generally occurs with indices of less than 0.8. Values less than 0.5 are frequently associated with rest pain or a threatened limb; one can expect that any ulcers present will be, at best, difficult to heal. In patients with ulcers who have indices in this range, revascularization may well be mandatory for the lesions to heal.

Measurement of *toe pressures* is necessary in some patients, most notably those patients with diabetes mellitus and patients with atherosclerosis because arteries in the calf can become calcified and stiff and are not compressible. The pressure cuff is not able to compress the artery to closing in these cases or can do so only at external pressures higher than the intraarterial pressure. The measured pressure reading in the cuff is therefore falsely elevated as compared with the true arterial pressure and is deceptive in that it makes the perfusion pressure appear better than it actually is. In these patients, incompressibility usually does not occur to so great a degree below the ankle; therefore pressures in the toes may be better indicators of perfusion than the pressures at the ankle.

Small cuffs are available for use on the toes, and systolic pressure can be determined by use of one of several instruments: the same ultrasonic Doppler probe as used in the segmental pressure measurements, a strain gauge, or a photoplethysmograph. These all generally work equally well, and whichever is most convenient can be used. The measurement is obtained in the same way as one obtains pressures at the other locations.

Pressures in the toes are normally about 60% of those in the brachial artery. Pressures in the range of 35 mm Hg are considered very low and are consistent with the presence of rest pain as well as being a good indication that healing of wounds or ulcers will either not occur or be prolonged.

Ultrasonic Doppler waveforms are used in patients with incompressible arteries. The waveform obtained from the ultrasonic Doppler probe may also serve as an indicator of the presence or absence of occlusive vascular disease and can give a semiquantitative appreciation of the severity of stenosis because it is not affected by calcified or noncompliant arteries.

To correctly perform this test, the ultrasonic Doppler instrument should have an output that can be recorded on a strip-chart recorder, though with a little practice one can easily differentiate between triphasic and monophasic waveforms using the ear alone. The Doppler probe is held at an angle of approximately 60 degrees to the skin to obtain a good signal, as should be done with any test using the Doppler instrument.

The normal Doppler waveform seen at the ankle is either triphasic as seen in Fig. 6-3 or biphasic with a sharp initial upslope. In the triphasic waveform there is a sharp initial upstroke followed by a downstroke that passes through zero and shows the reverse flow

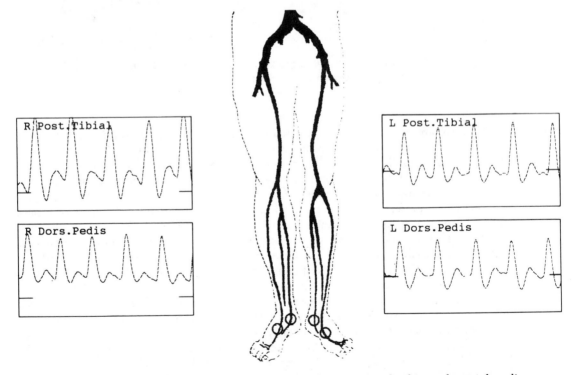

Fig. 6-3   Normal ultrasonic Doppler waveforms from a normal subject taken at dorsalis pedis (anterior tibial) and posterior tibial arteries. Signal is triphasic signal with a normal, narrow first phase of waveform.

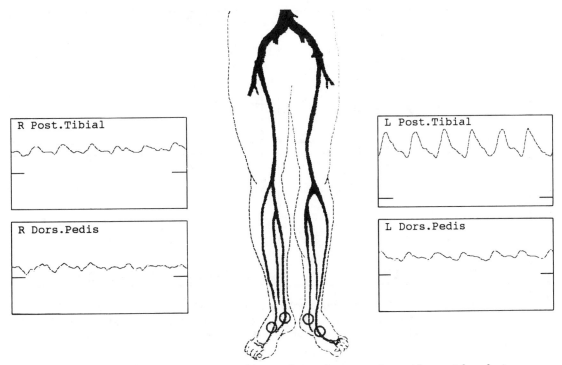

Fig. 6-4   Abnormal ultrasonic Doppler waveforms from a patient with arterial occlusive disease also taken at dorsalis pedis (anterior tibial) and posterior tibial arteries. Here the waveform is broadened with loss of negative second phase and positive third phase.

component, which occurs during early diastole in most subjects. The third phase of the triphasic waveform is the second positive waveform. As proximal narrowing increases, the waveform becomes damped and monophasic with a less sharp initial upslope and a broader duration with loss of the second and third phases. An example of a patient with severe proximal arterial disease is seen in Fig. 6-4. Although this waveform is not easily quantitated, it does give a good indication that relatively severe occlusive disease is present.

Pulse volume recording (PVR) is another commonly used, simple test of arterial sufficiency. Various commercially available instruments can be used. In this test, the moment-to-moment changes in the blood volume of an extremity are measured. A standard cuff is placed around the calf and inflated to 65 mm Hg where it is held. As blood enters the calf during the cardiac cycle, the volume of the calf changes causing transient small changes in the pressure in the cuff. These changes are recorded on a strip-chart recorder and represent changes in the blood volume of the limb with the different phases of the cardiac cycle. This is similar to the velocity waveform seen with the ultrasonic Doppler instrument except for not having the reverse flow as the second component. It is interpreted in a similar, semi-quantitative way. Fig. 6-5 shows both a normal tracing and one obtained from a patient with severe arterial disease. In the latter, the delayed, slow upstroke and the broadened prolonged waveform of arterial obstruction can be noted.

Transcutaneous oxygen tension is the actual measurement of the oxygen tension on the skin surface. The oxygen measured is that which has been delivered to the dermis by capil-

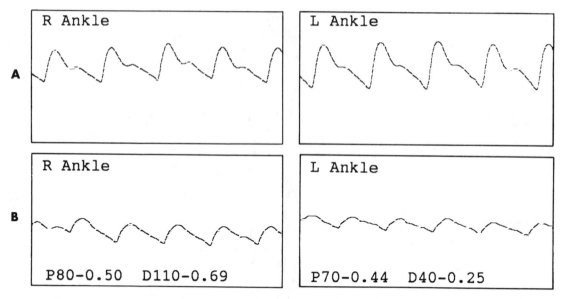

Fig. 6-5 Normal and abnormal pulse volume recorder (PVR) waveforms. **A,** In normal tracings the initial upslope is rapid and there is an anacrotic notch, whereas, **B,** in abnormal tracings taken from a patient with arterial occlusive disease, upslope is slower and notch is lost.

lary perfusion and has diffused through the nonvascular epidermis to the skin surface. Experience has shown that these levels do reflect perfusion to the skin and can be used to help determine the likelihood of a wound or ulcer healing.[107]

An oxygen-sensing electrode is attached to the skin in the area to be examined using double-sided adhesive tape. This is done both to secure the electrode to the skin and to prevent ambient air from leaking into the electrode and giving falsely elevated values. A heater is incorporated into the probe and is set to 44° Celsius. In some centers 45° C is used for a short time, frequently 10 minutes, but is then decreased to 44° C because a burn can result from prolonged exposure to 45° C. The heat stimulates capillary blood flow to the area. If heat is not used, the oxygen delivered by the blood flow is normally just enough to supply the tissue's nutritional needs and is consumed by the tissue, leaving little or none to diffuse to the skin surface for measurement. With heating, oxygen delivery far exceeds tissue requirements and most of the oxygen diffuses to the skin surface where it is measured. The several commercially available transcutaneous oxygen measurement systems are easy to use and the value is read directly from a digital readout or plotted on a strip-chart recorder.

Normal values for the transcutaneous oxygen levels are variable but are usually more than 40 mm Hg. Values less than 20 mm Hg have been shown to be associated with little or no healing and indicate the need for increased blood flow to the area. Values between 20 and 30 mm Hg fall into the gray area, and pressures of greater than 30 mm Hg are generally considered to indicate reasonable circulation. The user must be aware that transcutaneous oxygen levels are decreased in the presence of edema, and so low levels obtained when significant edema is present must be considered questionable. Edema should be treated and corrected and a repeat value obtained before the low value is used as a basis for any clinical decisions.

Invasive tests. *Angiography* is a procedure that involves visualization of parts of the vascular system after injection of radiopaque dye into the vessel of interest and taking cine-x-ray films to view the anatomy of the vessel in question. "Arteriography" is the name given to this procedure when arteries are being examined, and "venography" when applied to veins. This has been the standard for the evaluation of arterial and venous disease but has been overused as well. The information obtained is essentially anatomic data with only a minimum of physiologic data, but the study can complement the physiologic noninvasive studies discussed above. It does provide the map needed by vascular surgeons both in defining the extent of disease and possible options available for correction of the problem. Arteriography, however, can have complications and is not a totally benign procedure. Such problems as arterial perforation, intimal dissection, hematoma, and clotting can occur in the best of hands in a small percentage of cases and may require emergency surgical procedures to correct them. It is therefore generally believed that angiography should be performed only after the decision has been made to surgically approach the problem either with interventional radiology (such as balloon angioplasty) or surgical reconstruction. Because there is both morbidity and mortality associated with this invasive procedure, it should not be performed for diagnosis alone except in unusual circumstances.

The arteriogram is performed by insertion of a catheter into an artery, most commonly the femoral, brachial, or axillary, and advancement of the catheter to lie near or in the vessel or vessels of interest. The radiopaque dye is injected under high pressure using a power injector, and the cine-x-ray films are taken after injection at time intervals selected by the radiologist to best visualize the arteries in question. An example of an arteriogram of the lower aorta, iliac, and pelvic arteries is seen in Fig. 6-6.

In patients without extensive arterial occlusive disease this technique is adequate to visualize most arteries. However, with extensive or high-grade narrowing and very limited distal arterial blood flow, an adequate amount of dye may not get through the obstruction to visualize the distal vessels. This can be particularly true with diabetes; in patients with diabetes arterial occlusive disease commonly results in severe narrowing or occlusion of the three main arteries of the lower leg. To overcome this, some institutions are now using the "balloon inflow occlusion" technique. In this case, a balloon proximal to the end of the catheter is inflated so that it prevents blood from entering the artery to be examined. The dye is then injected through the distal end of the catheter and forced through the narrowed areas undiluted by inflowing blood. In good hands, excellent visualization of the distal arterial bed can be accomplished where it could not be with the standard technique. Although advocates of this method are highly enthusiastic, not everybody is in agreement. There are concerns related to inflation of a balloon in an artery with extensive atherosclerotic plaque and the potential for dislodgment of plaque with distal embolization.

Digital subtraction angiography involves taking a radiologic image both before and after an intervention and "subtracting" the first image from the second. Everything that remains the same between the two images is therefore removed, leaving an image of only the differences between the two films. The idea behind developing this technique was that, because of this image-enhancement capability, one would need a lesser concentration of contrast material, which would permit an intravenous injection rather than an intraarterial injection. Unfortunately its promise here has not come up to expectations, and most institutions have abandoned use of intravenous digital subtraction angiography.[95] The images obtained

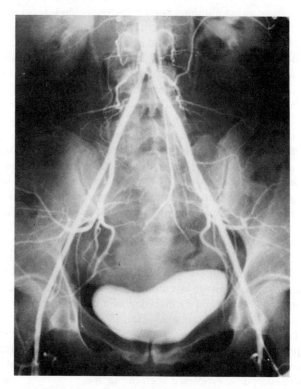

Fig. 6-6   Aortic injection contrast arteriogram of lower aorta, iliac, and pelvic arteries. There is narrowing at aortic bifurcation and proximal common iliac arteries.

have generally not been adequate and larger-than-desired doses of contrast material are required with the concomitant increased risk of renal toxicity. The equipment is also expensive and some hospitals are not equipped to perform digital subtraction procedures.

Because the standard dye contrast arteriogram discussed above uses intraarterial injection, digital subtraction can be a useful adjunct to this technique and is commonly used. The image of the preinjection film is subtracted from the image of the contrast film, which theoretically leaves only the image of the arteries filled with dye. This is generally true, but the images obtained are usually not as perfect as one would hope, and there are unanswered questions regarding arterial anatomy even with this technique. It is quite useful however in areas where many different layers of tissue and structures are superimposed in a normal arteriographic view. This is particularly valuable in looking at the carotid and intracerebral vascular systems as well as the arterial system in the extremities. An example of this technique is seen in Fig. 6-7, which is the result of subtraction derived from Fig. 6-6.

Management of Arterial Ulcers

Arterial ulcers often require months to heal, when wound closure is a reasonable goal. Close surveillance is essential, and the patient needs considerable education and encourage-

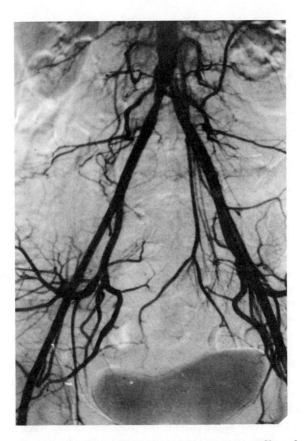

Fig. 6-7 Subtraction film made by subtracting the preinjection film of same area from image in Fig. 6-6. Arterial tree is seen in greater contrast than in Fig. 6-6, but one can see that other structures are not totally subtracted.

ment to comply with recommended life-style changes. Arterial ulcers present complex management problems because the patient usually has coexisting medical diseases; therefore collaboration of a multidisciplinary team is critical. Consultation with health care professionals such as those listed in Box 6-5 should be routine when one is managing arterial ulcers.

As with all wounds, the goals of a comprehensive management plan for arterial ulcers are to (1) reduce or eliminate the cause, (2) optimize the microenvironment, (3) support the host, and (4) provide education. In keeping with the multidisciplinary approach that is critical to arterial ulcer management, interventions are discussed as they pertain to the goals of therapy instead of by who performs the intervention.

Reduce or Eliminate the Cause. For the patient with PVD who acquires a lower extremity ulcer, improved circulation and perfusion are essential to healing. However, the likelihood that an ulcer will heal depends on (1) perfusion of the ulcer site (not necessarily the extent of the ulcer) and (2) the ability to regulate coexisting conditions that alter heal-

---

Box 6-5   MULTIDISCIPLINARY TEAM NECESSARY FOR ARTERIAL OR NEUROPATHIC ULCERS

Diabetes nurse specialist	Orthotist
Diabetologist	Podiatrist
Dietician	Physical therapist
ET (enterostomal therapy) nurse	Primary physician
Home care nurse	Interventional radiologist
Infectious disease specialist	Vascular surgeon
Orthopedist	Social service

---

ing. It may be wise to remember that healing is a process during which many factors interrelate and can change over time; for example, collateral circulation develops and edema can be regulated.

To reduce or eliminate the cause of arterial ulcers, one must enhance arterial perfusion by managing contributing factors or by administering pharmacotherapy, or by restoring perfusion through invasive procedures. Invasive procedures are the mainstay in arterial ulcer management.

Invasive procedures are used in an attempt to restore blood flow in the extremity. Attempts have been made to predict the potential for arterial ulcers to heal without surgical intervention. Although, historically, palpable pulses or the presence of runoff vessels on arteriography were used as predictive criteria,[110] today ankle and toe pressure measurements and perfusion scans have better predictive ability.[89,99] Vascular surgery may be required when blood flow is significantly compromised or conservative therapy fails.

It is difficult to state what patient populations should have revascularization surgery. Indicators that a revascularization procedure may not be necessary include brisk capillary refill, healthy-appearing lower extremity skin or ulcer, absence of rubor, and minimal delay in venous filling on dependency.[3] Rutherford[94] describes those patients who are not candidates:

1. Patients whose symptoms are not severe enough (that is, claudicators)
2. Patients who have experienced a very recent onset of symptoms so that the effect of collateral circulation cannot yet be assessed
3. Patients whose distribution of arterial problems is so peripheral that reconstruction would be impossible
4. Patients in whom reconstructive surgery has already been attempted but failed

Criteria for vascular surgery in the patient with diabetes are listed in Box 6-6. Unfortunately, vascular surgery for arterial insufficiency in the patient with diabetes is more difficult. First, involved arteries are usually the smaller tibial and peroneal vessels. Second, the vessels above and below the block may be abnormal. Finally, the collateral circulation may be involved. However, the presence of these conditions should not rule out a surgical procedure because repair of an obstruction may improve blood flow to distal vessels by increasing the head of pressure. Additionally, certain surgical techniques have proved effective with the smaller vessels below the knee.[61] Unfortunately, revascularization does not alter the pathogenesis of PVD for either patient populations, diabetic or nondiabetic.

Box 6-6   INDICATIONS FOR PERIPHERAL VASCULAR SURGERY IN THE DIABETIC

1. Nocturnal pain
2. Rest pain
3. Foot ulcers that do not respond to treatment
4. Infection that does not respond to treatment

5. Incipient gangrene
6. Severe disabling intermittent claudication (in select cases)

From Levin M: The diabetic foot: pathophysiology, evaluation, and treatment. In Levin ME and O'Neal LW, editors: The diabetic foot, ed 4, St. Louis, 1988, Mosby–Year Book, Inc.

Revascularization procedures for PVD are successful when the patient is judiciously evaluated, meticulous attention is given to technical details, and the appropriate operative procedure is chosen.[46] Optional techniques for revascularization include bypass procedures and angioplasty.

Bypass procedures are done to redirect arterial blood flow around the obstruction. The superficial femoral and popliteal arteries are the most common sites for obstruction in lower extremity PVD.[98]

Femorotibial or femoroperoneal bypass is generally indicated for rest pain, a persistent or progressing ischemic ulcer, and gangrene limited to toes and distal foot where major amputation would otherwise be certain.[3] The functional result should be a foot restored to optimal function with no more than débridement or minor amputation. The procedure involves using the patient's saphenous vein, removing it, and reversing it to align the one-way valves so that they do not obstruct the new arterial flow as shown in Fig. 6-8. Four conditions have been recognized as necessary for a successful bypass outcome: (1) unobstructed flow from the aortoiliac area to the site of proximal anastomosis, (2) a patent distal artery, (3) sufficient run-off capacity to maintain graft patency, and (4) a reliable graft.

Results of this revascularization procedure vary from 40% to 72% patency at 5 years.[3] Such variation reflects the differences in patients' conditions; patients with claudication alone have far better success than those patients with rest pain or arterial ulcers.

The in situ saphenous vein bypass technique was developed to avoid the risk inherent in removal of the vein from its normal physiologic environment before it is reimplanted in a reversed position. Leaving the vein in its normal alignment, or in situ, requires that the valves be defunctionalized so that arterial flow can progress unimpeded (Fig. 6-9). This is accomplished with valve cutters and special technique.[58] Since the vein is left in its normal tapered position, the distal anastomosis results in easier matching of two smaller vessels and in better patency than if the vein is reversed.

Results of a prospective, randomized comparison of the reversed technique and the in situ technique for limb salvage showed such a clear advantage to patency for the in situ group that the study was discontinued.[8] However, sentiment currently remains even for both types of bypass procedures.

Percutaneous transluminal angioplasty (PTA) is a nonoperative treatment option for patients with localized occlusions or patients with more extensive disease who are poor surgical candidates. A balloon catheter is passed, under fluoroscopy, into the artery, and the

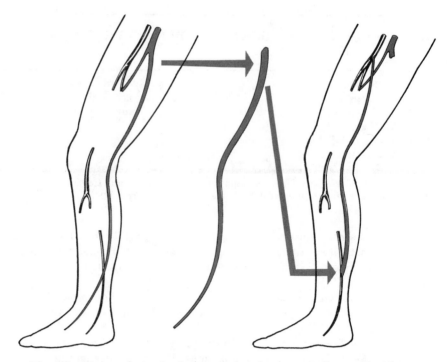

Fig. 6-8   Revascularization by reversed saphenous vein femorotibial bypass

balloon is inflated to shear or split the plaque lining the artery. Since the vessel lining is disrupted, platelets accumulate and antiplatelet aggregating agents are prescribed for several months after the procedure. Close follow-up observation with noninvasive vascular testing is necessary to monitor for any recurrence of the stenosis.[55]

Angioplasty is a technically demanding procedure and results are dependent on the skill of the angiographer.[55] This notwithstanding, results are best in larger vessels with short stenoses, less than 5 cm.[55] Patency rates decline in more distal vessels.[85] This procedure is difficult in patients who have diabetes and have diffuse disease of popliteal arterial branches (tibial and peroneal), but it has been used for limb salvage. Comparison with in situ bypass grafting needs to be done.[85] Even with small vessel disease associated with diabetes, angioplasty in the more proximal vessels can improve the pressure head to the more distal arteries.[85]

Laser thermal angioplasty is an experimental intervention designed to remove atherosclerotic plaque by heat vaporization, similar to PTA. Laser angioplasty has been attempted because of the rate of recurrent stenoses after PTA and in cases of total arterial obstruction.[23]

Lumbar sympathectomy has been employed historically in an attempt to increase the normal, resting blood flow to the lower extremity. However, in the group of patients who may benefit, more conservative measures have shown improvement.[97] In addition, many patients with diabetes already have an autosympathectomy secondary to their autonomic neuropathy and still experience foot ulcers. Today, lumbar sympathectomy is of little value in patients with diabetes and limb-threatening ischemia.[93,97,98]

Pharmacotherapy agents (vasodilators, a rheologic agent, anticoagulants, and anti-

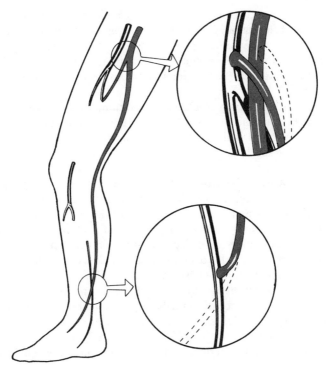

Fig. 6-9   Revascularization by in situ saphenous vein femorotibial bypass

platelet drugs) have been used in an attempt to improve tissue perfusion.

Vasodilators are a group of drugs believed to be effective at enhancing blood flow in patients' PVD. However, in a study by Coffman[14] this group of drugs proved to be of little if any benefit to the patient with PVD. He concluded that no known agent would selectively dilate arteries in exercising muscle or ischemic tissue. Other physiologic considerations against the use of these drugs in the patient with PVD are (1) the lack of response in rigid, atherosclerotic arteries, (2) a reduction in blood pressure, which can further diminish blood flow to ischemic tissues, (3) induction of the steal effect where healthy vessels do dilate and divert blood from already ischemic areas, and (4) possible autonomic peripheral neuropathy in the diabetic having already accomplished maximal arterial dilatation.[2,23,61]

The rationale for use of vasodilators is based on two unsubstantiated theories: (1) vasospasm occurs in ischemic extremities and (2) the drug helps to develop collateral circulation.[2] In fact, none of the vasodilators are approved for use in PVD by the Food and Drug Administration (FDA).

As a *rheologic agent,* pentoxifylline (Trental) has three actions that facilitate microcirculation by reducing blood viscosity: (1) increased red blood cell flexibility, (2) decreased platelet aggregation by stimulating production of prostacyclin, a powerful vasodilator and most potent known inhibitor of platelet aggregation, and (3) ability to increase deformation of white blood cells.[87] It is currently the only drug approved by the FDA for the treatment of intermittent claudication in the U.S.

Anticoagulants are rarely indicated in the treatment of atherosclerotic disease including chronic, lower extremity ischemia.[23,63]

Antiplatelet drugs are also used to alter platelet function. Platelet adhesion and aggregation are part of the pathogenesis of atherosclerosis. Therefore the use of antiplatelet drugs such as aspirin, dipyridamole (Persantine), and nonsteroidal antiinflammatory agents might mitigate the development of atheromatous plaques or thrombi. Diabetes affects platelet function, and this effect may be critical in the pathogenesis of vascular lesions and microthrombi.[61]

Clinical trials are being conducted to examine the effect of different specific drugs, such as prostacyclin, on atheromatous lesions.[22] Prostacyclin is produced by the endothelial surface of the vessel and is the most potent known inhibitor of platelet aggregation as well as being a potent vasodilator.

Optimize Wound Environment. Often the progress with which an arterial ulcer heals is attributed to the wound dressing's ability to achieve an optimal microenvironment. In fact, topical therapy may rivet the attention of the nurse and patient. However, it is important to put topical therapy and the microenvironment into perspective.

Successful local ulcer care depends, first, on recognizing the cause and pathogenesis of the lesion. For example, a neuropathic ulcer on the plantar surface of the foot of a patient with diabetes is not of ischemic origin. Second, an understanding of the patient's entire medical condition is crucial. And third, an assessment of the patient's self-care potential and the presence of contributing risk factors will afford the most beneficial and realistic plan of care. Well-known impediments to wound repair such as infection, pooled exudate, and necrotic tissue must be eradicated. To create an optimal microenvironment, topical therapy should then be selected to create a favorable environment for cellular repair (Table 6-3).

Débridement. "A little neglect may breed mischief" and "fools rush in where angels fear to tread" (Benjamin Franklin and Alexander Pope) should serve as caveats to the practitioner. Recommendation for débridement involves two dilemmas: when and how much. In an extremity with an adequate vascular supply, ridding the ulcer of necrotic debris will hasten healing. Although autolysis can achieve this assistance in the form of conservative therapy, sharp instrumental débridement lessens the patient's energy expenditure. Chemical debriding agents are frequently used, and insurers will reimburse for these medications. Unfortunately, chemical debriders may elicit sensitivity reactions with resultant hyperemia, and tissue necrosis may occur if blood supply is already marginal. However, many clinicians find autolysis or sharp débridement more effective and much faster than chemical debriding agents.[1,61,82]

Débridement is contraindicated in the presence of dry gangrene or a stable, dry, ischemic wound until vascular status is evaluated. Removal of eschar results in an open wound, which could easily become infected when the blood supply is diminished. Once the vascular supply is reestablished, the necrotic portion may demarcate and self-amputate with less tissue loss than if debrided. Otherwise appropriate amputation procedures can be performed.[80] Of course, the possibility of infection exists at any time, and the patient with dry gangrene must be closely monitored.

Eradicate infection. As described in Chapter 2, although all ulcers are contaminated, most are not infected. Wound infection is a multifactorial event where ultimately the pathogens' numbers overwhelm the host's ability to conquer them. When examination of the ulcer and the tissue surrounding the ulcer area reveals cellulitis (inflammation, warmth, and edema) or lymphangitis, a culture should be obtained; results will direct appropriate

Table 6-3 Topical dressing* algorithm for ischemic ulcers

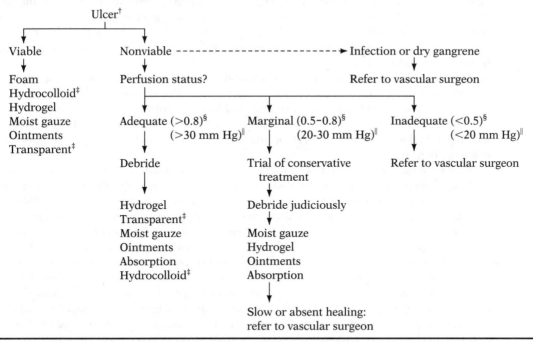

*Dressing selection is based on assessment of all wound parameters; therefore, not all options listed will be appropriate for each ulcer in the category. Options listed are not intended to be an exhaustive listing.
†Wound bed assessed after thorough cleansing.
‡Must consider bacterial flora and circulation changes in the diabetic.
§Segmental pressure: ankle/brachial index.
‖Transcutaneous oxygen tension.

systemic antibiotic therapy. However, it is important to remember that both local and systemic symptoms (fever, pain, and leukocytosis) of an infection may be absent in the patient with diabetes.

Infection must be promptly eradicated because bacteria compete with the host for the limited supply of oxygen and nutrients and thereby impair wound healing.[42] The role of oxygen in proper leukocyte phagocytosis is well established.[36,43] Furthermore, poorly perfused tissues appear to become infected more often than adequately perfused tissues.[68,108] In addition, the thickened capillary basement membrane that occurs in diabetes and with aging becomes a barrier for diffusion of oxygen to tissue.[100] Finally, since delivery of oxygen to the wound is dependent on adequate blood flow, the patient with PVD or diabetes mellitus is at particular risk for tissue hypoxia.

Cultures are indicated for any draining ischemic ulcer. Both aerobic and anaerobic cultures, as well as Gram's stain findings, should be obtained. Optimal microbiologic technique for obtaining anaerobic cultures as described by Louie[69] involves (1) a vigorous saline scrub, (2) débridement of superficial exudate using sterile instruments, and (3) scraping the ulcer base or the deep portion of the wound edge with a sterile curette. When curettage, surface swabs, and needle aspiration methods of obtaining cultures were compared in diabetic foot lesions,[96] none of the collection methods showed perfect agreement with the surgical specimen. However, curettage showed the best correspondence, and surface swabs were the least reliable. Additionally, needle aspiration from the ulcer is probably the best nonsurgical method of obtaining a deep culture specimen though the numbers of organisms may be underestimated.

Osteomyelitis is a concern when an ulcer lies over a bony prominence, especially a chronic ulcer in the foot of a patient with diabetes and PVD. In one study[106] approximately one third of 247 patients with osteomyelitis had diabetes with the osteomyelitis described as a bone infection associated with vascular insufficiency. Chronic ulcers become populated with bacteria that, with time, neglect, or improper care, can invade soft tissues and fascia to reach the bone.

Conventional radiography is a cost effective way to evaluate osteomyelitis, but neither clinical, radiographic, or radionuclide studies can consistently distinguish between osteomyelitis and the bony destruction that occurs in severe peripheral neuropathy.[30] When the skin is intact over a bony lesion, the bone destruction observed is more likely attributable to diabetic osteopathy than to osteomyelitis.[35] Radionuclide studies (bone scans), computerized tomography (CT scan), and magnetic resonance imaging (MRI) have their own strengths in further refining a diagnosis of osteomyelitis with diabetes.[35]

Sugerman and others[101] prospectively evaluated 28 pressure ulcers (extended to or beneath subcutaneous tissue) in spinal cord–injured patients that did not respond to 2 weeks of local therapy. As a result they suggest obtaining a bone scan alone or in addition to a radiologic exam; negative scans and x-ray films indicated osteomyelitis to be unlikely. If either or both tests are abnormal, however, further study is recommended; a bone biopsy with histologic examination of bone is suggested. The histology sample would correct for any infection or contamination resulting from passing the biopsy needle through soft tissue.

Topical antibacterials are of questionable efficacy in wound care. Different practice patterns persist, but many clinicians question the efficacy of topical antibacterials. In a predominantly granular wound they are unnecessary, since the inflammatory response has already succeeded in producing a clean wound. In a predominantly necrotic wound antibacterials will not penetrate the dead tissue present. Removal of dead tissue is most important in controlling bacteria. Furthermore, topical antibacterials can elicit sensitivity reactions in ischemic skin thereby raising demand for blood in compromised tissue.[66] If infection is suspected and confirmed, oral or parenteral antibiotics are indicated depending on perfusion status of the ulcer area. Topical medications (creams and ointments) that contain steroids and anesthetic agents are contraindicated because they trigger vasoconstriction.[44]

Finally, it should be remembered that the only topical antibacterial with the ability to penetrate avascular tissue is mafenide acetate (Sulfamylon Cream). However, its use in burn therapy, where infection is an ever-present threat, should not be compared to the isolated, ischemic ulcer.

Topical dressings require judicious use in the management of ischemic ulcers as outlined in Table 6-3. Dressings should be selected based on moist wound–healing principles, the severity of the ischemia, and the underlying pathologic reason for ischemia. In general, occlusive dressings should be used with caution. With occlusion, bacteria and small vessel disease can combine to produce cellulitis, particularly in the patient with diabetes.

When the ulcer base is predominantly nonviable, the perfusion status must be ascertained. Suspected inadequate perfusion, infection, or dry gangrene warrant a referral to a vascular surgeon. When vascular studies indicate that perfusion is marginal, a trial of conservative therapy may be instituted. In this case, débridement is essential to create an optimal wound-healing environment.[44] The nurse is often in the position to provide education and advocacy for what many clinicians describe as "aggressive" débridement. Dressings should be selected to facilitate the débridement process and must be monitored closely (weekly if not more often).

To prevent the creation of a new wound around an arterial ulcer, special attention should be given to the integrity of the surrounding epidermis. Topical therapies that may potentially macerate fragile epidermis should be avoided. Similarly, adhesives may be contraindicated because of their potential to strip the epidermis.

Growth factors have been used to stimulate wound repair. Derived from the patient's blood, growth factors interact with cells at the ulcer site through a chemotactic or mitogenic effect.[53] However, growth factors are not effective in the presence of ischemia or necrotic tissue. Topical application of growth factors for wound repair is discussed in more detail in Chapter 10.

Regular, systematic (bimonthly to monthly) evaluation of the ulcer is essential. Photographs can assist in monitoring progress or the lack thereof. Topical therapy should reflect the changes that occur in the ulcer. If the healing curve regresses or plateaus, careful scrutiny of contributory factors (edema, osteomyelitis, cellulitis, bacterial overload, or changes in perfusion) should ensue before therapy is changed. Because wounds are dynamic, no one type of topical dressing will be appropriate from onset of the ulcer to closure.

Support the Host. To support the patient with an arterial ulcer, it is important to support nutrition, control edema, and regulate diabetes (if present). Risk factors should be monitored and reduced or eliminated.

Nutrition needs vary widely between patients with arterial ulcers. Because these patients often have concurrent cardiovascular disease or diabetes mellitus, nutritional needs are complex and may be confusing to the patient. Nutritional needs should be based on a medical evaluation and a consideration of the patient's entire health history as discussed in Chapter 9. Dietary recommendations should be practical to enhance compliance. Frequent follow-up observation with the dietician is indicated not only to monitor the ability of the patient to incorporate the dietary recommendations, but also for support and encouragement.

Control of edema is essential to facilitate wound healing. Edema will intrinsically increase pressure on the vessels and therefore increase the diffusion distance for nutrients.

Dependent edema often develops as a consequence of keeping the legs in a dependent position to control pain. Other potential causes of edema (such as renal disease, hypoalbuminemia) should be investigated.

Patients should be instructed to (1) avoid sitting postures that put pressure on the popliteal vessels; (2) avoid crossing the legs; (3) discard, alter, or replace tight clothing and footwear; and (4) elevate feet periodically throughout the day but never above heart level. Compressive therapy is generally contraindicated in an ischemic extremity; however, when elevation is not possible or realistic, below-the-knee therapeutic support stockings should be prescribed in consultation with the patient's physician. In general, compressive stockings that provide safe support range from 18 to 30 mm Hg.

Regulation of diabetes has been demonstrated to be essential because hyperglycemia and ketosis may impair leukocyte function, particularly phagocytosis and chemotaxis.[73]

However, there is little convincing evidence to support that patients with diabetes are more susceptible to infection, have impaired immunologic competence, and experience an increased growth rate of common bacterial pathogens because of hyperglycemia.[68] Clinicians do, however, agree that good metabolic control is essential to sound medical management especially in any illness or stress state.

Control of contributing factors such as smoking, hypertension, and incidental trauma should be attempted. Some of these risk factors require behavioral modifications, and although support and encouragement can be offered, responsibility rests with the patient.

The patient's awareness of traumatic events should be heightened. Although tissue can die spontaneously from hypoxia, more often the ulcer is precipitated by some type of traumatic event: thermal, mechanical or chemical. All three have a common pathogenesis: increased metabolic demand from the injury cannot be met by the patient's limited vascular supply and tissue dies. The potential for such injuries to continue or recur must be eliminated for wound repair to ensue.

Provide Education. Medical and surgical therapies that restore the blood supply are crucial if the arterial ulcer is to heal. However, because many factors are known to contribute to ischemia, the patient must also understand what actions and life-style changes he can control and self-administer. Patient, family, and staff education is essential to maximize healing potential and minimize recurrences. In addition, education is needed regarding traumatic events that can precipitate ulcer formation. Nurses are in a position in which they can and must provide this information.

Environmental issues that might interfere with maximum blood flow should be brought to the patient's attention. The ischemic lower extremity that has difficulty delivering sufficient blood flow during resting, nonstress situations is particularly vulnerable. Constrictive clothing such as socks must be eliminated from the wardrobe.

To minimize further vasoconstriction, cold temperatures should be avoided. The patient's room should be kept warm. Cotton or wool socks should be used to warm cold feet, and heating devices or topical hot liquids should be assiduously avoided.

Positioning the bed in reverse Trendelenburg with the head of the bed on 6- to 8-inch blocks may facilitate distal blood flow and allow the patient to lie in bed at night. Many patients habitually sleep in chairs because the resulting dependent position for their legs relieves pain. Chronic pedal dependency can lead to edema formation, which further aggravates PVD; the increased pressure in the tissues occludes arterioles and increases the diffusion distance for nutrients. If the weight of bed linens creates discomfort, a bed cradle can be used.

Risk-factor control (blood pressure, glucose, smoking, and hyperlipidemia) must be understood by the patient and perceived as a priority so that the necessary life-style changes become a reality. The patient with an ischemic ulcer who smokes must be advised that he is courting potential disaster; if that patient happens to have diabetes, disaster may be imminent. Sound medical management is imperative to prevent hyperglycemia and ketosis. The health education literature is replete with education and life-style programs that focus on smoking cessation and relaxation.

Exercise and *activity* should be curtailed if an ischemic ulcer is to receive maximum perfusion. Although bedrest provides maximum perfusion to an ischemic lower extremity, it is usually not realistic or in one's best interest for general health. The severity of the patient's

PVD and ischemic ulcer must be assessed with regard to the patient's overall health. Recommendations for activity limitations are often warranted and are quite subjective.

Trauma must be avoided, and the patient must be taught to recognize potential sources of trauma. For example, fissures between the toes can develop primarily as a result of moisture entrapment and friction; lamb's wool or gauze woven between the digits may diminish these problems. Bony deformities may require surgical evaluation if severe. The diabetes literature outlines appropriate care of the feet; this information also applies to the nondiabetic patient with PVD (Box 6-7).

Ultimately, the patient with lower extremity ischemia needs to understand that there is no cure for PVD, that PVD is a progressive disease, and that treatment aims at control, not cure. The patient's active participation in self-care is crucial. Unfortunately, even with high compliance, the patient may not see the benefits of his efforts and may not be able to prevent problems.

Probably the major impediments for a patient trying to manage PVD are issues of chronicity. The long-term nature of the disease, slow treatment progress, and dependency on others are situations that must be borne day after day after day. Necessary treatment may make the patient dependent on others; even to the extent that he may need to leave his home environment. Financial limits may be readily exceeded by hospitalizations, outpatient monitoring, topical therapies, and orthotics. The nurse must help the patient chose a path through his maze of personal variables, often altering the best treatment plan for the more realistic or financially feasible one.

Summary

The patient with an ischemic ulcer of the lower extremity presents a challenge to the entire health care team. Sound knowledge of the pathophysiology of PVD and the pathogenesis of the ulcer is essential before one begins appropriate therapy. Armed with this knowledge, the nurse must be able to discriminate and prioritize the physical and psychosocial aspects of each patient's situation even as they change over the often lengthy course of treatment.

Box 6-7 SKIN CARE PROTOCOL FOR THE LOWER EXTREMITY WITH ARTERIAL INSUFFICIENCY

Wash daily with mild soap and rinse thoroughly.

Moisturize after bathing and, as necessary, with a nonirritating agent such as lanolin, petrolatum (Vaseline), and Eucerin (xipamide with water). Avoid agents with fragrance or other sensitizing agents.

Do not use moisturizers between toes.

Inspect skin daily and report any lesions to the health care team. Corns and calluses are the result of friction and pressure from footwear and are precursors of potential ulceration.

File calluses daily to prevent thickening and cracking. This prevents infection and reduces pressure on underlying subcutaneous tissue.

Wear supportive shoes that fit properly with cotton or wool socks because these wick away moisture.

Seek care from a podiatrist if toenails, corns, or calluses are thick, if vision is poor, or if patient can't perform safe care.

PERIPHERAL NEUROPATHY

Pathogenesis

Peripheral neuropathy can accompany diseases such as diabetes mellitus and Hanson's disease. Diabetic peripheral neuropathy will be the focus of this discussion. The cause of diabetic peripheral neuropathy is unknown but probably multifactorial. Ischemic injury to nerves and hyperglycemia have been implicated.[32] Diabetic peripheral neuropathy tends to be bilateral and symmetric. Patients complain of pain, paresthesias, and, paradoxically, diminished or absent ability to feel pain and temperature. Neuropathic pain, however, must be distinguished from ischemic pain and can be determined when the patient is asked if the pain is relieved by walking; neuropathy is the presumed cause when pain is relieved by ambulation.[61] The neuropathic foot is often termed the "insensate foot."

Types

Three types of neuropathy occur: sensory, motor, and autonomic. These can occur in isolation or together.

Sensory neuropathic changes are by far the most disastrous because the loss of sensation puts the patient at risk for mechanical, chemical, and thermal trauma. These are the unfortunate and preventable instances of stepping on nails, using a heating pad to warm cold feet, or using chemical callus and corn removers. As mentioned previously, the extremity with PVD can maintain a resting blood flow, but when presented with an increased demand, the system cannot respond and tissue malnourishment, or even death, occurs. Levin[62] provides the following cogent scenario:

At an ambient foot temperature of 70° F, a patient requires one milliter of blood flow per 100 grams of tissue per minute. A patient with even moderate PVD can manage this. Soaking the foot in hot water can quickly raise the skin temperature to 104° F. This requires an increase of 10 times the flow of blood. A patient with PVD cannot achieve this. The results: blistering, ulceration, infection and/or gangrene, and, not infrequently, amputation.

Motor neuropathy results in muscular atrophy in the foot and creates two basic problems. Foot deformities such as cocked-up toes, or hammertoes, develop and the patient's gait changes. These gait changes cause repetitive stresses on areas of the foot, usually a metatarsal head, rather than distributing the stresses of walking more uniformly. Callus buildup is the first sign of repetitive stress and will progress to ulceration if the weight is not properly redistributed with special shoes (orthotics).[15] These ulcers are sometimes referred to as neuropathic, neurotrophic, trophic, perforating, or malperforans ulcers (Plates 20 and 21).

Autonomic neuropathy is the third category of peripheral neuropathy. A principal symptom is distal anhydrosis, the absence of sweating. Anhydrosis results in xerosis (dry skin) and predisposes the patient to develop cracks and fissures. A chronically dry or moist interdigital environment on the foot favors selective bacterial or fungal flora (Plate 22). These bacteria or fungi that gain entry to soft tissues through the cracks and fissures penetrate further into the soft plantar tissues with repetitive stresses of ambulation and may cause infection, gangrene, and even ultimately amputation.

Management

When one is managing ulcers on the lower extremity, it is essential that the nurse be able to distinguish between ulcers caused by trauma in the patient with peripheral neuropathy and those caused by arterial insufficiency (Table 6-2). Furthermore, the nurse should understand the impact that peripheral neuropathy has on PVD. According to Levin,[60] three times more patients with diabetes are admitted to a hospital for foot ulcers caused by an insensitive, neuropathic foot than patients admitted because of ischemic pain.

The ulcer of neuropathic origin may be in a well-perfused extremity; but if PVD coexists, the diminished blood supply prevents oxygen and antibiotics from reaching the ulcer, which retards or prevents healing. In summary, the signs and symptoms of ischemia must be differentiated from peripheral neuropathy caused by diabetes. However, the nurse must keep in mind that it is entirely possible for the patient to have a combination of both PVD and neuropathy.

Trauma from chemical, thermal, and mechanical sources must be avoided when the patient has neuropathy because this insensate state is frequently seen with diabetes mellitus, a disease known to impair wound repair. Box 6-8, patient instructions for care of the diabetic foot, provides an excellent guide to enhance recognition of common sources of trauma and hence facilitate prevention.

Avoidance of trauma when the patient has arterial insufficiency is not difficult because the pain in the extremity serves as a reminder to be cautious. However, in the presence of peripheral neuropathy, ischemic tissues may not always be painful. The hospitalized patient with neuropathy serves as an excellent example. A patient with diabetes and coexisting peripheral neuropathy who finds himself in bed, in surgery, or otherwise supine for a period of time (recuperating from an illness) will not sense the discomfort of pressure-induced ischemia to his heels and hence the need for a position change. If PVD is also present, tissue damage can be swift and limb threatening.

Providing complete pressure relief by elevating heels entirely off the mattress is essential. Care should be taken to avoid elevating the heels too high for such a position would compromise blood flow. Furthermore, it should be reinforced that heel protectors do not reduce pressure. Finally, operating room staff and radiology staff should be alerted to the role they play in preventing trauma so that they may position and transfer the patient safely.

The neuropathic extremity is also more vulnerable to trauma because neuropathy makes temperature sensation difficult, if not impossible. Although the patient with arterial insufficiency may complain of cold legs or feet, the patient with neuropathy may not feel temperature changes. Patients with diabetes should never use hot-water bottles, heating pads, or foot soaks to "warm up" the feet; warmth increases the demand for blood. If neuropathy is present with arterial insufficiency and this increased demand for blood cannot be met, tissue injury results.

Orthotics are indicated to prevent mechanical trauma from shear and repetitive stress to the foot. As neuropathic bone and muscle changes develop and callous tissue forms, the foot becomes increasingly vulnerable to ulcerations. Orthotics are specially fit shoes that are intended to redistribute the weight of the foot, thus preventing traumatic ulcerations.[15,60]

Total contact casting is a temporary intervention that redistributes the weight of the foot and increases the surface area of contact[16] when an ulcer is present. Originally the contact cast was used for the insensate foot in patients with Hansen's disease (leprosy).[16] Unfortunately, the insensate foot lacks the sensory signals that prompt the person to shift gait patterns, remove a rock from the shoe, or rest. Consequently, ulcers largely the result of repetitive stress and shear develop on the plantar or dorsal surface of the foot. Because the contact cast reduces the pressure of walking to an insignificant amount,[16,37] it can be applied when the patient already has a plantar ulcer.

Box 6-8 PATIENT INSTRUCTIONS FOR CARE OF THE DIABETIC FOOT

1. Do not smoke.
2. Inspect the feet daily for blisters, cuts, and scratches. A mirror can aid in seeing the bottom of the feet. Always check between the toes.
3. Wash feet daily. Dry them carefully, especially between the toes.
4. Avoid temperature extremes. Test water with elbow before bathing.
5. If feet feel cold at night, wear socks. Do not apply hot water bottles or heating pads. Do not soak feet in hot water.
6. Do not walk on hot surfaces such as sandy beaches or on the cement around swimming pools.
7. Do not walk barefooted.
8. Do not use chemical agents to remove corns and calluses. Do not use corn plasters. Do not use strong antiseptic solutions on the feet.
9. Do not use adhesive tape on the feet.
10. Inspect the inside of shoes daily for foreign objects, nail points, torn linings, and rough areas.
11. If your vision is impaired, have a family member inspect your feet daily, trim the nails, and buff down calluses.
12. Do not soak feet.
13. For dry feet, use a very thin coat of lubricating oil such as baby oil. Apply the oil after bathing and drying the feet. Do not put oil or cream between the toes. Consult your physician for detailed instructions.
14. Wear properly fitting stockings. Do not wear mended stockings. Avoid stockings with seams. Change stockings daily.
15. Do not wear garters.
16. Shoes should be comfortable at the time of purchase. Do not depend on shoes to stretch out. Shoes should be made of leather. Running shoes may be worn after you check with your physician.
17. Do not wear shoes without stockings.
18. Do not wear sandals with thongs between the toes.
19. In winter take special precautions. Wear wool socks and protective footgear, such as fleece-lined boots.
20. Cut nails straight across.
21. Do not cut corns and calluses. Follow special instructions from your physician or podiatrist.
22. Avoid crossing your legs. This can cause pressure on the nerves and blood vessels.
23. See your physician regularly and be sure that your feet are examined at each visit.
24. Notify your physician or podiatrist at once if you develop a blister or sore on your feet.
25. Be sure to inform your podiatrist that you are a diabetic.

From Levin ME: The diabetic foot: pathophysiology, evaluation and treatment. In Levin ME and O'Neal LW, editors: The diabetic foot, ed 4, St. Louis, 1988, Mosby–Year Book, Inc.

To apply the cast, one should debride the ulcer, remove any callous tissue, and let the edema resolve. Contact casting is contraindicated in the presence of cellulitis, sinus tracts, or profuse drainage.[16,37]

With the patient in a prone position and the leg bent so that the foot is in the air, the cast material is wrapped carefully around the leg. Application begins at the toes, encloses the toes, and continues up the foot and leg to the knee. Wrapping should be loose and without wrinkles. Loose application allows the plaster to be molded over prominences and into uneven skin surfaces. Once applied and as the cast is drying, the plaster is massaged to enhance conformance of it to the shape of the extremity. To prevent the soiling of clothing from the plaster as it dries, self-adherent tape can be applied to the surface of the cast once it is in place.

Contact casts are left on for 3 to 7 days depending on the amount of drainage from the wound. Patients can walk with the cast in place, once it dries, approximately 24 hours.

A nonadherent dressing and topical antiseptics have been used to cover the wound in preparation for the cast.[16] To prevent interdigital maceration, cotton padding or lamb's wool is applied between the toes.

Summary

Peripheral neuropathy places the patient at risk for ulceration attributable to mechanical, thermal, or chemical trauma. Management of ulcers in the neuropathic or insensate foot has many similarities to the management of ulcers on the extremity with arterial insufficiency. However, the neuropathic foot also has some unique care requirements, which primarily focus on prevention of injury through diligent foot care and orthotics.

Peripheral neuropathy may occur with or without arterial insufficiency. Effective management can occur only when the dangers of neuropathy are appreciated and the status of arterial perfusion is appropriately evaluated.

VENOUS ULCERS

Venous ulcers of the lower extremities afflict 1% of the general population and 3.5% of persons over 65 years of age, with a recurrence rate approaching 70%.[11] Estimates indicate the cost of care for a patient with chronic venous insufficiency at $40,000, with costs expected to escalate despite cost-containment measures.[41] Among older persons, women are affected three times more often than men,[11] with the number of ulcers expected to rise as the population ages. Unfortunately, venous ulcers are subjected to numerous treatments, which often impede healing, potentiating functional impairment. Nurses caring for patients with venous ulcers must be cognizant of the concepts of wound management and devise a unified approach that appreciates the pathogenesis of venous ulceration and the biology of wound healing.

Pathophysiology

Venous ulcers (Plate 23) result from disorders of the deep venous system; however for a better understanding of the pathophysiology of venous ulceration, an understanding of normal venous anatomy of the lower extremities is imperative.

The venous system of the legs comprises three parts: (1) the deep venous system, which includes the femoral, popliteal, and tibial veins; (2) the superficial system, composed of the greater and lesser saphenous veins; and (3) the perforator veins that join the deep and superficial systems (Fig. 6-10). Normally, venous valves allow unidirectional blood flow from superficial veins to deep veins, advancing the return of blood from the capillary system to the heart.[76] When the forward flow of venous blood is significantly disturbed or impaired, venous dysfunction ensues. Venous disease consequently initiates a cascade of deleterious events that result in increased hydrostatic pressure, venous hypertension, and, ultimately, dermal ulceration.

Numerous disorders are capable of inducing venular dysfunction and include thrombosis of the deep venous system, postphlebitic syndrome, congestive heart failure, incompetent valves, obesity, pregnancy,[76] superficial vein regurgitation, and muscle weakness secondary to paralysis and arthritis;[41] all increase venous pressure, resulting in edema and ulceration.[9]

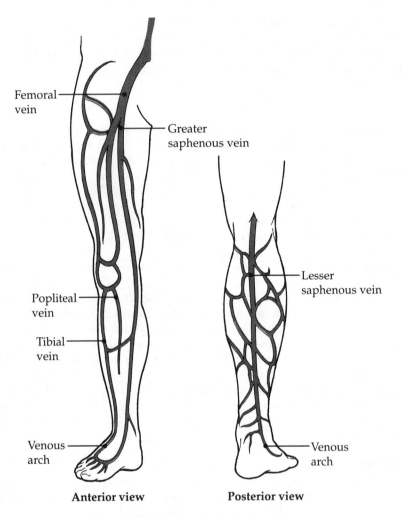

Fig. 6-10   Venous system in leg.

Until recently, stasis of blood was considered the primary culprit in the development of venous ulcers, a theory fostered by Homans[40] in 1917, who suggested that tissue anoxia and ulceration occurred secondary to stagnant venous circulation. This concept gained acceptance when low oxygen content was noted in varicose veins.[71] Homan's hypothesis was repudiated by Blalock[4] and Piulacks and Barraquer,[86] who demonstrated a higher oxygen content and faster circulation time in the veins of persons with venous disease.[25]

Subsequently, Browse and Burnand[5] formulated the current postulate for venous ulceration, work that is supported by Landis's[57] microinjection studies of capillary blood pressure in human skin. Their research indicates that excessive venous pressure may provoke extravasation of erythrocytes and fibrinogen. The erythrocytes release hemoglobin, which is converted to hemosiderin, producing the brownish discoloration characteristic of venous disease.

Fibrinogen, which is polymerized to fibrin and deposited around capillaries, then forms pericapillary fibrin cuffs, which impede the diffusion of oxygen and nutrients, promoting venous ulceration. Fibrin cuffs may also be encouraged by a reduction in tissue plasminogen activity (TPA),[7,8,112] a rise in TPA inhibitors,[9] and an elevated plasma fibrinogen level described in patients with venous disease.[7]

Additionally, white blood cells become entrapped in areas of reduced venous flow, causing capillary occlusion[75,76] and release of proteolytic enzymes and oxygen metabolites, further impairing capillary function and permitting fibrinogen leakage[76] (Fig. 6-11). Although the fibrin cuff theory must receive definitive in vivo affirmation, Falanga and Eaglstein[25] have demonstrated by direct immunofluorescence that pericapillary fibrin staining is a unique feature of venous ulcers and is not detected in normal skin or skin with arterial ulcers or ulcers of other causes.

Contributing Factors

Aside from the previously mentioned disorders capable of producing venous dysfunction, several contributing factors may encourage and assist in the formation of venous ulceration. These include malnutrition, hypoalbuminemia, immobility, and trauma.

The importance of nutrition in wound healing is indisputable; however malnutrition may also promote disruption of normal dermal integrity.[71] Vitamins C and A and the mineral zinc are necessary for the maintenance of dermal health. Vitamin C participates in the hydroxylation of lysine and proline during collagen synthesis,[11,71,26] vitamin A directs the differentiation of epithelium,[50] and zinc supports protein synthesis;[71] these are cardinal nutrients in the prevention and treatment of venous ulcers. Although deficiencies of vitamin

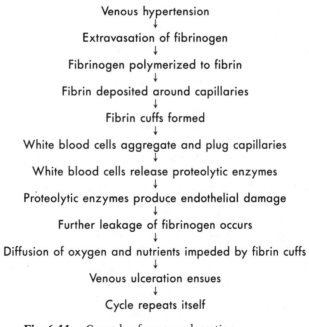

Fig. 6-11   Cascade of venous ulceration.

C are uncommon, many elderly and debilitated patients are reportedly at risk for subclinical or marginal deficits.[78] However, supplementation without demonstrable deficiencies does little to promote the healing of venous wounds. Deficiency of zinc among the general population is rare; however, once again there is evidence that the older populace may not receive adequate amounts.[78] Zinc status is associated with total caloric intake and is consequently of concern among patients with diabetes or cirrhosis and patients consuming diuretics, all such conditions being comparatively common in old age.[13] In a study by Hallbook and Lanner[33] zinc sulfate was shown to improve the healing of venous ulcers among zinc-deficient subjects, whereas Reed[90] suggested that elevated zinc levels produced by supplementation may actually impede wound healing and disturb immune function. There is conjecture that hypoalbuminemia may also peripherally contribute to venous wounds by increasing interstitial edema and extending the distance between blood vessels and dermal surface; however prospective, controlled studies are necessary to inculpate low albumin levels in the genesis of venous ulcers.

Contraction of calf muscles assists in the return of venous blood to the heart; however immobility impedes muscle function and promotes the development of thrombophlebitis and edema of the lower extremities.[71] Immobility may also induce muscular atrophy, negative nitrogen balance, impaired glucose tolerance, and reduced plasma volume, further contributing to the incipience of venous ulceration.[45]

Mechanical, thermal, or chemical trauma to extremities predisposed to venous ulcers often assists in the evolution of venous ulceration. Unintentional injuries such as hitting the leg on a car door or chair, soaking the foot in hot water, or topical application[71] of various store-bought or homemade compounds can initiate the emergence of dermal irritation and venous ulcer formation.

Assessment Parameters

History and Physical Examination. The clinical diagnosis of venous ulceration is often elementary when accompanied by a careful review of the patient's medical history and a focused physical examination. The medical history may reveal prior pregnancy, leg trauma, cardiac disease, nutritional ailments, or deep venous thrombosis. Interestingly, 20% to 70% of postphlebitic patients do not describe a history of venous thrombosis, since the initial episode of thrombosis was silent or undiagnosed.[46]

Physical examination of a patient with venous disease usually discloses lipodermatosclerosis and edema of the lower extremity. Lipodermatosclerosis, an induration and erythematous hyperpigmentation of the leg[11,71,76] is a preulcer dermal change that is often mistaken for cellulitis and forebodes impending ulceration. Deposition of hemosiderin ultimately contributes a brown discoloration to the affected area, whereas chronic dryness with epithelial scaling promotes scratching, excoriations, and eczematous changes.[41]

Combined, the preceding changes are commonly referred to as "stasis dermatitis," though Falanga and Eaglstein[25] suggest "venous dermatitis" is more appropriate, since the concept of stasis in venous disease is clearly erroneous. Additionally, the "ankle flare" sign, a collection of small venular channels inferior to the medial malleolus extending onto the medial foot, may also be observed and is indicative of chronic venous insufficiency.[41]

When venous wounds develop, ulcer characteristics are unique, though confusion with other causes of lower extremity ulcers may occasionally exist and necessitate biopsy (Table 6-2). Venous ulcers are commonly found on the medial aspect of the leg, just superior to the medial malleolus where the great saphenous vein is located.[41,71,76] Ulcers on the plantar aspect of the foot, interdigitally, or on bony prominences such as the toes, tibial surfaces,[25] or lateral malleolus should prompt a search for arterial disease, since such locations are rare sites for venous wounds.

In addition, up to 21% of patients with venous ulcers experience concomitant arterial disease, with the risk of coexisting arterial dysfunction increasing with age.[12] Consequently, diminished arterial pulses, though of benefit, do not necessarily justify a diagnosis of arterial ulceration or negate a venous cause. Venous ulcers generally have irregular borders that are flat and slope into a shallow crater,[71,76] exhibit surrounding lipodermatosclerosis and edema, and are painless unless infected or desiccated.[76] Exudation is usually present and varies from a small amount to significant quantities (Table 6-2).

The Trendelenburg test also assists in the physical evaluation of venous valvular competence in the perforators and saphenous system.[29] To perform this maneuver, the patient is placed in a supine position with the leg elevated for 5 to 10 minutes allowing venous blood to empty. A tourniquet is then placed above the knee to occlude venous circulation and prevent retrograde flow. The patient then stands, and the manner in which the veins refill is noted, with normal veins filling from below in approximately 30 seconds. If the superficial veins fill rapidly with the tourniquet in place, the perforator valves are incompetent. The tourniquet is then released, and if sudden additional filling occurs, the valves of the saphenous vein are incompetent.

Diagnostic Tests. Although the diagnosis of venous ulcers is frequently determined by physical assessment, further diagnostic maneuvers may be necessary to assist in the identification of lower extremity ulcers.

Doppler ultrasonography provides a noninvasive means of ascertaining the status of the deep venous system, and although accuracy is limited as secondary to the subjective quality of operator interpretation, it is an ideal technique for establishing the absence or presence of venous reflux and obstruction.[41] If diminished arterial flow is suspect in the pathogenesis of leg ulceration, the ankle-brachial index (ABI) can be computed by use of Doppler ultrasonography, with a ratio of less than 0.9 being indicative of underlying arterial disease.[11,72]

One can also use *impedance plethysmography* (IPG) to assess the venous outflow of the lower extremities by measuring variations in electrical impedance that accompany changes in blood volume. Although IPG is most reliable for venous occlusions above the knee,[29] it is reportedly more accurate than Doppler ultrasound in detecting changes in the deep veins of the calf.[70]

Photoplethysmography (PPG) utilizes a transducer with infrared light to measure vascular volume and provide an index of valvular incompetence. One can determine the venous refill time by employing PPG and by measuring after calf muscle exercise empties the veins. Normal venous refill is greater than 20 seconds, with values less than 20 seconds being indicative of incompetent valves. In addition, persons with refill times of less than 10 seconds take considerably longer to heal and exhibit a greater chance of ulcer recurrence.[46]

Duplex scanning with color-flow imaging can reportedly locate venous reflux in the superficial, deep, and perforator systems.[41] In patients without venous ulcers, duplex scanning may foretell the probability of lipodermatosclerosis and venous ulceration.[79]

Radionuclide venography (RV), utilizing the radiopharmaceutical technetium 99m, can be performed to assess the venous system, and although tibial veins are not well visualized, RV may be useful in persons with renal disease.[70] Although the sensitivity of RV for deep thrombophlebitis is high, the low specificity with false-positive results has raised concern among clinicians.[48]

Finally, *contrast venography* can provide a radiographic picture of the venous system by injection of radiopaque dye into a pedal dorsal vein. Unfortunately, it is not without significant side effects, including allergic reactions, renal dysfunction, and thrombophlebitis[48] and, as such, has limited usefulness (as when one considers surgical options).

Management

The management of venous ulceration is directed at reduction of venous hypertension and eradication of pericapillary fibrin.[25,26] Management involves four basic doctrines: (1) control of underlying medical and nutritional disorders, (2) elimination of edema, (3) stimulation of fibrinolysis, and (4) maintenance of a moist wound environment.

Control of Underlying Medical and Nutritional Disorders. Proper wound healing necessitates correction of underlying contributing factors. Although select disorders are not amenable to medical intervention, most can be improved or eliminated.

Congestive heart failure, a common malady among the elderly, should be appropriately managed to reduce the extent of venous hypertension and lower extremity edema. Nutritional deficiencies should be addressed, particularly total caloric intake and the status of vitamins C and A and zinc. However, one should keep in mind that vitamin and mineral supplementation does little to promote wound healing in the absence of deficiencies. Consultation with a dietician may be necessary, particularly when moderate to severe malnutrition is evident.

If obesity is evident, a weight reduction regimen should be initiated, including limited caloric intake and appropriate exercise. Walking is probably the best form of physical activity, since ambulation expends calories and encourages venous return through muscular contraction.

Arthritic complaints should be treated utilizing correct footwear, physical therapy, and pain-relieving medications. Most patients with arthritis consume nonsteroidal antiinflammatory agents (NSAID) for pain reduction, however, Velasco and Guaitero[105] suggest NSAIDs may be detrimental to wound healing, at least in early or acute wounds. If patients with difficult or refractory venous ulcers take NSAIDs, it may be worthwhile to discontinue the medication and substitute plain acetaminophen or acetaminophen with codeine for a period of time and observe the effect on wound healing.

Similarly, patients with arthritis and pulmonary disease occasionally use corticosteroids. Like NSAIDs, prednisone in doses exceeding 10 mg per day delays wound healing and should be discontinued after appropriate tapering.[25,76,81]

Patients who expend considerable time in wheelchairs with their legs in a dependent position (patients with arthritis or who are paralyzed) must be encouraged to elevate the ulcerated leg as much as possible during the day and raise the foot of the bed while sleeping. In fact, all patients with venous ulcers should be encouraged to elevate their legs unless significant arterial disease is present.

Patients with diabetes frequently develop ischemic or neuropathic ulcers; however venous wounds are not uncommon.[25] Accordingly, blood glucose should be adequately controlled by use of diet, exercise, oral hypoglycemics, and insulin therapy. For ambulatory homebound patients, home glucose monitoring is useful but should be limited to reliable and compliant patients.

Elimination of Edema. Elimination of edema is accomplished by two mechanisms: elevation of the legs and use of compressive therapy. As previously mentioned, patients with venous ulcers should elevate their legs as often as possible and raise the foot of the bed while sleeping. Although such treatment is often coupled with diuretic therapy, diuretics are generally unsuccessful in chronic venous insufficiency and are not indicated unless congestive heart failure is evident.

The amount of external compressive pressure necessary to heal a venous ulcer is unknown, though Mulder and Reis[76] and Hendricks[38] relate that as little as 24 mm Hg at the ankle and 16 mm Hg at the calf will assist the healing of most venous wounds. Current compressive modalities include elastic wraps, elastic stockings, Unna boots, and mechanical pumps.

Elastic wraps are best used in patients who do not have access to mechanical pumps or who are unable to tolerate elastic stockings or Unna boots. Elastic bandages are most effective on early, small ulcers, with limited success being reported on large, chronic wounds.[76] Unfortunately, when elastic wraps are applied inappropriately, venous return can be further hindered. Lippmann and Briere[67] allude that elastic wraps do little if anything to assist the reduction of edema, since repeated contractions of calf muscles stretch the wrap and reduce compressive abilities. Additionally, Mulder and Reis[76] suggest such wraps are contraindicated when concomitant arterial occlusive disease, weeping venous dermatitis, and venous ulcers with infectious complications are present. If utilized, elastic wraps should be placed on the leg when edema is absent or minimal to afford maximal compression and venous return, with highest pressures applied at the foot and ankle and decreasing as the wrap proceeds toward the knee.

Graduated compression stockings do a commendable job of assisting venous return and reducing edema. However many patients who are disabled, have arthritis, or are elderly are unable to put compression stockings on. Nevertheless, they are of considerable benefit as confirmed in recent literature.[64,38]

Compression stockings probably reduce edema by maintaining empty periulcer venous channels, often with pressures as low as 18 mm Hg. If a patient is unable to tolerate high-pressure stockings, consideration should be given to low-pressure stockings. Ideally, all patients with venous disease should wear compression stockings; however they should not be measured and fitted until edema has resolved. These stockings are put on before the patient gets out of bed and are worn all day. They are effective for prevention as well as treatment of venous ulcers.

The *Unna boot* is one of the more popular compressive therapies that not only aids venous return but may also stimulate epithelialization.[76] The boot, initially developed by the German physician Paul Gerson Unna in the 1880s, consists of cotton gauze or white cloth impregnated with a moist paste of zinc oxide, gelatin, and glycerin. One applies the boot in a circular fashion, not the customary figure-of-8 method, starting from the foot and terminating just below the knee. The wrap can be cut, folded, or pleated to ensure a snug but not tight fit.[74]

Unna boots should be applied in the morning when edema has subsided,[41] with an expected wear time of 4 to 7 days, though more frequent changes may be necessary with heavy exudation. Once the boot is in place, it should be covered with a gauze or compression wrapping (Ace or Coban) to protect the patient's clothing. The boot is particularly useful for patients who are unable to comply with other modalities but should be avoided in patients with poor personal hygiene[76] and significant arterial disease. Unna boots are contraindicated in patients with friable, sensitive tissue, since the presence of moisture may irritate surrounding skin and contribute to worsening of the wound. The boot should not cause discomfort, and the patient should be instructed to report any pain or significant toe changes such as swelling, loss of feeling, or blue or purple coloration.[74]

Intermittent pneumatic sequential compression devices (SCD) are becoming more popular among clinicians and reportedly aid venous return, reduce edema, stimulate fibrinolysis,[76] and heal refractory ulcers even after other measures have failed.[83] As described by Mulder and Reis,[76] each leg sleeve of the SCD is divided into six chambers, with peak pressures of 45 to 60 mm Hg at the ankle. The two ankle chambers inflate, followed 2½ seconds later by the calf chambers, and then 3 seconds later by the thigh chambers, the latter inflating to a pressure of 25 to 30 mm Hg. All chambers remain inflated for 5½ seconds and then simultaneously deflate, with the cycle repeated every 71 seconds. Treatment varies from 1 to 2 hours per session[71,77] and may be completed morning and evening on a daily basis.[77]

Mulder and associates[77] evaluated the Sequential Compression Device Therapeutic System (SCD) (Kendall Healthcare Products, Mansfield, Mass.) in a study of eight patients with venous ulcers and noted that venous wounds, particularly chronic, resistant ulcers, responded well to sequential compression therapy. Two of the patients discontinued SCD therapy after their wounds healed but subsequently became reulcerated at 3 and 6 months. SCD treatment was reinstituted, resulting in closure of the ulcers, an indication that SCD may also be valuable as a preventive modality. As evidenced by other clinicians,[54,83] sequential compression therapy is an important tool in combating the underlying pathophysiologic condition of venous ulcers; however it is not a cure and must be used chronically in patients with venous dysfunction. Furthermore, it is not clear that sequential compression is better than nonsequential (or graduated) compression, and the latter is much less expensive.

Stimulation of Fibrinolysis. If the theory of Browse and Burnand[5] is accepted as the cause of venous ulceration, a crucial component of wound management is the stimulation of fibrinolysis. As previously mentioned, compression therapy probably encourages fibrin degradation, as occlusive dressings do. However, in recurrent or refractory ulceration, which results in significant morbidity, a trial of stanozolol (Winstrol) may be considered. Stanozolol, an anabolic steroid, enhances the activity of tissue plasminogen activator[20] but is not approved by the Food and Drug Administration for use in venous ulcers; furthermore, definitive studies confirming its effectiveness are lacking.[25] Side effects, which include polycythemia, sodium retention, liver abnormalities, and azotemia,[25,26] limit usefulness, and as such, stanozolol should not be prescribed for patients with heart failure or liver or renal disease. If stanozolol is utilized, recommended dosage varies, ranging from 2 to 10 mg per day; however one protocol[11] suggests 10 mg daily until lipodermatosclerosis is reduced and then 2 mg per day for 1 to 3 months.

Topical Therapy. Local wound care encompasses a variety of topical preparations, including antiseptics, antibiotics, and occlusive dressings. Principles of moist wound healing as outlined in Chapter 2 provide fundamental guidance.

Wound cleansing. Wounds should be cleansed with normal saline or a noncytotoxic commercial cleanser. Unfortunately, many clinicians insist on cleaning and packing a wound with deleterious topical antiseptics. Povidone-iodine, hydrogen peroxide, sodium hypochlorite, and acetic acid are frequently employed; however all are toxic to fibroblasts at normal-to-high concentrations and are of dubious value.[65] Moreover, povidone-iodine is readily inactivated by serum proteins, further negating its use in exudative wounds.[27]

Saline-moistened gauze may be used to liquefy necrotic tissue and to encourage granulation. Since gauze is placed in the wound while moist, the periulcer tissue must be protected from maceration by means of a moisture-barrier ointment or skin sealant.

Topical Antibiotics or Antibacterials. Topical antibiotics are also popular but of little or no benefit.[76] Although they are used to eradicate ulcer bacteria, surface contaminants do not present a high risk of infection, and their elimination does little to promote wound healing; moreover, topical antibiotics may merely serve to select out resistant organisms. Topical antibacterials may also induce allergic reactions, further abrogating their utility.

Two antibiotics deserve special mention, however, both for what they can and cannot do. Silver sulfadiazine (Silvadene) is a commonly used antibacterial agent, and although epithelialization is reportedly 28% faster when compared with untreated wounds, the healing effects are not related to antimicrobial activity.[27] In fact, silver sulfadiazine probably exerts its healing ability through maintenance of a moist wound environment. On the other hand, topical nitrofurazone (Furacin) significantly retards epithelialization, and such retardation implies epidermal cytotoxicity[27] and precludes its use in venous ulceration.

If periulcer cellulitis is present, topical antibiotics do little to suppress the infection; instead, oral or parenteral antibiotics are recommended. Suggested agents include a penicillinase-resistant penicillin, erythromycin, or cephalosporin.[41] If cellulitis develops while an occlusive dressing is in place, systemic antibacterials covering aerobic and anaerobic organisms are recommended.[10]

Venous dermatitis may be managed with topical emollients or lotions that contain lactic acid or urea;[41] however topical corticosteroids may be helpful in severe cases. Low- to intermediate-strength agents such as 1% hydrocortisone are recommended, with use being limited to 1 to 2 weeks, since chronic application promotes dermal thinning and further injury to the periulcer environment. Interestingly, ointments containing petrolatum have been shown to impede healing[24] and should be avoided when one is treating venous dermatitis.

Dressings. Occlusive dressings are efficacious in the management of venous ulceration and work primarily by maintenance of a moist wound environment. Occlusive dressings also protect the wound from external contaminants, encourage débridement,[76] promote granulation, reduce pain,[11] accelerate wound healing time up to 50%[39,111] and reduce nursing costs secondary to a dressing change regimen of 3 to 7 days. Polyurethane or transparent dressings are not recommended in venous wounds because their ability to absorb sufficient exudate is limited. Hydrocolloid dressings are preferable for venous ulcers because they are able to absorb significant amounts of wound drainage. Such dressings gently debride venous ulcers thus avoiding traumatic and painful surgical or gauze débridement.[26]

When a hydrocolloid is applied to a venous ulcer, excessive exudation often results. Absorptive products can be used with the hydrocolloid to control the exudate. If the volume of exudate requires daily hydrocolloid dressing changes, topical therapy should be re-evaluated. Care must also be exercised to prevent periulcer maceration by large amounts of wound exudate; more frequent dressing changes and the use of skin sealants help avert such problems.

Nonadhesive, nonocclusive dressings, such as foam dressings, hydrogels, and calcium alginates, are useful for venous ulcers with considerable venous dermatitis or friable periulcer tissue. Also, because occlusive dressings are contraindicated in ulcers that extend to the muscle or bone, or in infected wounds evidenced by purulent drainage, surrounding cellulitis, fever, chills, and leukocytosis, nonocclusive dressings should be used.

Calcium alginate dressings are particularly useful in wounds with excessive drainage.[103] The dressing, a soft, naturally occurring polysaccharide found in brown seaweed, is placed directly into the wound and secured with a secondary bandage. When exudate is absorbed, the alginate forms a gel that is readily removed by saline lavage, necessitating dressing changes every 1 to 3 days.

Growth factors are a new and fascinating topical therapy that will undoubtedly become more popular and available in the near future. Multiple agents are under study (at least 36), including platelet-derived growth factor, epidermal growth factor, fibroblast growth factor, insulin-like growth factor, and transforming growth factor-beta.[51,52] Although there are available several nonrandomized trials that allow one to evaluate growth factors, Knighton and associates[52] reported on a double-blind, randomized, crossover, placebo-controlled trial of platelet-derived growth factors. Thirty-two patients were randomized into treatment and control groups. In the placebo group, 15% of wounds healed, whereas all wounds healed after crossover to growth factor treatment, clearly a statistically significant occurrence ($P = 0.0002$).

In addition, Brown et al.[6] in a prospective, randomized, double-blind clinical trial, studied the use of epidermal growth factor on skin-graft donor sites and noted that donor sites treated with epidermal growth factor had an accelerated rate of epidermal regeneration, with an average reduction of healing time of 1 to 1.5 days ($P < 0.02$). Further clinical experience with growth factor wound healing was described by Fylling,[31] who suggests that growth factor technology accelerates wound healing, reduces recurrent ulcers and inpatient lengths of stay, and is cost effective, ensuring significant growth factor–related pharmaceutical sales in the near future. Currently, however, growth factor technology has been researched primarily in neuropathic and arterial ulcers.

Surgical options. Approximately 85% of venous wounds respond to nonsurgical management;[41] however in ulcers resistant to conservative therapy, surgical intervention may be considered. Various modalities are available, including split- and full-thickness skin grafts, pinch biopsy grafts, xenografts, and punch-biopsy grafts. Although all have their proponents, punch-biopsy and split-thickness grafts are preferable. However, application of cultured epidermal allografts utilizing neonatal foreskin has proved successful in recent studies.[59,84,102] Phillips and associates[84] have considerable experience with cultured allografts and conclude that the procedure is most successful in patients with chronic ulcers that are not deep or associated with connective tissue disorders.

SUMMARY

Ulcerations on the lower extremities can present a confusing array of intervening variables. Although at first glance it seems easy to distinguish between an arterial ulcer and a venous ulcer based upon the characteristics of the ulcer and the extremity, coexisting pathologic conditions such as peripheral neuropathy can cloud the assessment.

Management of lower extremity ulcers requires aggressive débridement, clear delineation of cause by diagnostic studies, correction of the underlying cause, appropriate topical therapy, sensitive supportive counseling, and routine follow-up observation. Collaboration of a multidisciplinary team is critical. A thorough understanding of the pathogenesis of lower extremity ulcers, risk factors, and treatment is the necessary foundation to provide the state of the art in the care that patients with these ulcers require.

SELF-EVALUATION

QUESTIONS AND PROBLEMS

1. Explain how atherosclerosis and arteriosclerosis contribute to arterial insufficiency.
2. Rest pain is indicative of:
   a. 70% occlusion.
   b. 55% occlusion.
   c. 90% occlusion.
   d. motor neuropathy.
3. Identify at least two ways in which PVD in the diabetic differs from PVD in the nondiabetic.
4. Briefly explain how the following factors contribute to PVD:
   a. Smoking
   b. Hyperlipidemia
   c. Hypertension
   d. Diabetes mellitus
5. Explain the physiologic basis for intermittent claudication and nocturnal pain in the patient with PVD.
6. Identify the four lower extremity pulses that should be palpated during circulatory assessment of the patient with PVD.
7. Identify signs of arterial insufficiency in the lower extremity.
8. Identify three types of diabetic neuropathy and the impact of each on skin integrity.
9. Identify key components of nursing assessment for the patient with an ischemic ulcer.
10. Segmental pressures are a noninvasive diagnostic test for arterial competence. In a comparison of lower extremity pressures to upper extremity pressures, which of the following is associated with a poor prognosis in terms of healing?
    a. Ankle/brachial index of 1.1
    b. Ankle/brachial index of 0.9
    c. Ankle/brachial index of 0.8
    d. Ankle/brachial index of 0.4
11. Normal values for transcutaneous oxygen tension readings are:
    a. 60 to 80 mm Hg.
    b. >40 mm Hg.
    c. 30 to 40 mmHg.
    d. 20 mm Hg.
12. Patients with PVD are believed to be at greater risk for infection than patients with normal perfusion.
    True
    False
13. In culturing diabetic foot lesions, needle aspiration provides more accurate results than a swab culture.
    True
    False

14. Which of the following may indicate osteomyelitis?
    a. Abnormal bone scan
    b. Nonhealing ulcer
    c. Abnormal x-ray film findings
    d. All of the above

15. Which of the following is the *most* significant factor in healing an ischemic ulcer?
    a. Nutritional status
    b. Perfusion status
    c. Topical therapy
    d. Adequate débridement

16. Identify surgical, pharmacologic, and nursing interventions that may be used to improve the blood supply to an ischemic limb.

17. Identify the factors other than topical therapy that must be addressed in the management plan for an ischemic ulcer.

18. Explain why and when débridement is contraindicated in the management of an ischemic ulcer.

19. Identify routine precautions that one should include in teaching the patient with PVD.

20. State four factors that predispose the patient to develop venous ulcerations.

21. Which of the following provide compressive therapy?
    a. Elastic wraps, intermittent pneumatic sequential compression, and orthotics
    b. Unna boot, contact cast, and graduated compression stockings
    c. Antiembolism stockings, Unna boot, and orthotics
    d. Intermittent graduated compression stockings, Unna boot, and elastic wraps

22. All of the following surgical procedures may be indicated for venous ulcerations *except:*
    a. full-thickness graft.
    b. myocutaneous flaps.
    c. punch biopsy.
    d. split-thickness graft.

SELF-EVALUATION

ANSWERS

1. Atherosclerosis refers to the accumulation of plaque along the walls of the arteries; this narrows the lumen of the vessel. Arteriosclerosis refers to thickening and reduced elasticity of the arterial walls; this further narrows the lumen and reduces the vessel's ability to dilate. The narrowed lumen and loss of elasticity results in decreased resting blood flow and a loss of ability to provide increased blood flow during times of increased need (such as exercise).

2. c

3. PVD occurs at a younger age and advances more rapidly in the diabetic.
   In diabetics, PVD is almost as common in women as it is in men.
   In the diabetic, involvement is usually bilateral.
   The diabetic is likely to have involvement of the vessels below the knee as well as the larger more proximal vessels.

The diabetic is likely to have multisegmental occlusion.

The diabetic is likely to have patchy areas of gangrene.

4. a. Smoking decreases blood flow to the extremities and promotes atherosclerosis and platelet aggregation.

b. Hyperlipidemia promotes plaque accumulation in the arterial walls.

c. Hypertension damages vessels and promotes plaque formation.

d. Diabetes mellitus is known to increase the risk of PVD, but the exact initiating mechanism is unknown.

5. The patient with intermittent claudication has enough blood flow to meet metabolic demands at rest. With exercise, however, metabolic demands increase, and the compromised vasculature is unable to meet these increased demands. As a result, the muscle becomes ischemic, which produces cramping, burning, and aching in the feet and legs. Nocturnal pain occurs because with sleep and a recumbent position the blood pressure drops and perfusion of the extremities is reduced. This causes ischemic neuritis, which causes the patient to wake with pain.

6. Femoral, popliteal, posterior tibial, dorsalis pedis

7. Reduced temperature; elevational pallor and dependent rubor; shiny, smooth, thin skin; hair loss; subcutaneous tissue loss and muscle atrophy; necrosis (gangrene)

8. 1. *Sensory neuropathy.* Reduced sensitivity to pain and temperature changes results in increased susceptibility to injury.

2. *Motor neuropathy.* Loss of innervation to the muscles causes foot deformities and changes in gait, which alter weight bearing and result in repetitive stress. These predispose the patient to callus formation and ulceration, unless weight is properly redistributed.

3. *Autonomic neuropathy.* Loss of sweating, which leads to chronically dry skin and predisposes the skin to "cracking."

9. *History:* Previous vascular work-up or surgery, diabetes mellitus or other systemic medical conditions, smoking history, ulcer history (onset and any initiating event), previous treatment of ulcer

Physical examination: Blood pressure (brachial and ankle), inspection of skin (color, temperature, lesions), palpation of lower extremity pulses, assessment of blanching and capillary refill

Ulcer: Location, appearance (depth, status of ulcer base, presence or absence of sinus tracts and foreign bodies, signs of infection), surrounding tissue (such as erythema or induration)

10. d

11. b

12. True

13. True

14. d

15. b

16. *Surgical:* Bypass procedures, angioplasty

Pharmacologic: Pentoxifylline, antiplatelet drugs

Nursing: Avoidance of constrictive agents (nicotine, caffeine, cold, constrictive garments), maintenance of normal blood pressure, neutral or dependent position for legs, titrated activity

17. Causative factors, vascular status, infection, osteomyelitis, necrotic tissue, diabetes mellitus, edema, nutritional status.

18. Débridement is contraindicated in a wound with dry gangrene or a dry ischemic wound until vascular status has been evaluated. Débridement would produce an open wound with significant potential for overwhelming infection in the presence of poor perfusion.

19. 1. Daily washing with mild soap and thorough rinsing.

  2. Lubrication after bathing and as needed with a nonirritating agent such as lanolin, petrolatum, or Eucerin. Agents with fragrance should be avoided, and lubricants should not be applied between the toes.

  3. Daily skin inspection and prompt reporting of any skin lesions to the health care team. Corns and calluses are precursors of potential ulceration and should be reported.

  4. Calluses should be filed daily to prevent thickening and cracking.

  5. Cotton or wool socks should be worn to wick away moisture, and shoes must fit properly. Appropriate footwear provides protection from injury; going barefoot is never appropriate.

  6. A podiatrist should be consulted if toenails, corns, or calluses are thick, or if the patient is unable to provide safe self-care because of poor vision or the inability to bend over.

20. 1. Thrombophlebitis

  2. Congestive heart failure

  3. Obesity

  4. Superficial vein regurgitation

  5. Paralysis

21. d

22. b

REFERENCES

1. Alterescu V: Debriding enzymes, J Enterostom Ther 11(3):122, 1984.
2. Baur GM and Porter JM: Vasodilating agents in peripheral arteriosclerotic ischemic disease. In Rutherford RB, editor: Vascular surgery, ed 2, Philadelphia, 1983, WB Saunders Co.
3. Bernhard VM: Bypass to the popliteal and infrapopliteal arteries. In Rutherford RB, editor: Vascular surgery, ed 2, Philadelphia, 1983, WB Saunders Co.
4. Blalock A: Oxygen content of blood in patients with varicose veins, Arch Surg 19:898-905, 1929.
5. Browse NL and Burnand KG: The cause of venous ulceration, Lancet 2:243-245, 1982.
6. Brown GL, Nanney LB, Griffen J, et al: Enhancement of wound healing by topical treatment with epidermal growth factor, N Engl J Med 321:76-79, 1989.
7. Browse NL, Gray L, Jarrett PE, and Morland M: Blood and vein wall fibrinolytic activity in health and vascular disease, Br Med J 1:478-481, 1977.
8. Buchbinder D et al: Comparison of patency rate and structural change of "in-situ" and reversed vein arterial bypass, J Surg Res 30:213, 1981.
9. Burnand KG: Aetiology of venous ulceration, Br J Surg 77:483-484, 1990.
10. Burnand KG, Whimster I, Naidoo A, and Browse NL: Pericapillary fibrin in ulcer-bearing skin of the leg: the cause of lipodermatosclerosis and venous ulceration, Br Med J 285:1071-1072, 1982.
11. Callam MJ, Eaglstein WH, and Lynch DJ: Meeting the challenge of leg ulcers, Patient Care 22(9):24-34, 1988.
12. Callam MJ, Harper DR, Dale JJ, et al: Arterial disease in chronic leg ulceration: an underestimated hazard? Lothian and Forth Valley leg ulcer study, Br Med J 294:929-931, 1987.
13. Cape RDT: Malnutrition, weight loss, and anorexia. In Abrams WB, Berkow R, and Fletcher AJ, editors: The Merck manual of geriatrics, Rahway, NJ, 1990, Merck Sharp & Dohme.

14. Coffman JD: Vasodilator drugs in peripheral vascular disease, N Engl J Med 300:713, 1979.
15. Coleman WC: Footwear in a management program of injury prevention. In Levin ME and O'Neal LW, editors: The diabetic foot, ed 4, St. Louis, 1988, Mosby–Year Book, Inc.
16. Coleman WC, Brand PW, and Birke JA: The total contact case: a therapy for plantar ulceration on insensitive feet, J Am Podiatr Assoc 74(11):548+, 1984.
17. Colwell JA et al: New concepts about the pathogenesis of atherosclerosis in diabetes mellitus. In Levin ME and O'Neal LW, editors: The diabetic foot, ed 4, St. Louis, 1988, Mosby–Year Book, Inc.
18. Connor J, Wilson SE, and Williams RA: The clinical examination of the vascular system. In Wilson SE et al, editors: Vascular surgery: principles and practice, New York, 1987, McGraw-Hill Book Co.
19. Couch, NP: On the arterial consequences of smoking, J Vasc Surg 3:807, 1986.
20. Davidson JF, Lochhead M, McDonald GA, and McNicol GP: Fibrinolytic enhancement by stanozolol: a double blind trial, Br J Hematol 22:543-559, 1972.
21. DePalma RG: Medical management of atherosclerotic vascular disease. In Wilson SE et al, editors: Vascular surgery: principles and practice, New York, 1987, McGraw-Hill Book Co.
22. DeWeese JA: Antiplatelet agents. In Wilson SE et al, editors: Vascular surgery: principles and practice, New York, 1987, McGraw-Hill Book Co.
23. Doyle JE: Treatment modalities in peripheral vascular disease, Nurs Clin North Am 21(2):241, 1986.
24. Eaglstein WH and Mertz PM: Effect of topical medicaments on the rate of repair of superficial wounds. In Dineen P, editor: The surgical wound, Philadelphia, 1981, Lea & Febiger.
25. Falanga V and Eaglstein WH: A therapeutic approach to venous ulcers, J Am Acad Dermatol 14:777-784, 1986.
26. Falanga V and Eaglstein WH: Management of venous ulcers, Am Fam Physician 33(2):274-281, 1986.
27. Feedar JA and Kloth LC: Conservative management of chronic wounds. In Kloth LC, McCulloch JM, and Feedar JA, editors: Wound healing: alternatives in management, Philadelphia, 1990, FA Davis.
28. Fenn JE: Reconstructive arterial surgery for ischemic lower extremities, Nurs Clin North Am 12(1):129, 1977.
29. Friedman SA: Peripheral vascular disease. In Abrams WB, Berkow R, and Fletcher AJ, editors: The Merck manual of geriatrics, Rahway, NJ, 1990, Merck Sharp & Dohme.
30. Friedman SA and Rakow RB: Osseous lesions of the foot in diabetic neuropathy, Diabetes 20:302, 1971.
31. Fylling CP: A comprehensive wound management protocol including topical growth factors, Wounds 1(1):79-86, 1989.
32. Greene DA: Neuropathy in the diabetic foot: new concepts in etiology and treatment. In Levin ME and O'Neal LW, editors: The diabetic foot, ed 4, St. Louis, 1988, Mosby–Year Book, Inc.
33. Hallbook T and Lanner E: Serum zinc and healing of venous leg ulcers, Lancet 2:780-782, 1972.
34. Hallett JW, Brewster DC, and Darling RC: Manual of patient care in vascular surgery, Boston, 1982, Little, Brown & Co.
35. Hardy DC et al: Imaging of the diabetic foot. In Levin ME and O'Neal LW, editors: The diabetic foot, ed 4, St. Louis, 1988, Mosby–Year Book, Inc.
36. Harkless LB and Dennis KJ: The role of the podiatrist. In Levin ME and O'Neal LW, editors: The diabetic foot, ed 4, St. Louis, 1988, Mosby–Year Book, Inc.
37. Helm PA, Walker SC, and Pullium G: Total contact casting in diabetic patients with neuropathic foot ulceration, Arch Phys Med Rehabil 65:691+, 1984.
38. Hendricks WH and Swallow RT: Management of stasis leg ulcers with Unna's boots versus elastic support stockings, J Am Acad Dermatol 12:90-98, 1985.
39. Hinman CC, Maibach HI, and Winter GD: Effect of air exposure and occlusion on experimental human skin wounds, Nature 200:377-378, 1963.
40. Homans J: The aetiology and treatment of varicose ulcers of the leg, Surg Gynecol Obstet 24:300-311, 1917.
41. Hurley JP: Chronic venous insufficiency: venous ulcers and other consequences. In Krasner D, editor: Chronic wound care, King of Prussia, Penn, 1990, Health Management Publications.

42. Hunt TK et al: Oxygen tension and wound infection, Surg Forum 23:47, 1972.

43. Hunt TK et al: The effect of differing ambient oxygen tensions on wound infection, Ann Surg 181:35, 1975.

44. IAET: Standards of care: dermal wounds, leg ulcers, 1987, International Association for Enterostomal Therapy, 2081 Business Center Dr., no. 290, Irvine, CA 92715.

45. Kane RL, Ouslander JG, and Abrass IB: Essentials of clinical geriatrics, ed 2, New York, 1989, McGraw-Hill Book Co.

46. Karp DL: Venous ulceration: assessment, healing prediction and treatment, SPVN 5(3):14-15, Norwood, Mass, 1987 (now called Journal of Vascular Nursing).

47. Kempczinski RF and Bernhard VM: The management of chronic ischemia of the lower extremities: introduction and general considerations. In Rutherford RB, editor: Vascular surgery, ed 2, Philadelphia, 1983, WB Saunders Co.

48. Kidawa AS: Vascular disorders. In Levy LA and Hetherington VJ, editors: Principles and practice of podiatric medicine, New York, 1990, Churchill Livingstone.

49. Klein P: Vitamin A acid and wound healing, Acta Dermatol 74 (suppl):171-173, 1975.

50. Klemp P and Staberg B: Smoking reduces insulin absorption from subcutaneous tissue, Br Med J 284:237, 1982.

51. Knighton DR, Fiegel VD, and Doucette MM: Wound repair: the growth factor revolution. In Krasner D, editor: Chronic wound care, King of Prussia, Penn, 1990, Health Management Publications.

52. Knighton DR, Fiegel VD, Doucette MM, et al: The use of topically applied platelet growth factors in chronic nonhealing wounds: a review, Wounds 1(1):71-78, 1989.

53. Knighton DR et al: Stimulation of repair in chronic, nonhealing, cutaneous ulcers using platelet-derived wound healing formula, Surg Gynecol Obstet 170(1):56, 1990.

54. Kolari PJ and Pekanmäki K: Intermittent pneumatic compression in healing of venous ulcers, Lancet 2:1108, 1986.

55. Kumpe DA: Percutaneous transluminal angioplasty for lower extremity ischemia. In Rutherford RB, editor: Vascular surgery, ed 2, Philadelphia, 1983, WB Saunders Co.

56. Kwiterovich, PO: Beyond cholesterol, Baltimore, 1989, Johns Hopkins University Press.

57. Landis EM: Microinjection studies of capillary blood pressure in human skin, Heart 15:404-453, 1930.

58. Leather RP and Karmody AM: "In-situ" saphenous vein arterial bypass. In Rutherford RB, editor: Vascular surgery, ed 2, Philadelphia, 1983, WB Saunders Co.

59. Leigh IM, Purkis PE, Navsaria HA, and Phillips TJ: Treatment of chronic venous ulcers with sheets of cultured allogenic keratinocytes, Br J Dermatol 117:591-597, 1987.

60. Levin ME: Diabetic foot lesions: pathogenesis and management, J Enterostom Ther 17(7):29, 1990.

61. Levin ME: The diabetic foot: pathophysiology, evaluation and treatment. In Levin ME and O'Neal LW: The diabetic foot, ed 4, St. Louis, 1988, Mosby–Year Book, Inc.

62. Levin ME and Sicard GA: Evaluating and treating peripheral vascular disease, part I, Clinical Diabetes, pp 62-70, May/June 1987.

63. Lewis JL and Salzman EW: Antithrombotic therapy. In Rutherford RB, editor: Vascular surgery, ed 2, Philadelphia, 1983, WB Saunders Co.

64. Lewis CE, Antoine J, Mueller C, et al: Elastic compression in the prevention of venous stasis: a critical reevaluation, Am J Surg 132:739-743, 1976.

65. Lineaweaver W, Howard R, Soucy D, et al: Topical antimicrobial toxicity, Arch Surg 120:267-270, 1985.

66. Lippmann HI: The foot of the diabetic. In Brodoff BM and Bleicher SJ, editors: Diabetes mellitus and obesity, Baltimore, 1982, Williams & Wilkins.

67. Lippman HI and Briere JP: Physical basis of external supports in chronic venous insufficiency, Arch Phys Med 52:555-559, 1971.

68. Little JR and Kobayashi GS: Infection of the diabetic foot. In Levin ME and O'Neal LW, editors: The diabetic foot, ed 4, St. Louis, 1988, Mosby–Year Book, Inc.

69. Louie TJ et al: Aerobic and anaerobic bacteria in diabetic foot ulcers, Ann Intern Med 85:461, 1976.

70. MacKinnon J: Doppler ultrasound assessment in peripheral vascular disease. In Krasner D, editor: Chronic wound care, King of Prussia, Penn, 1990, Health Management Publications.

71. McCulloch JM and Hovde J: Treatment of wounds due to vascular problems. In Kloth LC, McCulloch JM, and Feedar JA, editors: Wound healing: alternatives in management, Philadelphia, 1990, FA Davis.
72. McCulloch JM and Kloth LC: Evaluation of patients with open wounds. In Kloth LC, McCulloch JM, and Feedar JA, editors: Wound healing: alternatives in management, Philadelphia, 1990, FA Davis.
73. McIntyre, KE: Control of infection in the diabetic foot: the role of microbiology, immunopathology, antibiotics, and guillotine amputation, J Vasc Surg 5(5):787, 1987.
74. Mignor D: The Unna boot makes a comeback, Home Healthcare Nurse 8(5):22-25, 1990.
75. Moosa HH, Falanga V, Makaroun MS, et al: Oxygen diffusion in chronic venous ulceration, J Invest Dermatol 84:358, 1985.
76. Mulder GD and Reis TM: Venous ulcers: pathophysiology and medical therapy, Am Fam Physician 42(5):1323-1330, 1990.
77. Mulder GD, Robison J, and Seeley J: Study of sequential compression therapy in the treatment of non-healing chronic venous ulcers, Wounds 2(3):111-115, 1990.
78. Nelson RC and Franzi LR: Nutrition and aging, Med Clin North Am 73(6):1531-1550, 1989.
79. Nicolaides AN: Diagnostic evaluation of patients with chronic venous insufficiency. In Rutherford RB, editor: Vascular surgery, Philadelphia, 1989, WB Saunders Co.
80. O'Neal LW: Debridement and amputation. In Levin ME and O'Neal LW, editors: The diabetic foot, ed 4, St. Louis, 1988, Mosby–Year Book, Inc.
81. Oxlund H, Fogdestam I, and Viidik A: The influence of cortisol on wound healing of the skin and distant connective tissue response, Surg Gynecol Obstet 148:876-880, 1979.
82. Pecoraro R: Diabetic ulcers of the foot, International Association for Enterostomal Therapy national conference presentation, Las Vegas, Nevada, June 13, 1990.
83. Pekanmäki K, Kolari PJ, and Kiistala U: Intermittent pneumatic compression treatment for post-thrombotic leg ulcers, Clin Exp Dermatol 12:350-353, 1987.
84. Phillips TJ, Kehinde O, Green H, and Gilchrest BA: Treatment of skin ulcers with cultured epidermal allografts, J Am Acad Dermatol 21:191-199, 1989.
85. Picus D et al: Radiographic imaging and treatment of vascular disease in the diabetic patient. In Levin ME and O'Neal LW, editors: The diabetic foot, ed 4, St. Louis, 1988, Mosby–Year Book, Inc.
86. Piulacks P and Vidal Barraquer F: Pathogenic study of varicose veins, Angiology 4:59-100, 1953.
87. Porter JM et al: Pentoxifylline therapy in intermittent claudication, Am Heart J 104:66, 1982.
88. Potter DA and Rose MB, editors: Cardiovascular system. In Assessment, Springhouse, Penn, 1983, Intermed Communications, Inc.
89. Raines J: Segmental plethysmography. In Rutherford RB, editor: Vascular surgery, ed 2, Philadelphia, 1983, WB Saunders Co.
90. Reed JW. Pressure ulcers in the elderly: prevention and treatment utilizing the team approach, Md State Med J 30:45-50, 1981.
91. Ross R: Pathophysiology of atherosclerosis. In Wilson SE et al, editors: Vascular surgery: principals and practice, New York, 1987, McGraw-Hill Book Co.
92. Ross R: The pathogenesis of atherosclerosis—an update, N Engl J Med 314:488, 1986.
93. Rutherford RB: Lumber sympathectomy: indications and technique. In Rutherford RB, editor: Vascular surgery, ed 2, Philadelphia, 1983, WB Saunders Co.
94. Rutherford RB: Nonoperative management of chronic peripheral arterial insufficiency. In Rutherford RB, editor: Vascular surgery, ed 2, Philadelphia, 1983, WB Saunders Co.
95. Rutherford R: Hemodynamics and diagnosis of arterial disease. In Rutherford R, editor: Vascular surgery, ed 3, Philadelphia, Penn, 1989, WB Saunders Co, vol 1, Sect II, pp 17-177.
96. Sapico FL et al: The infected foot of the diabetic patient: quantitative microbiology and analysis of clinical features, Rev Infect Dis 6(suppl 1):S171, 1984.
97. Scher LA, Samson RH, and Veith FJ: Combined aortoiliac and femoropopliteal occlusive disease. In Wilson SE et al, editors: Vascular surgery: principles and practice, New York, 1987, McGraw-Hill Book Co.
98. Sicard GA, Walker WB, and Anderson CB: Vascular surgery. In Levin ME and O'Neal LW, editors: The diabetic foot, ed 4, St. Louis, 1988, Mosby–Year Book, Inc.

99. Siegel ME et al: A new objective criteria for determining, noninvasively, the healing potential of an ischemic ulcer, J Nucl Med 22(2):187, 1981.
100. Strauss MB: Wound hypoxia, Curr Concepts Wound Care 9(4):16, 1986.
101. Sugarman B et al: Osteomyelitis beneath pressure sores, Arch Intern Med 143:683, 1983.
102. Teepe RGC, Koebrugge E, Ponec M, and Vermeer BJ: Fresh vs cryopreserved cultured allografts for the treatment of chronic skin ulcers, J Invest Dermatol 92:530, 1989.
103. Thomas S and Tucker CA: Sorbsan in the management of leg ulcers, The Pharmaceutical Journal 243:706-709, 1989.
104. Turner J: Nursing intervention in patients with peripheral vascular disease, Nurs Clin North Am 21(2):233, 1986.
105. Velasco M and Guaitero E: A comparative study of some antiinflammatory drugs in wound healing of the rat, Experientia 29:1250-1251, 1973.
106. Waldvogel FA, Medoff G, and Swartz MN: Osteomyelitis: a review of clinical features, therapeutic considerations and unusual aspects, N Engl J Med 282:198, 260, 316, 1979.
107. White RA and Klein SR: Chapter 6, Amputation level selection by transcutaneous oxygen pressure determination. In Moore WS and Malone JM, editors: Lower extremity amputation, Philadelphia, 1989, WB Saunders Co.
108. Whitney JD: Physiologic effects of tissue oxygenation on wound healing, Heart and Lung 18(5):466, 1989.
109. Williams GM: Peripheral vascular disease. In Harvey AM et al, editors: The principles and practice of medicine, ed 20, New York, 1980, Appleton-Century-Crofts.
110. Winston MA: Radioisotopes and their application to the study of peripheral vascular disease. In Wilson SE et al, editors: Vascular surgery: principles and practice, New York, 1987, McGraw-Hill Book Co.
111. Winter GD. Formation of scab and rate of epithelialization of superficial wounds in the skin of the domestic pig, Nature 193:293-294, 1962.
112. Wolfe JH, Morland M, and Browse NL: The fibrinolytic activity of varicose veins, Br J Surg 66:185-187, 1979.
113. Young JR: Differential diagnosis of leg ulcers, Cardiovasc Clin 13:171, 1983.

7 Management of Percutaneous Tubes

MICKEY YOUNG
ELAINE McCLURE
KATHI THIMSEN-WHITAKER

OBJECTIVES

1. Identify two primary reasons for use of percutaneous tubes.

2. List major content areas to be included in education for the patient with a percutaneous tube.

3. Describe the percutaneous endoscopic gastrostomy procedure and explain its advantages as compared to standard operative gastrostomy.

4. Explain the rationale for use of polyethylene or silicone tubes as opposed to latex tubes.

5. List advantages and disadvantages of the gastrostomy button.

6. Discuss guidelines for gastrostomy site selection.

7. Explain why tube stabilization is a priority in management of the patient with percutaneous tubes.

8. Describe at least two options for stabilization of gastrostomy or jejunostomy tubes.

9. Describe at least one option for management of persistent leakage around a percutaneous tube.

10. Identify two safe measures for preventing obstruction of gastrostomy and jejunostomy tubes.

11. Identify features of an effective pouching system for the patient with an empyema tube.

12. List the three most common complications associated with percutaneous nephrostomy tubes.

13. Describe at least two options for stabilization of a percutaneous nephrostomy tube.

14. Identify measures the nurse may utilize to prevent nephrostomy tube obstruction.

15. Describe measures that can be utilized to reduce the risk of infection in the patient with a percutaneous nephrostomy tube.

16. Describe routine site care for the patient with a percutaneous nephrostomy or biliary tube.

17. Identify at least two potential complications for the patient with a percutaneous biliary tube.

The use of tubes into the gastrointestinal tract for the purposes of feeding, decompression, or drainage was first described in the thirteenth century, though successful performance was not recorded until 1876 by Verneuil.[7] Today the use of tubes is commonplace; they may be placed on a temporary or a long-term basis, for the purposes of drainage and decompression, or for nutritional support.

Effective nursing management of the patient with tubes placed percutaneously requires an understanding of the anatomy and physiology of the affected body system, the pathology involved, and the rationale for tube placement. Although specific care procedures vary depending on the body system involved and the purpose of tube placement, management should always include routine care designed to maintain tube function, education for the patient or caregiver, and ongoing surveillance for early detection of complications. Comprehensive care is best provided with a collaborative team approach involving but not limited to the interventional radiologist, gastroenterologist, surgeon or internist, and nurse.

Patient education is a major nursing responsibility. Since the hospitalization period after tube placement may be brief, education is essential and outpatient follow-up care is usually required. The transition to self-care may be facilitated by home health care in addition to outpatient management. The nurse must continually assess the knowledge and self-care level of the patient or caregiver and provide additional teaching as indicated. Key content areas to be included in a patient teaching plan are listed in Box 7-1.

Another general concern in percutaneous tube management is prevention of complications, most notably infection. There is some controversy as to whether the use of preoperative antibiotics, administered either intravenously or orally, reduces the incidence of postoperative infection; therefore usage varies with body system involved, the patient's status and physician preference.[7] Postoperative measures to reduce the risk of infection are listed in Box 7-2.

Box 7-1   KEY CONTENT FOR PATIENT EDUCATION

Purpose and procedure for tube insertion	Signs and symptoms of complications,
Normal tube function	and appropriate response
Tube stabilization	Tube feeding schedule and procedure
Routine care and hygiene	(when applicable)

Box 7-2   MEASURES TO REDUCE INFECTION

Minimize handling and manipulation of tubes.

Use gloves and aseptic technique when handling the tube, dressings, or stabilization devices.

Teach the patient aseptic technique for self-care. In the home setting, gloves may or may not be required depending on the tube site and the patient's overall health status.[10]

Follow universal precautions when providing percutaneous tube care.

GASTROSTOMY AND JEJUNOSTOMY TUBES

A gastrostomy is an opening into the stomach, whereas a jejunostomy is an opening into the jejunal portion of the small intestine. These procedures may be used to provide gastric or small bowel decompression, or to provide enteral support for a patient unable to ingest adequate nutrients orally.[25]

Placement Procedures

Gastrostomy procedures were first performed successfully from 1875 to 1877.[6,7,12] For over a century, gastrostomy and jejunostomy required a surgical intervention involving anesthesia and the traditional preoperative preparation for abdominal surgery. Historically, in the immediate postoperative period, gastrostomy and jejunostomy tubes were immobilized by placement of a suture around the base of the tube near the skin level and suturing of the tube to the skin. Gastrostomy tubes were usually connected to suction for 12 to 24 hours for the purpose of reducing tension on the suture line. Feedings were delayed until bowel sounds, tube patency, and proper placement of the tube were confirmed.[21]

Presently, a gastrostomy or jejunostomy is created by means of a surgical, endoscopic or radiologic approach. The numerous techniques available are summarized in Table 7-1. The two most common surgical techniques are known as the Stamm and the Janeway. A Stamm gastrostomy is created when one makes a "stab wound" surgical incision over the body of the stomach; a catheter is then inserted through this incision and placed inside the stomach (Fig. 7-1). Although the Stamm gastrostomy is easy to create and remove, it is frequently difficult to manage and is plagued with peritubular leakage.[32]

A Janeway gastrostomy is a surgically constructed mucosa-lined gastrostoma that is intubated as needed for feeding or decompression. Fig. 7-2 illustrates how the Janeway is constructed. This type of permanent gastrostomy requires more operative time than the Stamm gastrostomy and results in many similar complications. Surgical construction of a jejunostomy is quite varied; a more comprehensive review of jejunostomy construction can be found in the literature.[6]

Although the placement and care of a gastrostomy or jejunostomy tube may appear to be relatively simple, such tubes are associated with numerous significant complications (Table 7-2). The types of patients who typically require these tubes is a major reason for the high morbidity; patients are commonly debilitated and malnourished.[6,32] For these reasons, the surgical approach is quickly being replaced by the endoscopic or radiographic approach.[16,20]

Text continued on p. 221

Table 7-1 Descriptive summary of common gastric and jejunal tube feeding enterostomies (TFEs): techniques, advantages/disadvantages, and nursing care considerations.[*][†]

Type	Placement technique	Advantages	Disadvantages	Tube/skin care
Stamm gastrostomy (temporary)	Subcostal incision through abdominal wall creating serosa-lined tract; stomach sutured to wall for stabilization; balloon-tipped catheter passed through tract and sutured in place; after inflation, balloon rests snugly against abdominal wall for additional stabilization	• Simple surgical procedure requiring limited operating room time • Can be performed under local anesthesia • Large-diameter feeding tube reduces incidence of tube occlusion	• Spontaneous tract closure after tube removal or dislodgment • Potential deflation of catheter balloon permits tube migration or dislodgment • High incidence of peritubular leakage with rapid skin destruction r/t enlargement of enterostomal opening associated with large-diameter feeding tube	• Observe daily for tube dislodgment, leakage, and skin irritation • Daily cleansing of skin with H_2O_2 followed by NS rinse or per hospital routine; if unpouched, cover with small fenestrated dressing • If leakage develops, pouching is recommended • External anchoring of feeding tube is recommended • HOB at 30 degrees for feedings to prevent gastroesophageal reflux

*From Bodnar B and Fraher J: Tube feeding enterostomies: indications, techniques and management strategies. In Engelking C, editor: Progressions: Developments in Ostomy and Wound Care 1(2), [8], summer 1989, Mosby-Year Book (Journal Dept.), St. Louis.

†Data from (1) Jarvis-Perrault J et al: Ostomy Wound Management 21:60-63, 1988; (2) Brewer C: J Enterostom Ther 14:163-167, 1987; (3) and (4) McGee L: J Enterostom Ther 14:73-78 and 201-211, 1987.

HOB, Head of bed; *NS*, normal saline; *r/t*, related to; *PEG*, percutaneous endoscopic gastrostomy (or jejunostomy); *S&S*, signs and symptoms.

Table 7-1 Cont'd

Type	Placement technique	Advantages	Disadvantages	Tube/skin care
Percutaneous endoscopic gastrostomy (temporary)	Gastroscope inserted through mouth into stomach; stomach inflated with air and transilluminated at desired puncture site; No. 16 needle passed through abdominal wall at identified site into stomach; suture wire passed through needle into stomach and grasped by endoscopy snare; gastroscope and suture removed from stomach; suture tied to distal end of feeding tube and pulled through alimentary tract and abdominal wall; anchored with internal and external bridges	• Simple procedure performed nonsurgically in endoscopy suite or at bedside • General anesthesia avoided • More cost-effective and less morbidity than surgically created TFE	• Spontaneous tract closure after tube removal or dislodgment • High incidence of tube occlusion r/t small-diameter feeding tube lumen	• Observe daily for tube dislodgment, leakage, skin irritation, S&S infection • Daily cleansing of skin with H_2O_2 followed by NS rinse or per hospital routine; be sure to slide external bridge away for cleansing and then reposition; no dressing required after cleansing • Avoid tube occlusion by regular flushing; administering low-viscosity viscosity feedings with enteral feeding pump and medications in liquid preparations • HOB at 30 degrees for feedings to prevent gastroesophageal reflux

Table 7-1 Cont'd

Type	Placement technique	Advantages	Disadvantages	Tube/skin care
Janeway gastrostomy (permanent)	Rectangular mucosal flap cut from mid-anterior stomach wall; stomach defect closed; flap used to construct mucosa-lined tube; end of tube pulled through rectus muscle and brought out onto abdomen; stoma constructed	• Permanent stoma; risk of tube dislodgment eliminated; intubated for feedings only • Simplest surgical technique for establishing permanent gastrostomy	• Requires surgical procedure under general anesthesia • High incidence of leakage and subsequent peristomal skin erosion r/t gastric incontinence	• Observe daily for reflux and peristomal skin irritation; report occurrence of reflux • Daily cleansing with soap and water • Apply 2 by 2 gauze dressing when not in use for feedings • If leakage develops, pouching is recommended • Feeding tube remains in place until tract heals (1-2 wk); teach patient and family to intubate stoma intermittently for feedings once healing has occurred • HOB at 30 degrees for feedings to prevent gastroesophageal reflux

Table 7-1 Cont'd

Type	Placement technique	Advantages	Disadvantages	Tube/skin care
Spivak gastrostomy (permanent)	Similar to Janeway procedure with surgically created valve to achieve continence; accomplished by fundoplication at base of gastric tube	• Permanent stoma; risk of tube dislodgment eliminated; intubated for feedings only • Continence mechanism reduces incidence of leakage and subsequent peristomal skin erosion	• Requires complex surgical procedure under general anesthesia	See Janeway
Percutaneous endoscopic jejunostomy (temporary)	Extension of PEG procedure; small feeding tube passed through PEG into duodenum via endoscope; tube propelled by peristalsis into jejunum; anchored with internal and external bridges	See PEG ↓ Incidence of gastroesophageal reflux phenomenon and potential for aspiration	See PEG	See PEG
Witzel jejunostomy (temporary)	Subserosal tunnel constructed in jejunum by placing catheter in jejunum, folding exterior serosa over catheter and suturing it in place; distal end of catheter is brought out through a stab wound onto the abdomen and sutured in place; jejunum is then fixed to the abdominal wall	• Can be performed either as adjunctive procedure during abdominal surgery or as primary procedure under local anesthesia • Permits use of a larger feeding tube (i.e., 12-16 Fr), which reduces incidence of tube occlusion	• Spontaneous tract closure after tube removal or dislodgment	• Observe daily for S&S infection, tube dislodgment, leakage, and/or skin irritation • Cleanse skin with H_2O_2 followed by NS rinse or providone-iodine every 48 hr and apply gauze dressing, or apply transparent occlusive dressing for 5-7 days to anchor catheter; if gauze dressing used, tape catheter securely to abdomen

Table 7-1 Cont'd

Type	Placement technique	Advantages	Disadvantages	Tube/skin care
Needle catheter jejunostomy (temporary)	Similar to Witzel except jejunum accessed percutaneously via large-bore hollow needle through which small catheter is threaded; needle is removed once catheter is in place	• Performed as an adjunctive procedure during abdominal surgery, adding little additional operating time	• Spontaneous tract closure after tube removal or dislodgment • High incidence of tube (catheter) occlusion r/t small luminal diameter	See Witzel
Roux-en-Y (permanent)	Jejunum is severed; distal end brought out onto abdomen through stab wound stoma created; proximal portion looped up and sewn to abdominal wall; end anastomosed to distal portion	• Permanent stoma; risk of tube dislodgment eliminated; intubated for feedings only • ↓ Incidence of gastroesophageal reflux phenomenon and potential for aspiration	• Requires complex surgical procedure under general anesthesia	See Janeway and Spivak • Also observe for fistula formation and wound dehiscence

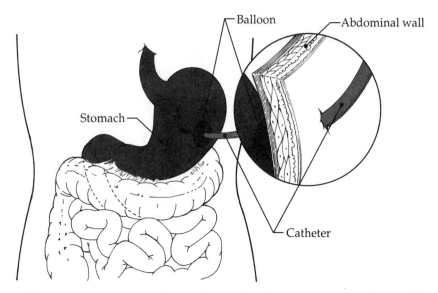

Fig. 7-1 Stamm gastrostomy, oblique view. An incision is placed through the abdominal wall into the stomach, through which a catheter is passed.

The endoscopic approach to gastrostomy tube placement was first reported in 1980; by the late 1980s, percutaneous endoscopic gastrostomy (PEG) had become the procedure of choice[6,16,20] (Fig. 7-3). After application of a topical pharyngeal anesthetic and sedation, an endoscope is passed into the stomach. With the Gardner-Ponsky method of placement, the stomach is distended with air and the proposed gastrostomy site is transilluminated.[14] A small incision is made over the illuminated site and a large-gauge Medicut catheter is inserted into the stomach. The needle is then withdrawn and 60 inches of silk suture are passed through the cannula into the stomach. The endoscopist then grasps the silk suture and pulls one end up and out through the mouth while the endoscope is removed. During this step the other end of the silk suture is held by an assistant so that the silk suture now passes through the oral cavity and esophagus and out through the stomach. The proximal (oral) end of the silk suture is then secured to the distal (external) end of the gastrostomy tube. The silk suture and attached tube is then pulled down through the esophagus, stomach, and abdominal wall until the gastrostomy tube is correctly positioned within the stomach (that is, snugly against the anterior stomach wall). These tubes are equipped or fashioned with an internal "bumper," which helps stabilize the tube. At this point, the endoscope is again inserted, and the endoscopist verifies appropriate placement.[6,20] Once placement is confirmed, the tube is secured to the abdominal wall with an external "bumper," fixation disk, or tube attachment device.

Recent advances have led to the development of a radiographic approach to percutaneous gastrostomy tube placement. In the radiographic approach the stomach is dilated with air and a needle is percutaneously inserted into the stomach. A J-wire is threaded into the stomach under fluoroscopic guidance, and the needle is then withdrawn. A 1 cm long incision is made into the skin at the exit site of the wire. When entry into the stomach has been determined, the tract is slowly dilated and the permanent catheter is inserted. These

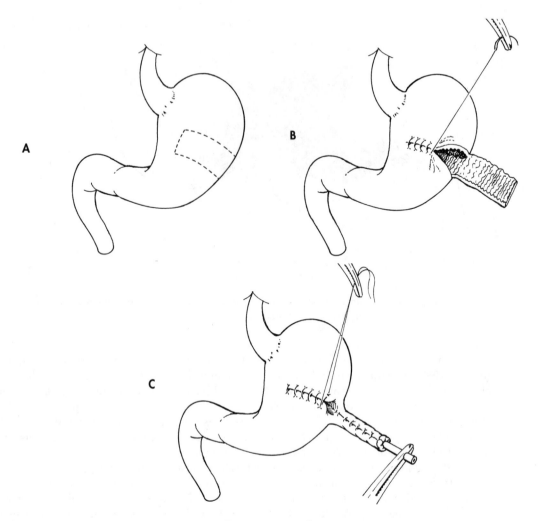

Fig. 7-2   Diagram of construction of Janeway gastrostomy.

catheters usually have a balloon, which is inflated and positioned snugly against the gastric wall; stabilization at the skin surface is achieved by use of a suture or a tube stabilization device.

As noted in Table 7-2, these nonsurgical approaches have a lower complication rate and are more cost effective than surgical methods and can be performed on an outpatient basis.[16]

Types of Tubes

Gastrostomy and jejunostomy tubes have traditionally been made of latex. More recently, polyurethane and silicone have been used; these materials are associated with less soft-tissue reaction and longer wear time. Table 7-3 summarizes advantages and disadvantages of various tube materials.[8] Table 7-4 describes the products.

Table 7-2 Complications of surgical versus percutaneous gastrostomy placement

	Surgical (N = 100)	Percutaneous (N = 1471)
30-day mortality	12 (12%)	10 (0.6%)
Morbidity	8 (8%)	2 (0.0%)
Intraperitoneal leak	1 (1%)	1 (0.06%)
Infusion of enteral nutrient	—	1 (0.1%)
Wound infection	5 (5%)	53 (0.3%)
Aspiration requiring tracheal intubation	10 (10%)	0
Stomal leaks	14 (14%)	24 (1.6%)
Pneumoperitoneum	0	23 (1.5%)
Tube dislodgment	12 (12%)	22 (1.4%)
Perforation and peritonitis	0	6 (0.4%)
Myocardial infarct	3%	—
Bleeding	—	6 (0.4%)
Gastrocolic fistula	—	5 (0.3%)
Aspirations	—	40 (2.7%)
Placement failure	—	4 (0.2%)
Ileus	—	4 (0.2%)

From Ho CS, Yee AC, and McPherson R: Gastroenterology 95(5):1206, 1988, and Molnar W and Stockum AE: Am J Roentgenol 122:35-367, 1974.

The triple-lumen gastrostomy tube may be indicated for patients who require both proximal decompression and enteral feeding. There are three outlets to this tube: a gastric lumen for gastric suction, a proximal duodenal lumen for duodenal suction, and a distal duodenal lumen for feeding. There is a gastric balloon, which is inflated with sterile water; this helps to maintain proper tube placement. Placement is further enhanced when the tube is secured at skin level with a retaining disk.

Recently a device that is flush with the abdominal surface known as a gastrostomy "button" has been developed. The button was first developed for use in children who require long-term gastrostomy feedings. It is a short silicone tube with a flip-top opening, a one-way antireflux valve (to prevent leakage of stomach contents around the tube) and a radiopaque dome that fits snug against the stomach wall[11-13] (Fig. 7-4).

To administer feedings, an adapter is passed through the one-way valve and connected to a feeding catheter. When the feeding is completed, the tube is flushed with water, the adapter is removed, and the flip-top opening is closed.

A button can be inserted in a clinic setting and does not require anesthesia. To have a button inserted, the patient must have a well-established gastrostomy tract with at least an 18 to 20 French diameter. The device is available in different "shaft" lengths and diameters. Correct shaft length is critical to ensure the proper position of the dome of the button against the anterior stomach wall, hence preventing gastric reflux around the button. By insertion of a special measuring device into the tract, the appropriate shaft length is determined. An obturator is then inserted into the button to straighten the dome of the button making insertion of the button into the tract possible. The button should be lubricated to facilitate insertion. Once it is in place, the obturator is removed and the flip-top opening closed.

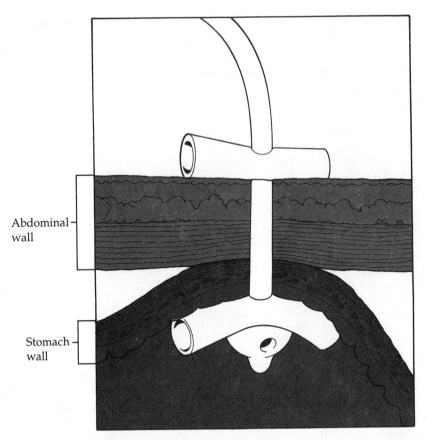

Fig. 7-3   Percutaneous endoscopic gastrostomy (PEG). Notice internal bumper against anterior stomach wall and external bumper at skin level.

Disadvantages of the button include expense, the potential for dysfunction of the antireflux valve with subsequent leakage, the need for replacement every 3 to 4 months, and the inability to provide adequate decompression when necessary. Studies and refinements of the device are ongoing; current reports demonstrate good success, few complications, and high user satisfaction.[10,13]

Nursing Management

Optimal management for patients requiring long-term gastrostomy or jejunostomy tubes begins in the preplacement phase. Assessment of each patient should include the reason for the tube alternatives, risks and benefits associated with various treatment options, and the commitment of the patient or caregiver to long-term management. It is important to provide preplacement instruction and to discuss the above issues with the patient and family.

When possible, the site for tube placement is selected preoperatively to reduce the potential for complications and to facilitate self-care. Site selection is based on the following principles:

Table 7-3   Types of gastrostomy and jejunostomy tubes

Type	Advantage	Disadvantage	Examples
Latex	Inexpensive Easily replaced Comfortable Easily cleaned Inflatable balloons	Inflation port weakens with bending of tube Balloon deflates easily Retains odors 3 to 6 months use	Foley catheters
Polyurethane	Inflatable balloons Moderately priced Easily cleaned Large inner diameter (good flow rate) Replaced easily	Expensive	Ross Sacks-Vine Sheridan-Moss Silk
Silicone	Comfortable Does not retain odors Easily cleaned Long term use over 6 months	Expensive, small inner diameter (slow flow rate) Cannot piggyback fluids Reduces peristomal skin inflammation	MIC (Medical Innovations Corp.); Silastic Foley

Table 7-4   Description of products

Brand name	Length (inches)	Diameter (French)	Balloon (ml)
LATEX TYPE			
Bard	10-16	8-30	3, 5, 10, 30
Biosearch: Entri-replacement	37, 16	12, 16	30
POLYURETHANE TYPE			
Biosearch PEG	30, 38	16, 20	—
Ross:			
Sacks–Vine G	17, 18	14, 18	NA
Sacks–Vine J	30, 36	9, 12	NA
Sacks–Vine G-J	36	18(G), 9(J)	NA
Sheridan-Moss	18	18	NA
Silk	22	6, 8, 10	NA
SILICONE TYPE			
Button, Stomate	0.6, 0.7, 0.9, 1.1, 1.3, 1.7	18, 24, 28	NA
MIC: G-Tube	9	12-24	5-28
Ross:		18	NA
Replacement G	7.5		

NA, Not applicable.

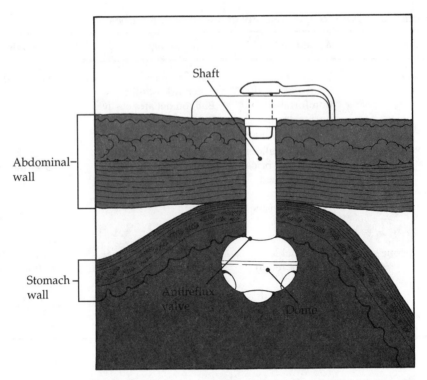

Fig. 7-4 Gastrostomy button demonstrating how stability is achieved by use of correct shaft length so that dome is positioned against anterior stomach wall. (Modified from Foutch PG, Talbert GA, Gaianes JA, and Sanowski RA: Gastrointest Endosc 35:41, 1989.)

- Position the site approximately 5 cm to the left of the midline and 5 cm below the left costal margin.
- Avoid the costal margin to reduce discomfort from tube migration with normal respiratory excursion.
- Avoid the umbilicus, the vertical dropoff of the costal margin, the belt line, and any folds, creases, and wrinkles. (The patient should be assessed in both the lying and the sitting positions.)
- Locate and avoid the left lobe of the liver.[20]

The most common complications related to gastrostomy or jejunostomy placement are leakage of gastric or jejunal contents around the tube onto the skin and tube dislodgment (Table 7-2). These complications are frequently attributed to the failure to adequately stabilize the tube. Therefore postplacement nursing management must include measures to stabilize the tube.[21,31]

Adequate tube stabilization is characterized by three objectives: (1) ensure proper balloon placement against the anterior stomach wall; (2) minimize lateral movement in the tube at skin level; and (3) prevent tube migration (in and out movements). Proper balloon placement is essential to prevent reflux of contents around the tube onto the skin and is achieved when (1) the balloon is inflated with an adequate volume of water or air (in accordance with the manufacturer's guidelines and institutional protocols), and (2) the balloon is snugly positioned against the anterior wall of the stomach. The balloon on catheters placed in the jejunum, however, is not inflated; an inflated balloon within the jejunum is sufficient to obstruct the jejunum.

Lateral movement of the tube contributes to leakage of gastric contents onto the skin by eroding the tissue along the tract. Inflammation of the site can also develop from the presence of this chronic irritant. A stabilized tube should not allow lateral movement of the tube.

Migration of the tube in and out of the tract must be prevented. Nonstabilized tubes are subject to migration as a result of gastric motility and abdominal wall motion; the tube can actually migrate and obstruct the gastric outlet and compromise tube function.

Historically sutures have been used to stabilize tubes. Unfortunately sutures can cause tearing of the skin with subsequent inflammation and pain at the suture site. Although sutures prevent tube migration, sutures do not eliminate lateral tube movement.[27]

Baby nipples are also used to secure gastrostomy tubes. Typically the nipple is cut along one edge, wrapped around the tube, and secured with tape as the tube exits from the nipple. Although quite popular and readily available, this technique, in isolation, is not completely effective at preventing lateral movement or tube migration. Effective tube stabilization can be accomplished only with a baby nipple when it is used with tape to secure the nipple to the abdomen (Fig. 7-5) or with a skin-barrier flange (Fig. 7-6). Box 7-3 describes these two methods of tube stabilization.

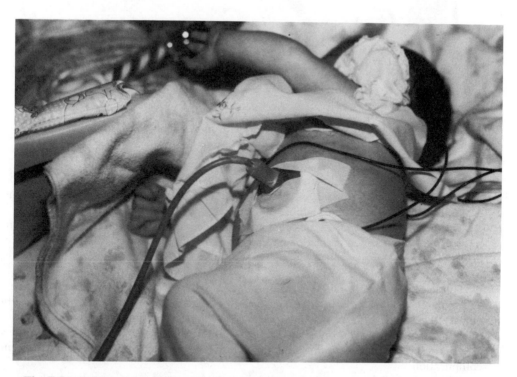

Fig. 7-5   Appropriate stabilization of gastrostomy tube using a nipple that is taped to the skin; gauze has been place between the skin and the nipple though a solid-wafer skin barrier could also be used. (Courtesy Abbott Northwestern Hospital, Minneapolis.)

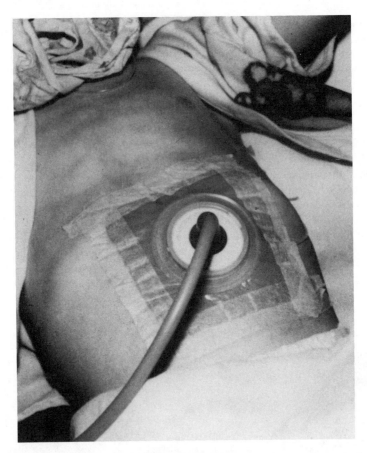

Fig. 7-6   Gastrostomy tube secured in place with baby nipple and skin-barrier wafer flange with convex insert. (Courtesy Abbott Northwestern Hospital, Minneapolis.)

Commercial external tube stabilization devices are also available. Table 7-5 compares the advantages and disadvantages of the commercial stabilization devices. Fig. 7-7 shows examples of commercial tube stabilization devices.

The tube stabilization system is changed as needed: frequency is determined by the need to assess the tube site or provide site care. When frequent site care is required (as with newly placed tubes), a stabilization system that allows easy visualization of the site without removal of adhesives is desirable.

For selected patients the stabilization system may be discontinued once the tube site and tract are well healed (Fig. 7-8). This usually occurs in 5 to 6 weeks after tube placement unless the patient is receiving corticosteroids, is immune compromised, or is malnourished.[9] Before discontinuing stabilization measures, the nurse must assess the site to ensure that the tract is well granulated and that tube migration is no longer a potential complication.

Many tubes are being created specifically as gastrostomy tubes complete with stabilization features inherent in the design, thereby eliminating the need for external stabilization

Box 7-3 METHODS OF TUBE STABILIZATION WITH BABY NIPPLE

USE OF BABY NIPPLE WITH SKIN-BARRIER WAFER

Cut skin-barrier wafer to size of stomal opening at tube exit site.

Slit skin-barrier wafer along one edge so that wafer can be positioned around tube.

Remove protective paper backing and apply wafer to skin.

Slit baby nipple along one side and position baby nipple around tube.

Secure baby nipple to wafer and tube with tape.

USE OF BABY NIPPLE WITH SKIN-BARRIER FLANGE AND CONVEX INSERT

Cut opening in 1½-inch skin-barrier flange the size of stomal opening at tube exit site.

Peel off protective paper backing and apply barrier flange to skin.

Slit baby nipple along one side and position baby nipple around tube so that the wide part of the nipple fits inside the flange.

Feeding the tube through the center of a convex insert (1¼-inch internal diameter), snap the convex insert into place inside the flange, securing the nipple. For ease of application, the convex insert can be applied so that the curve projects *away* from the patient's skin.

Tape baby nipple to tube.

NOTE: A 1¼-inch skin-barrier flange can also be used. The wide end of the baby nipple will fit into the flange and is then secured with tape instead of a convex insert.

---

devices. For example, the button has a dome, limited shaft length, and flip-top cap to ensure stabilization of the tube. The internal and external bumper present with percutaneous endoscopic gastrostomies provide tube stabilization. A few Silastic catheter feeding tubes (with a balloon to secure the tube against the anterior stomach wall) have an adjustable external "flange" (Fig. 7-9). Once the Silastic catheter is in position and the balloon is inflated, the "flange" is slid down against the skin, hence stabilizing the catheter without the use of adhesives.

As stated previously, leakage around the tube site is a frequent complication. Leakage warrants a thorough evaluation of the adequacy of tube stabilization, appropriate balloon placement, and tube patency. Steps must be taken to correct any possible cause for the leakage. When drainage is persistent, methods to contain the drainage and protect the skin must be implemented. Hydrocolloids and absorbent dressings are not appropriate because they will trap drainage against the skin and cause chemical irritation. Plate 2 demonstrates chemical irritation from reflux of gastric contents onto the skin.

To manage drainage around a tube site, one can apply an ostomy pouch and catheter port. By attaching a catheter port to the pouch, one can have the tube exit the wall of the pouch through the port and allow feeding, suction, or gravity drainage to continue; the pouch then contains the peritubular drainage (Fig. 7-10). Such a pouching system is cost effective and allows collection, identification, and measurement of the drainage as well as skin protection. Instructions for containing peritubular leakage are outlined in Box 7-4.

Table 7-5 External tube stabilization devices

Device trade name	Advantages	Disadvantages
Hollister: Drain/Tube Attachment Device	Accommodates tube sizes 12 to 22 French Attached skin barrier Easy to apply	Will not accommodate very small or large tubes Securing clamp difficult to adjust Drainage will not be contained or absorbed Cannot be reused
VPI: Edelman Device	Flexible Accommodates wide variety of tube sizes Securing device easy to adjust Reusable Durable construction Range of sizes can accommodate a wide variety of tube sizes including very small or large tubes	No attached skin barrier Must obtain appropriate-size device if tube size is changed Not adjustable
Kells: Tube Anchor	Will accommodate a variety of tube sizes Durable construction Inexpensive Easy to apply	No attached skin barrier Drainage will not be contained or absorbed Cannot be reused

Frequency of pouch change is determined by the duration of the pouch seal, with an average frequency being every 4 to 7 days.

The care plan should also incorporate measures to prevent or manage tube obstruction, such as selection of a formula with the appropriate viscosity for the intraluminal diameter of the tube, thorough flushing after administration of medications or feedings, and irrigation with a 30 to 50 ml of diet carbonated beverage every 4 hours and as needed to promote tube patency.[8,23] In the past, the use of meat tenderizers and bicarbonate solution was common; however, recent controversy over this practice has emerged after reports of life-threatening electrolyte shifts after instillation of these substances.[23] The insertion site and surrounding tissue should also be monitored for signs and symptoms of infection (that is, erythema, induration, and pain). Soft-tissue infections should be managed with culture-based antibiotics.

EMPYEMA (CHEST) TUBES

Empyema is defined as the presence of pus in a body cavity, particularly the presence of a purulent exudate within the pleural cavity. This complication occurs in the postoperative phase of thoracic procedures such as pneumonectomy.

Symptoms of empyema include dyspnea, coughing, unilateral chest pain, malaise, and fever. Diagnostic tests involve chest computerized tomography (CT) scan and thoracentesis

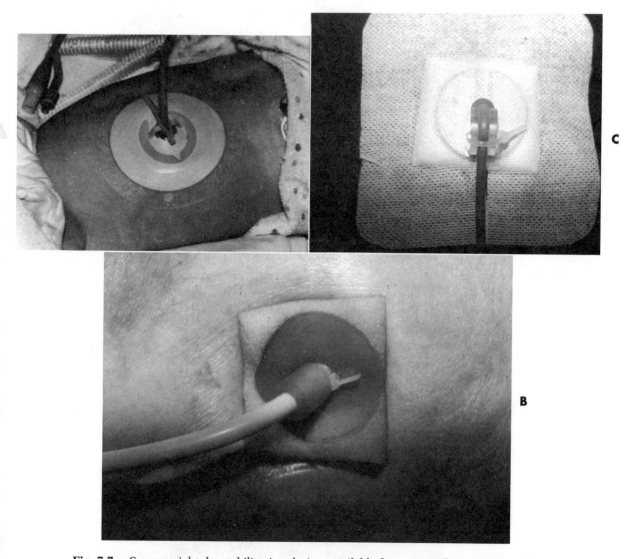

Fig. 7-7   Commercial tube stabilization devices available from, **A,** Hollister, Chicago; **B,** Cook Urological/Vance Products, Inc., Spencer, Indiana; and, **C,** Kells Medical Inc., Burr Ridge, Illinois.

or needle aspiration to determine the specific causative organism. Medical management includes rest, antibiotic therapy, and continuous drainage of the chest cavity by intubation. The chest catheter is connected to a waterseal drain for several days to provide adequate drainage and promote lung expansion. Successful drainage of the empyema may eliminate the need for a thoracotomy.[1,4]

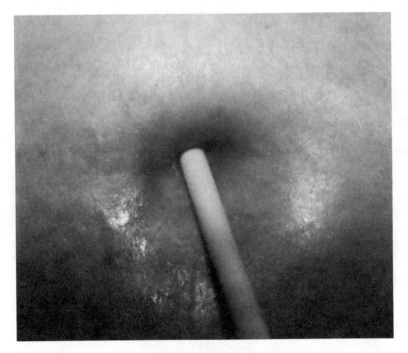

Fig. 7-8   Established (matured) gastrostomy tube site. (Courtesy Nancy Faller, Mendon, Vermont.)

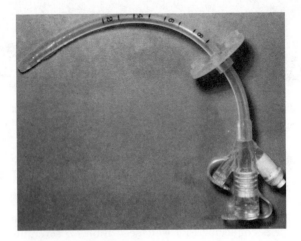

Fig. 7-9   Silicone elastic (Silastic) feeding tube with an adjustable external "flange" that stabilizes the tube against the skin.

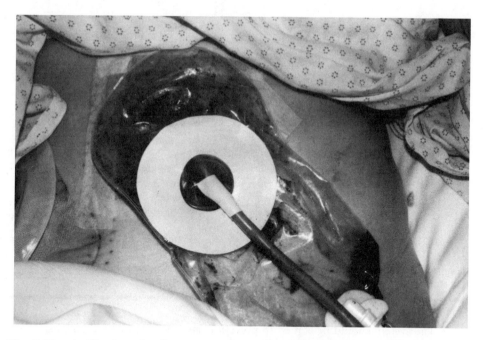

Fig. 7-10   Application of catheter access device to an ostomy pouch to manage peritubular drainage. (Courtesy Abbott Northwestern Hospital, Minneapolis.)

Placement Procedures

An empyema tube may be required for long-term use if the pyogenic infection becomes chronic and surgical intervention is contraindicated. Insertion of a 28 to 32 French chest tube can be performed with local anesthesia. The tube is made of a firm plastic material; approximately 1 to 3 inches of the external portion of the tube protrudes from the chest wall. This length may be shortened to promote comfort and to facilitate drainage.[30] To stabilize the tube and to prevent migration or retraction into the chest cavity, a safety pin or a 2-inch plastic rod should be inserted through the tube. (Safety pins must be replaced regularly because they will rust.) The plastic rod can be cleansed with soap and water when the drainage collection pouch is replaced.

When water-seal drainage is discontinued, application of a drainable stoma pouch is recommended to protect the skin and clothing, control odor, and facilitate resumption of daily activities (Fig. 7-11). The following factors should be considered when one is selecting an appropriate pouching system:

- The pouch should be drainable so that it can be emptied as needed. If a urinary pouch is used, the antireflux valve must be removed or inactivated to facilitate drainage of thick exudate.
- A skin-barrier wafer should be used; a skin-barrier wafer with low meltdown potential is recommended because it will provide greater protection and prolong wear time.[18,30] An additional skin-barrier ring may be applied around the tube and under the skin barrier to act as a cushion and increase comfort.

Box 7-4   POUCHING PROCEDURE FOR LEAKAGE AROUND TUBE

1. Assemble pouch and catheter access device.
   - Cut opening in barrier and pouch to accommodate tube site.
   - Make small slit in anterior surface of pouch.
   - Attach an access device to the anterior surface of the pouch.
   - Tear paper backing on pouch or wafer but leave in place.
2. Prepare skin.
   - Clean and dry skin.
   - Treat any denuded skin (skin-barrier powder to denuded area; water or skin sealant if needed to make powder tacky).
   - Apply thin layer of skin-barrier paste to skin around insertion site, if needed.
3. Disconnect and plug tube.
4. Feed catheter through opening in pouch. Use water-soluble lubricant to pass tube, and use hemostat to pull tube through the pouch or barrier opening, anterior wall of the pouch, and the access device.
5. Reconnect tube.
6. Assure dry skin; remove paper backing from wafer and secure pouch to skin.
7. Secure tube to stabilization device with tape.

- The system should be vented to prevent excessive inflation and collapse of the pouch with normal respirations. Options for venting include use of a filtered pouch, addition of an adhesive filter to the pouching system (Fig. 7-11), or use of a small flexible "vent" catheter inserted into the superior aspect of the pouch.

The pouch should be changed frequently enough to prevent erosion of the skin barrier with resulting skin breakdown and leakage. Optimal frequency must be determined for the individual patient, but the range is usually 4 or 5 days.

Nursing Management

The patient with an empyema tube requires meticulous nursing care to maintain tube patency, control odor, promote comfort, and provide needed emotional support. The nurse must closely monitor the patency of the tube and volume of the drainage so that any suspected obstruction can be promptly reported. Irrigation of empyema tubes is usually not recommended. Measures to control odor include use of an odorproof pouch, a deodorizing filter to "vent" the pouch, meticulous hygiene, and a pouch or room deodorizer. Comfort measures are of particular importance because of the tube's rigid construction and intercostal location. Soft rolled gauze may be taped in place around the tube to provide support and to limit tube manipulation with patient movement. Two small pillows (not to exceed 3 inches in thickness) may be placed under the shoulder and directly under the tube to facilitate rest and sleep. Foam wedges are another option for positioning. Emotional support is critical because most patients with empyema have been critically ill as a result of the underlying disease or trauma. Patients and families need support to deal with the empyema and the pouching system, as well as practical instruction in self-care and tube management.

PERCUTANEOUS NEPHROSTOMY TUBES

Percutaneous nephrostomy tubes are inserted to provide temporary or permanent drainage of the urinary collection system in the presence of obstructive uropathy of the

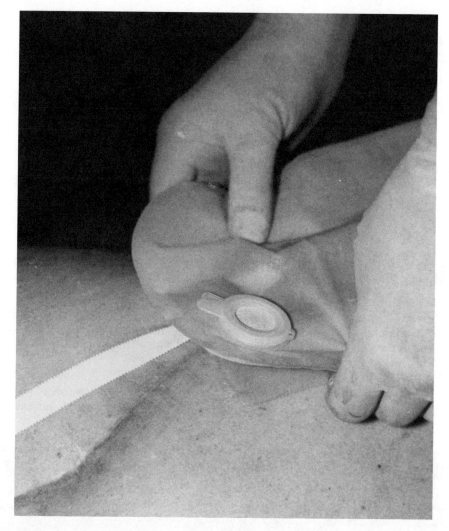

Fig. 7-11   Drainage around an empyema tube managed with pouch; gas filter acts as a vent. (Courtesy Phyllis Kohlman, Newport News, Va.)

lower urinary tract. Percutaneous nephrostomy tubes are also utilized after surgical stone extraction to ensure low intrapelvic pressure in the kidney and to promote healing of urinary tract injuries such as tears and perforations.[26]

Placement Procedures

Placement of nephrostomy tubes is usually performed by a radiologist under fluoroscopy. Under local anesthesia the nephrostomy tube is inserted through the patient's side or back and is positioned in the renal pelvis of the kidney (Fig. 7-12).

Percutaneous nephrostomy tubes are usually small-lumen polyethylene catheters (Fig. 7-13). However, Foley catheters are occasionally utilized and, less frequently, the U tube.

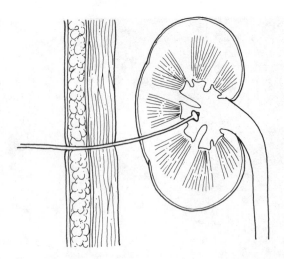

Fig. 7-12 Nephrostomy tube placed in renal pelvis. (From Broadwell DC and Jackson BS, editors: Principles of ostomy care, St Louis, 1983, Mosby–Year Book, Inc.)

When a Foley catheter is used, balloon inflation varies with physician preference and patient condition. The U-tube nephrostomy has an entry and exit point through the kidney as well as the skin, and the two ends are connected with a Y connector.

Nursing Management

Immediately after insertion of a new nephrostomy tube the patient should be monitored closely for gross hematuria. Small amounts of hematuria is expected, but frank bleeding

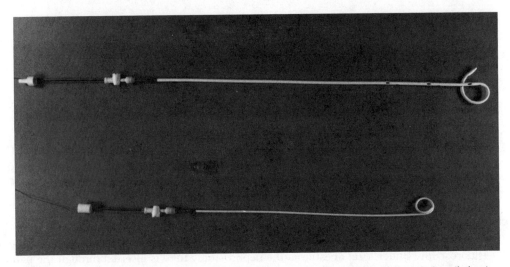

Fig. 7-13 Sample catheters commonly used for percutaneous nephrostomy tubes *(below)* and biliary tubes *(above)*.

usually indicates hemorrhage, a potential complication because of the high vascularity of the kidney. Monitoring should include vital signs and accurate intake and output. Leakage from the nephrostomy tract is normal until the tract heals and closes around the tube, which usually occurs in 7 to 10 days.

Stabilization of the percutaneous nephrostomy tube is essential to prevent dislodgment and trauma to renal tissue from catheter mobility. There are several methods utilized for tube stabilization. Nephrostomy tubes may be sutured to the skin by the physician; although this is acceptable as a temporary measure, use of sutures for more than a few weeks commonly results in local inflammation at the suture sites.[31] The sutures become painful, may pull loose from the skin, and can become infected; thus long-term stabilization requires alternative approaches.

Temporary nephrostomy tubes secured by sutures may be managed as follows: Cleanse the insertion site with an antiseptic solution, rinse and dry the area, apply an antibiotic or antiseptic ointment around the insertion site, and cover with a dry sterile dressing. If there is minor leakage around the tube in the first 7 to 10 days after tube placement, it may be helpful to apply a thin skin-barrier wafer (cut to fit around the tube) under the dressing to protect the skin. If leakage is severe, persistent, or recurrent, the patient *must* be carefully reevaluated for accurate tube placement and tube patency.

The most common complications of percutaneous tubes are dislodgment, blockage, and infection. Therefore, long-term management of percutaneous nephrostomy tubes should include measures to ensure catheter stabilization, prevent infection, maintain tube patency, protect the skin, and facilitate home care.

Tube stabilization prevents catheter mobility and migration, which can result in renal damage and infection and catheter dislodgment. There are several approaches that have been used to provide long-term stabilization of nephrostomy tubes (Box 7-5 and Figs. 7-14 and 15).[5,9,22,31] There are many variations on these approaches, with the goal being to devise a method that is effective and manageable for the patient and caregiver.

Box 7-5   STABILIZATION OPTIONS FOR PERCUTANEOUS NEPHROSTOMY TUBES

CONWILL'S TECHNIQUE[5] (Fig. 7-14)
- Supplies needed: skin barrier wafer with flange, convex insert, and suture
- Procedure:
  Cut wafer out to fit around tube and apply wafer to skin.
  Wrap the suture around the tube, and bring the two ends of the suture over the flange.
  Snap convex insert into flange to secure the suture.

MCKEE AND SHEER'S TECHNIQUE[20]
- Supplies needed: Two solid-wafer skin barriers
- Procedure:
  Cut one skin barrier wafer out to fit around tube and in a gasket shape $1^{3}/_{4}$ inches in diameter; apply to skin under disk.
  Cut second skin barrier out to fit around tube and about 4 inches in diameter; apply over disk.

COMMERCIAL TUBE STABILIZATION DEVICE (Fig. 7-15)
- Follow manufacturer's instructions.

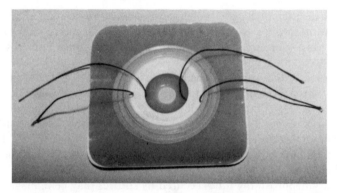

Fig. 7-14   Example of Conwill's technique using a skin barrier flange, convex insert, and sutures to secure nephrostomy tube. (Courtesy Jill Conwill, Corpus Christi, Texas.)

Stabilization systems are changed as needed, usually about every 5 to 7 days. The insertion site (and retention disk, if applicable) is cleansed with an antiseptic solution, rinsed, dried, and a new stabilization system is applied. Patients who are at home must be taught how to recognize and respond to inadvertent dislodgment of the catheter. Marking the catheter with an indelible marker at skin level (or just above the disk) will permit early

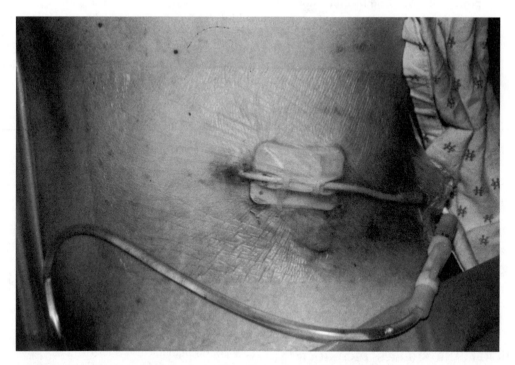

Fig. 7-15   Transparent dressing used over a commercial stabilization device to secure a nephrostomy tube. (Courtesy Abbott Northwestern Hospital, Minneapolis.)

detection of tube migration. The patient should be instructed to go to the emergency department promptly if dislodgment is suspected.

Tube obstruction is a serious complication that may quickly result in infection, pain, and fever. Adequate fluid intake is critical to maintenance of tube patency. Routine "milking" of the tube, that is, rolling the catheter between the fingers, may be recommended to prevent the buildup of urinary salt plugs.[17] Routine sterile irrigations with 5 ml of water or normal saline may be ordered if the catheter becomes occluded with any frequency. Sterile technique should be used, and the solution is allowed to return by gravity.

Tube patency may also be affected by positioning and taping. Kinks at connection sites must be eliminated, and the nephrostomy tube must be positioned to prevent tension. Guidos describes a taping technique that prevents kinking and effectively stabilizes the tube.[15] This technique involves use of a flexible skin-barrier wafer or hydrocolloid dressing cut to fit around the tube and applied to the skin; a soft 4 × 4-inch gauze pad is then rolled and wrapped around the base of the tube so that the tube curves over the roll of gauze. The gauze is taped securely into place. A strip of "bridging" tape is applied to secure the tube without tension just below the gauze roll; a second skin-barrier wafer is applied under the connector between the nephrostomy tube and the extension tubing; and the connector is taped securely to this barrier[15] (Fig. 7-16).

Patients with nephrostomy tubes are at risk for development of pyelonephritis. One can reduce the risk of infection by maintaining a patent, freely draining system; encouraging an adequate fluid intake; minimizing the number of interruptions in the closed drainage system; and using meticulous technique in the care of the site and the drainage system. Although maintenance of a closed system reduces the risk of infection, leg bags are commonly used to permit patients with long-term nephrostomy tubes to resume normal activities without the inconvenience and embarrassment of carrying a drainage bag and tubing.

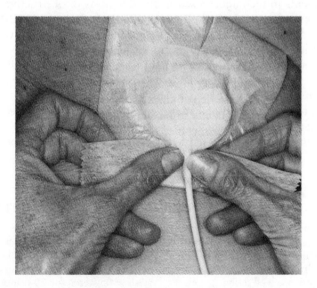

Fig. 7-16 Taping procedure to secure and stabilize a nephrostomy tube and tubing. (From Guidos B: J Enterostom Ther 15(5):189, 1988.)

In this situation, it is necessary to teach the patient to use strict aseptic technique when changing from one drainage system to another,[2] to keep the connecting ends of the system capped when not in use to prevent contamination, and to cleanse the drainage bags as detailed in Box 7-6. Finally, the patient is also taught the signs and symptoms of infection and how to monitor the color, odor, and clarity of the urine. Clinical signs of infection warrant a culture; treatment is based on results. Some physicians order prophylactic antibiotic therapy to reduce the incidence of pyelonephritis.

The nurse is frequently asked to devise an ambulatory drainage system that is simple, effective, and leakproof. When devising such systems for Luer-Lok tubes, the nurse should utilize drainage systems or adapters with Luer-Lok connectors, which are now available commercially (such as Cook Urological, Spencer, Indiana, and Marlen Manufacturing, Bedford, Ohio).

PERCUTANEOUS BILIARY CATHETERS

Improved diagnosis and management of biliary obstruction has led to increasing numbers of patients with percutaneous biliary tubes.

The hepatic cells of the liver secrete 600 to 1000 ml of bile daily. The bile flows from the bile canaliculi to the intralobular septa and then into the terminal bile ducts. The terminal bile ducts become progressively larger and terminate at the hepatic and common bile ducts. The common bile duct empties into the duodenum, where the bile mixes with chyme from the stomach and begins the emulsification of fats (Fig. 7-17). When biliary flow is obstructed, the bile will eventually infiltrate the blood vessels in the surrounding tissues, resulting in hyperbilirubinemia and jaundice. In addition to jaundice, hyperbilirubinemia may cause nausea, vomiting, pain, fever, and pruritus. If uncorrected, this condition can result in serious complications and death.

Advancements in techniques used in the diagnosis of obstructive biliary disease led to the development of percutaneous transhepatic biliary drainage (PTBD).[3] First described by Molnar in 1974, this procedure is a nonsurgical technique used to divert the flow of bile and decompress the engorged biliary system on either a temporary or a permanent basis.[19,24]

PTBD is indicated for patients with jaundice caused by any condition that obstructs the flow of bile to the small intestine. Patients with disease that can be surgically treated may require temporary PTBD to reduce severe hyperbilirubinemia (total bilirubin greater than 20 mg%) and to provide relief of symptoms until surgery is performed. Patients with biliary obstruction caused by malignancies can benefit greatly from PTBD. Permanent PTBD can significantly improve the quality of life for patients with incurable disease.

Box 7-6   NEPHROSTOMY DRAINAGE SYSTEMS: ROUTINE CARE

- Use aseptic technique when connecting or disconnecting nephrostomy tube.
- Cleanse drainage bags with warm soapy water and rinse well daily.
- "Cap" open ends of tubing when system not in use.

- Use white vinegar and water solution (1:1) or a commercial appliance-cleaning solution to soak the drainage systems for 20 minutes one or two times a week; follow with thorough rinsing.

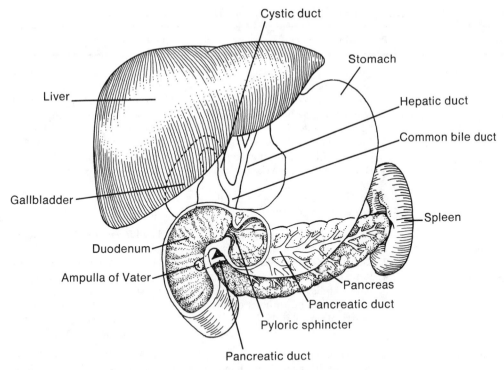

Fig. 7-17 Diagram of biliary tree demonstrating relationship of gallbladder, biliary ducts, hepatic duct, common bile duct, and duodenum. (From Broadwell DC and Jackson BS, editors: Principles of ostomy care, St Louis, 1983, Mosby–Year Book, Inc.)

Placement Procedures

Insertion of a biliary catheter is a multistep procedure. Percutaneous transhepatic cholangiography is performed initially for visualization of the biliary tree and location of the obstruction. A fine-bore cholangiogram needle is then inserted percutaneously through the liver and into a bile duct. Contrast medium is injected into the biliary tree, and visualization with fluoroscopy is obtained. A pigtail catheter such as that found in Fig. 7-13 is then threaded over a guidewire and inserted along the existing needle path. The catheter is then positioned so that the drainage holes are both above and below the obstruction. Removal of the guidewire allows the pigtail tip of the catheter to curl, thus securing the catheter within the biliary tree.[24,26,29,28] If possible, the catheter is advanced through the common bile duct and into the duodenum. This allows natural drainage of bile into the duodenum and is called "internal drainage."[3] If it is not possible to pass the catheter beyond the obstruction or to advance it into the duodenum, external drainage is required. (After decompression of the biliary tree, the radiologist may be able to reposition the catheter, which would then allow conversion to internal drainage.)

Once the catheter has been positioned within the biliary tree, it is secured at skin level by a variety of methods. The radiologist or physician may suture the biliary catheter to the patient's skin, thread it through a plastic disk, which is then sutured to the skin, or utilize a tube-stabilization device.

Table 7-6 Biliary catheter complications: identification and intervention

Problems	Presenting signs and symptoms	Intervention
Displacement of catheter	1. Decreasing bile drainage 2. Absence of bile drainage 3. Presence of blood in the drainage when drainage had previously been clear bile 4. Migration of catheter as evidenced by increasing length 5. Return of obstructive symptoms (jaundice) 6. Leakage around catheter of bile or irrigation solution	1. Hold irrigation. Consult with physician or radiologist. 2. Notify physician or radiologist immediately of findings. Catheter placement will need to be checked most likely with cholangiography.
Obstruction of catheter	1. Decreasing bile drainage 2. Absence of bile drainage 3. Resistance to irrigation 4. Return of obstructive symptoms 5. Fever, chills, hypotension 6. Leakage around catheter of bile or irrigation solution	1. Hold irrigation. Consult with physician. 2. Notify physician immediately of findings. Cholangiography is most likely required to check catheter patency and may require replacement or repositioning.
Sepsis	1. Fever, chills, hypotension 2. Purulent drainage through or around catheter 3. Local inflammation of insertion site	1. Notify physician immediately. May require cultures of blood and bile, antibiotic therapy. 2. More frequent dressing changes and assessments.
Bowel obstruction with retrograde flow of duodenal contents	1. Drainage from catheter of more than 1500 ml in 24 hours 2. Presence of undigested food particles in bile drainage 3. Hyponatremia	1. Notify physician immediately of findings. Cholangiography and evaluation of bowel status may be necessary.
Altered skin integrity	1. Erythema, maceration, ulceration of skin surrounding catheter 2. Skin denudation from adhesive tapes or dressings	1. Apply a skin barrier to heal and protect altered skin. 2. If fungal infection is suspected, obtain order to treat with an antifungal powder. 3. If allergy to adhesive or cleansing agents is suspected, substitute with comparable product. 4. If irritation is caused by leakage, notify physician for further evaluation of cause.

Nursing Management

The nurse should verify whether the tube is to be used for internal or for external drainage. Antibiotics are usually ordered on a prophylactic basis, and blood levels for bilirubin and liver enzymes are obtained to allow one to assess liver function and biliary drainage.[3]

Irrigation of the biliary tube is recommended to maintain patency.[3,29,33] The frequency and amount of irrigant should be specified by the physician, and only bacteriostatic normal saline solution should be used. Biliary tubes should never be aspirated because aspiration could cause contamination of the bile ducts with duodenal contents, resulting in infection and possible sepsis. However, Munn recommends aspiration of 10 ml of bile before one irrigates if the biliary tube is known to be positioned with the tip in the bile duct and is not extending into the duodenum.[29] Munn explains that instilling the irrigant without aspirating may cause excessive pressure, which could promote the occurrence of infection.

Dressings over the biliary tube insertion sites vary based on practitioner preference and institutional protocol. Sterile gauze dressings are used in some settings and require daily changes. Occlusive dressings require less frequent changes, usually 1 to 3 times per week. At each dressing change, the site is assessed for complications and the catheter is checked for evidence of migration. Site care usually involves cleansing with an antiseptic solution and application of an antibacterial ointment to the insertion site. The tube must be positioned without kinks and stabilized, either with gauze and tape or with tube-stabilization devices.

The importance of surveillance for complications related to biliary catheters cannot be overstressed. Although acute complications occur in less than 10% of patients undergoing transhepatic biliary catheter drainage, the complications are serious, and effective management is dependent on early detection.[24,31] Even biliary catheters that have been in place for a length of time can malfunction, and catheter malfunction can result in biliary peritonitis and sepsis.[24] Table 7-6 lists the possible complications, presenting signs and symptoms, and interventions.

The patient who is discharged home with a biliary catheter must be taught the principles and procedures for site care, dressing change, tube stabilization, catheter irrigation, signs and symptoms of complications, and appropriate response. Most patients will benefit from home health referral as well as routine outpatient follow-up observation.

SUMMARY

Percutaneous tubes are contributing both to quantity and quality of life for many patients. Nurses play a vital role in providing tube stabilization, maintaining tube patency, providing surveillance for complications, and teaching the patient self-care.

SELF-EVALUATION

QUESTIONS AND PROBLEMS

1. Identify two indications for use of percutaneous tubes.
2. List the major content areas to be included in a teaching plan for the patient with a percutaneous tube.
3. Describe measures to reduce the risk of infection in the patient with a percutaneous tube.
4. Define the following terms: Janeway gastrostomy; PEG; gastrostomy button.
5. Identify advantages and disadvantages of a gastrostomy button.
6. List factors to be considered in the selection of the optimal placement of a gastrostomy tube.
7. Explain the rationale for effective stabilization of percutaneous tubes.
8. List three options for stabilization of gastrostomy or jejunostomy tubes.
9. In managing peritubular leakage, the initial goal should be:
   a. determination of cause for leakage.
   b. initiation of skin-protection measures.
   c. establishment of an appropriate pouching system.
   d. cauterization of tract with silver nitrate.
10. Which of the following should *not* be used to clear obstructions in feeding tubes?
    a. Meat tenderizer
    b. Tap water
    c. Diet carbonated beverage
11. Explain why it is necessary to utilize a vented pouching system in the management of an empyema tube.
12. Mild hematuria and peritubular leakage is expected in the first 5 to 7 days after insertion of a nephrostomy tube.
      True
      False
13. Identify three common complications associated with the use of nephrostomy tubes and the nursing measures for prevention of each.
14. Identify at least two complications associated with use of percutaneous biliary tubes.
15. Percutaneous biliary drainage may be either "internal" or "external."
      True
      False

SELF-EVALUATION

ANSWERS

1. Drainage and decompression
   Nutritional support
2. Purpose and procedure for tube insertion
   Normal tube function
   Tube stabilization
   Routine care and hygiene

Signs and symptoms of complications and appropriate response

Tube feeding schedule and procedure (when applicable)

3. Minimize handling of tubes.

Use gloves and aseptic technique when handling the tube, dressings, or stabilization device.

Teach patient aseptic technique for self-care.

Follow universal precautions when providing tube care.

4. *Janeway:* Gastrostomy intended for long-term use, surgically constructed to provide mucosa-lined stoma, which can be intubated as needed.

PEG: Nonsurgical placement of gastrostomy tube; involves endoscopy to determine appropriate site; percutaneous insertion of needle or cannula; removal of needle and passage of silk suture into stomach, which is grasped with endoscope and pulled out through mouth (with other end still exiting stomach and controlled by endoscopy assistant); securing of distal end of gastrostomy tube to silk suture, which is then pulled down and out through small abdominal opening, seating gastrostomy tube against gastric or abdominal wall. Endoscope is then reinserted for verification of placement. Advantage is that this is a nonsurgical approach and has a lower complication rate than with surgery.

Gastrostomy button: Short silicone tube with flip-top opening and one-way valve, which prevents external reflux of stomach contents. Feedings are administered after an adapter is passed through the one-way valve. Insertion is through established gastrostomy site.

5. *Advantages:*

Low profile

Prevents many complications associated with gastrostomy tubes (migration, leakage, inadvertent removal, tissue reaction)

One-way valve allows feeding but provides continence

Disadvantages:

Requires well-established tract for insertion

Expensive

Potential dysfunction of antireflux valve with leakage

Need for replacement approximately every 3 to 4 months

6. Usual location (5 cm to left of midline; 5 cm below left costal margin)

Avoidance of costal margin to prevent discomfort

Avoidance of left lobe of liver

Flat surface to facilitate management (avoidance of umbilicus, vertical dropoff of costal margin, belt line, and folds, creases, wrinkles)

7. Tube stabilization reduces tube migration, which can cause gastric outlet obstruction (with gastrostomy tubes), compromised tube function, and tract erosion resulting in leakage and skin breakdown.

8. Use of tube-stabilization devices

Use of baby nipple placed around tube and secured to skin-barrier wafer

Use of baby nipple placed around tube and secured with convex insert snapped over nipple and inside flange of skin-barrier wafer with flange

9. a

10. a

11. To prevent excessive inflation and collapse of pouch with normal respirations

12. True
13. *Dislodgment:* Prevention involves tube stabilization.
    Obstruction: Prevention includes maintenance of adequate fluid intake; "milking" of tube to prevent buildup of urinary salts or mucus plugs; appropriate positioning and taping of tube to prevent kinking; sterile irrigations when ordered.
    Infection: Prevention includes maintenance of adequate fluid intake; maintenance of patent freely draining system; minimizing disruptions of closed system; careful aseptic technique in handling tubes and dressings; scrupulous hygiene in management drainage systems
14. Catheter displacement
    Catheter obstruction
    Sepsis
    Bowel obstruction with retrograde flow of duodenal contents
    Altered skin integrity
15. True

REFERENCES

1. Baldwin J and Baldwin MJ: Treatment of bronchopleural fistula after pneumonectomy, J Thorac Cardiovasc Surg 90:813, 1985.
2. Barr JE: Standards of care for the patient with a percutaneous nephrostomy tube, J Enterostom Ther 15(4):147-153, 1988.
3. Beaulieu J and Bernacki J: A nursing challenge: care of the patient undergoing percutaneous transhepatic biliary drainage, Oncol Nurs Forum 11(4):20-29, 1984.
4. Clemmer JP and Fairfax WR: Critical care management of chest injury, Crit Care Clin 2(4):759, 1986.
5. Conwill J: Management of long-term percutaneous catheters, J Enterostom Ther 13(4):163, 1986.
6. Deveney KE: Endoscopic gastrostomy and jejunostomy. In Rombeau JL and Caldwell MD, editors: Clinical nutrition: enteral and tube feeding, ed 2, Philadelphia, 1990, WB Saunders Co.
7. Ditesheim JA, Richards W, and Sharp K: Fatal and disastrous complication following percutaneous endoscopic gastrostomy, Am Surg 55(2):92, 1989.
8. Eisenberg P: Enteral nutrition, Nurs Clin North Am 24(2):315, 1989.
9. Faller N: Stabilizing tubes and catheters: a cost effective alternative: gastrostomy, suprapubic, ciliary or nephrostomy, Presented at 22nd annual conference of International Association for Enterostomal Therapy, Inc., Las Vegas, Nevada, June 1990.
10. Favero MS and Garner JS: CDC guidelines on infection control, Atlanta, Ga, 1986, Centers for Disease Control.
11. Foutch PG, Talbert GA, Gaines JA, and Sanowski RA: The gastrostomy button: a prospective assessment of safety, success and spectrum of use, Gastrointest Endosc 35(1):41, 1989.
12. Gauderer MWL and Stellato TA: Gastrostomies: evolution, techniques, indications and implications, Curr Probl Surg 23:657, 1986.
13. Gauderer M, Olsen M, Stellato T, and Dokler M: Feeding gastrostomy button: experience and recommendations, J Pediatr Surg 23(1):24, 1988.
14. Gauderer MWL and Ponsky JL: Gastrostomy without laparotomy: a percutaneous technique, J Pediatr Surg 15:872, 1980.
15. Guidos B: Preparing the patient for home care of the percutaneous nephrostomy tube, J Enterostom Ther 15(5):187, 1988.
16. Ho CS, Yee AC, and McPherson R: Complications of surgical and percutaneous nonendoscopic gastrostomy: review of 233 patients, Gastroenterology 95(5):1206 1988.
17. King AW: Nursing management of stomas of the genitourinary system. In Broadwell DC and Jackson BS, editors: Principle of ostomy care, St. Louis, 1983, Mosby–Year Book, Inc.
18. Kohlman PA: Managing a draining chest tube, Nursing88 18(8):58-59, 1988.

19. LaSala C: Caring for the patient with a transhepatic biliary decompression catheter, Nursing85 15(2):52-55, 1985.
20. Mamel J.: Percutaneous endoscopic gastrostomy, Am J Gastroenterol 84(7):703, 1989.
21. McGee L: Feeding gastrostomy, J Enterostom Ther 14(2):73 1987.
22. McKee MC and Sheer C: Maintaining percutaneous catheters and the management of intractable leakage at the insertion site, J Enterostom Ther 14(3):125, 1987.
23. Metheny N, Eisenberg P, and McSweeney M: Effect of feeding tube properties and three irrigants on clogging rates, Nurs Res 37(3):165-169, 1988.
24. Molnar W and Stockum AE: Relief of obstructive jaundice through a percutaneous transhepatic catheter—a new therapeutic approach, Am J Roentgenol Radium Ther Nucl Med 122:356-367, 1974.
25. Moran JR and Greene HL: Digestion and absorption. In Rombeau JL and Caldwell MD, editors: Clinical nutrition: enteral and tube feeding, ed 2, Philadelphia, 1990, WB Saunders Co.
26. Moskowitz GW, Lee WJ, and Pochaczevsky R: Diagnosis and management of complications of percutaneous nephrolithotomy, CRC Crit Rev Diagn Imaging 29(1):1-12, 1989.
27. Motta G: Cost saving alternative to stabilizing a Foley catheter used as a gastrostomy tube, Continuing Care J 8(6):11, 1989.
28. Mueller PR and Ferrucci JT: Percutaneous biliary drainage current techniques, Appl Radiol 12(3):53-64, 1983.
29. Munn N.: When the bile duct is blocked, RN 52(1):50-57, 1989.
30. Panzau KT: Management of a permanent indwelling empyema tube, J Enterostom Ther 9(4):36-37, 1982.
31. Powers ML et al: A clinical report on the comparison of a drain/tube attachment device with conventional suture methods in securing percutaneous tubes and drains, J Enterostom Ther 15(5);206-209, 1988.
32. Rombeau JL and Palacio JC: Feeding by tube enterostomy. In Rombeau JL and Caldwell MD, editors: Clinical nutrition: enteral and tube feeding, ed 2, Philadelphia, 1990, WB Saunders Co.
33. Stoker F: Improving biliary drainage management, Nurs Times 81(27):32-35, 1985.

8 Management of Drain Sites and Fistulas

RUTH A. BRYANT

OBJECTIVES

1. Identify factors contributing to fistula formation.

2. List three complications that contribute to mortality from fistulas.

3. Define the following terms:
   Internal fistula
   External fistula
   Low output fistula
   High output fistula
   Enterocutaneous fistula
   Colovesical fistula
   Vesicovaginal fistula
   Rectovaginal fistula
   Pancreaticocutaneous fistula

4. Identify the three phases of medical management for the patient with a draining wound or fistula.

5. Describe guidelines for providing nutritional support to the patient with a fistula to include amount of calories and protein needed and selection of route of nutritional support.

6. Identify common alterations in fluid and electrolyte balance produced by high-output small-bowel fistulas.

7. List factors known to impede spontaneous closure of fistula tracts.

8. Describe surgical procedures commonly used to close or bypass fistula tracts.

9. List seven goals for nursing management of the patient with a fistula.

10. Describe four factors to be considered when assessing the patient with a draining wound or fistula.

11. Explain the role of each of the following in providing a skin protection for the patient with a fistula:
    Skin-barrier powders
    Solid wafer skin barriers
    Skin-barrier pastes
    Skin sealants
    Ointments

12. Identify the criteria for appropriate use of gauze dressings.

13. Identify features to be considered when selecting a fistula pouch.

14. Identify at least two options for extending the adhesive area of a pouch.

15. Describe a routine pouching procedure for a draining wound or fistula.

16. Identify at least two alternatives for pouching a wound with very irregular contours or very limited pouching surface.

17. Briefly describe the "bridging" technique and identify indications for use.

18. Identify indications for the use of suction catheters.

19. Specify one method of stabilizing suction catheters when:
    • The suction catheter is used with a pouching system.
    • The suction catheter is used with a closed wound drainage system.

20. Describe options for management of vaginal fistulas.

21. Identify options for odor control in a wound managed with dressings and in a wound managed with pouching.

22. Describe one procedure for attaching a drainable fecal pouch to a bedside drainage system.

23. Describe the indications for silicone molds to contain fistula output.

24. Describe key elements to an organized discharge plan for a patient with a fistula or drain site.

The presence of a draining site or fistula can be a very frustrating and disheartening experience to the patient and family because it represents a major catastrophe. For the nurse, too, it may be a difficult experience; however, management can be quite rewarding when effluent is successfully contained, odor is controlled, the patient is comfortable, and realistic resolution is observed. Caring for this patient population requires astute assessment skills, knowledge of pathophysiology, competent technical skills, and knowledge of equipment alternatives.

INCIDENCE AND ETIOLOGY

The incidence of fistula formation is difficult to determine because it varies widely according to the involved organs, precipitating factors, and referral patterns of the surgeon and institution.[10,13] However, most enterocutaneous fistulas arise immediately after a surgical procedure.[10,30] Fistulas may also be a complication associated with an inflammatory bowel process (such as Crohn's disease, diverticulitis), malignancy, trauma, small bowel obstruction, and irradiation.[15,21] Patients who have been treated for a gynecologic malignancy are particularly vulnerable for fistula formation because of the increasingly aggressive nature of the treatment.[19,38]

Several factors are recognized as contributing to the development of a fistula in the immediate postoperative period.[4,21,27] These factors include (1) the presence of a foreign body close to the suture line, (2) tension on the suture line, (3) improper suturing technique, (4) distal obstruction, (5) hematoma or abscess formation in the mesentery at the anastomotic site, (6) the presence of tumor or disease in the area of anastomosis, and (7) inadequate blood supply to the anastomosis.

An inadequate blood supply can be a consequence of surgical procedures and of radiation therapy. Because surgical procedures require dissection and disruption of vascular structures, tissues can be left somewhat devitalized. Irradiation triggers occlusive vasculitis, fibrosis, and impaired collagen synthesis—a process termed "radiation-induced endarteritis." Unfortunately, because this endarteritis persists, complications may develop immediately after radiation or years later.[5,33,39] It is of interest to note that irradiation-induced fistulas most commonly occur when capillary perfusion is already compromised by processes such as atherosclerosis, hypertension, diabetes mellitus, pelvic inflammatory disease, and previous pelvic surgery.[5,39]

The patient with a fistula experiences a 6% to 20% mortality despite improvements made in intraoperative technique, sepsis diagnosis and management, perioperative care, and nutritional support.[10,30,34,35] Complications that contribute to this mortality are electrolyte imbalance, malnutrition, and sepsis.

Regardless of the cause, fistulas present a tremendous burden on the patient, family, health care system, and society in terms of cost, lost wages, and physical and emotional trauma. Prolonged hospital stays, nutritional support, diagnostic tests, additional pharmacologic interventions, surgical procedures, and additional nursing care whether home care or long-term care contribute to the costs of fistula management.

TERMINOLOGY

Definitions

A fistula is an abnormal passage between two or more structures or spaces. This can involve a communication tract from one body cavity or a hollow organ to another hollow organ or to the skin (Fig. 8-1). Fistulas typically develop in a dehisced wound or a surgical incision.

It is important to differentiate between a fistula and a wound dehiscence.[8] The dehiscence of an abdominal wound refers to the separation between the anterior fascial sheath and deeper tissue layers.[34] Although a dehisced wound may drain, it should drain only serosanguinous fluid.

It is also important to distinguish between a fistula and a drain site or draining wound. Not all wounds that drain are fistulas. The term "draining wound" commonly refers to surgical sites that are draining. Often these are surgical sites where drain tubes have been placed (such as Penrose drains or sump catheters) or fluid has been drained (such as paracentesis sites). For example, a drain tube, such as a Penrose or Jackson-Pratt, may be placed in a surgical incision to facilitate drainage of pooled fluid.

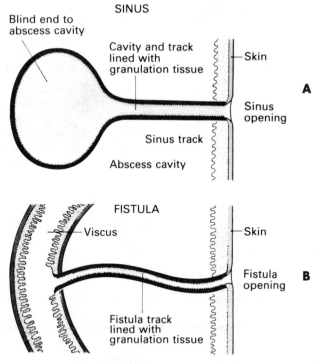

Fig. 8-1. Distinction between a sinus and a fistula. (From Everett WGL: Wound sinus or fistula? In Westaby S, editor: Wound care, St Louis, 1985, Mosby–Year Book, Inc.)

Surgically approximated wounds may superficially separate after surgical procedures and drain temporarily. These generally reepithelialize quickly; however, if sufficient predisposing factors are present, the wound may deteriorate into a fistula.

Classification

Fistulas may be classified according to location, involved structures, and volume of output (Table 8-1). An internal fistula is one where the fistula tract is located inside the body, whereas an external fistula exits cutaneously or within the vagina or rectum. More specific nomenclature is used to identify the involved structures (such as enterocutaneous or rectovaginal); thus the name specifies the structures that adjoin the fistula tract. Examples of such terminology are listed in Table 8-2.

Fistulas may be further subclassified by volume of output. High-output fistulas are defined as those producing more than 500 ml per 24-hour period and define a group of patients who experience a higher mortality.[9,15,30]

MANIFESTATIONS

The passage of gastrointestinal secretions or urine through an unintentional opening onto the skin heralds the development of a cutaneous fistula. Manifestations of a fistula exiting through the vagina (that is, rectovaginal or vesicovaginal) includes passage of gas, feces, or urine through the vagina. Irradiation-induced rectovaginal fistulas are often pre-

Table 8-1   Fistula classification

Location	Internal	Tract contained within body
	External	Tract exits through skin
Involved structures	Colo-	Colon
	Entero-	Small bowel
	Vesico-	Bladder
	Vaginal	Vagina
	Cutaneous	Skin
	Recto-	Rectum
Volume	High output	Over 500 ml per 24 hours
	Low output	Under 500 ml per 24 hours

From Boarini JH, Bryant RA, and Irrgang SJ: Semin Oncol Nurs, 2:287-292, 1986.

Table 8-2   Fistula terminology

From	To	Name	Internal/external
Pancreas	Colon	Pancreatico-colonic	Internal
Jejunum	Rectum	Jejunorectal	Internal
Intestine	Skin	Enterocutaneous	External
Intestine	Colon	Enterocolonic	Internal
Intestine	Bladder	Enterovesical	Internal
Intestine	Vagina	Enterovaginal	Internal
Colon	Skin	Colocutaneous	External
Colon	Colon	Colocolonic	Internal
Colon	Bladder	Colovesical	Internal
Rectum	Vagina	Rectovaginal	Internal
Bladder	Skin	Vesicocutaneous	External
Bladder	Vagina	Vesicovaginal	Internal

From Irrgang S and Bryant R: J Enterostom Ther 11:211-225, 1984.

ceded by diarrhea, the passage of mucus and blood rectally, a sensation of rectal pressure, and a constant urge to defecate.[32,13] Typically a rectovaginal fistula produces an odorous vaginal discharge. Fistulas between the intestinal tract and the urinary bladder (such as colovesical) present with passage of gas or stool-stained urine through the urethra.

MEDICAL MANAGEMENT

Goal of Management

The ultimate goal when managing the patient with a fistula is closure of the fistula either spontaneously or surgically. Such a goal requires patience, astute assessment skills, and the cooperation of many health care specialists. Comprehensive and effective medical management of the patient with a fistula requires attention to five objectives: fluid and electrolyte replacement, perifistular skin protection, infection control, adequate nourishment, and measures to enhance closure.[21,29]

Phases of Management

For convenience and practicality the medical management of patients with fistulas is divided into three phases: fluid and electrolyte stabilization, evaluation and treatment of sepsis, and definitive therapy. Within each phase, attention to fluid and electrolyte balance, skin protection, infection control, nutritional support, and closure plans is necessary.

Fluid and Electrolyte Stabilization. Approximately 5 to 9 liters of fluid rich in sodium, potassium, chloride, and bicarbonate are secreted into the gastrointestinal tract daily. The loss of fluid and electrolytes that accompanies the presentation of a high-output fistula may result in hypovolemia and circulatory failure. Such blood-volume imbalances must be corrected before further treatments can be instituted. Within 48 hours fluid and electrolyte imbalances should be resolved.[30]

Careful monitoring of intake and output is essential. Potential electrolyte imbalances should be anticipated and can be inferred when one knows the electrolyte composition of the gastrointestinal secretions (Table 8-3). The signs and symptoms of electrolyte imbalances should be familiar to the nurse (Table 8-4).

At times, it may be necessary to analyze the electrolyte composition of the fistula drainage in order to accurately calculate electrolyte-replacement needs. Upon occasion, refeeding of fistula effluent has been used to achieve fluid and electrolyte balance. This involves collection of fistula output, transfer of the contents to some type of feeding bag, and administration of the contents to the patient through a feeding tube placed in the jejunum, for example. Unfortunately, this procedure is not esthetically pleasant for the patient or the nurse.

Evaluation and Treatment of Sepsis. Sepsis is the major cause of death in patients with enteric fistulas.[10,11,42] Causative organisms are commonly of bowel origin: coliform, *Bacteroides,* and enterococci. Staphylococci may also be present. These bacteria proliferate rapidly in the poorly vascularized tissue typically surrounding fistulas[10].

The presence of systemic or local sepsis must be evaluated and treated with drainage and antibiotics. Effective drainage can be accomplished by use of surgical or radiographic techniques; the specific approach depends on abscess location, patient status, and available resources. Nutritional support is initiated during this phase. For purposes of this chapter, it is discussed in detail in the following section.

Definitive Treatment. Once fluid and electrolyte balance is achieved and sepsis is controlled or eliminated, a decision regarding definitive therapy must be made. Definitive therapy involves assessment of the potential for spontaneous closure of the fistula as opposed to the need for surgical closure. Nutritional support and a thorough investigation of the fistula tract are critical to the success of either definitive approach. The definitive therapy phase can last several weeks.

Nutritional support. It is well recognized that nutritional support has resulted in improved spontaneous closure rate of enterocutaneous fistulas.[2,25,31] However, the actual impact on mortality is controversial.[41] It is unclear whether the improved mortality that accompanied the introduction of nutritional support in the middle to late 1970s was the

Table 8-3   Characteristics of gastrointestinal secretions

Source	Secretions	pH	24-hour volume	Color	Electrolyte concentration			
					Na	K	Cl	HCO$_3$
Saliva	Ptyalin, maltase	6.0-7.0	1000-1200	Clear	20-80	16-23	24-44	20-60
Gastric juice	Pepsin, rennin (chymosin), lipase, hydrochloric acid	1.0-3.5	2000-3000	Clear/green	20-100	4-12	52-124	0
Pancreatic juice	Amylase, trypsin, chymotrypsin, lipase, sodium bicarbonate	8.0-8.3	700-1200	Clear/milky	120-150	2-7	54-95	70-110
Bile	Bile salts, phospholipids	7.8	500-700	Golden brown–greenish yellow	120-200	3-12	80-120	30-50
Duodenum Jejunum Ileum	Peptidase, trypsin, lipase, maltase, sucrase, lactase	7.8-8.0	2000-3000	Gold–dark gold	80-130	11-21	48-116	20-30
Colon		7.5-8.9	50-200	Brown	4	9	2	—

Modified from Given BA and Simmons SJ: Gastroenterology in clinical nursing, ed 4, 1984, St. Louis, Mosby–Year Book, Inc, and Rombeau J and Caldwell M: Clinical nutrition: enteral and tube feeding, ed 2, Philadelphia, 1990, WB Saunders Co.

result of nutritional support or the combined effects of multiple therapeutic advances (advanced surgical techniques, antibiotic therapy, resuscitation methods).[30,31]

Malnutrition is a significant complication that most patients with a fistula experience. Several factors contribute to the fistula patient's poor nutritional status. Often the patient is malnourished before the fistula develops. There are many factors contributing to malnutrition and negative nitrogen balance: reduced protein intake, inefficient nutrient use, excessive losses of protein-rich fluids (especially from pancreatic and proximal jejunal fistulas), and muscle protein breakdown that occurs with sepsis.

Adequate nutritional support is achieved when the patient is maintained in a state of positive nitrogen balance and receives adequate vitamin and trace mineral replacement. The amount of calories and protein required will depend on the patient's preexisting status, sepsis, and fistula output. Caloric needs can range from 37 to 45 calories/kg per 24 hours and protein requirements are estimated at 1.5 to 1.75 g/kg in 24 hours.[10] Fischer further states that much of the caloric needs will be met from stored fat but 20% will be in the form of body protein with the deficit accumulating at the rate of 1800 to 2700 calories/day.[11] Thus it is important to initiate nutritional support without delay. Although these ranges of caloric and protein needs help guide the practitioner in instituting nutritional support, a formal nutritional assessment is essential to confirm that the patient's nutritional requirements are adequately met.

The route of nutritional support is contingent upon the patient's ability to ingest sufficient quantities, the location of the fistula tract, the absorptive capacity of the bowel mucosa, and patient tolerance.[4] The preferred route of nutritional support is always the gastrointestinal tract. Continued use of the gastrointestinal tract has been shown to maintain the normal structure of the intestine and prevent atrophy of the villi.[25] Unfortunately, complications such as increased fistula output may develop with enteral nutrition.[25,30]

Guidelines for selecting the route for nutritional support are listed in Box 8-1. Enteral nutrition is appropriate when fistulas are located in the most proximal or distal gastrointestinal tract; however, the gastrointestinal tract must be functional and the patient cooperative. Many types of enteral solutions are available, and a dietician should be consulted to recommend the most appropriate solution and administration procedure so that negative sequelae (such as osmolar diarrhea) can be avoided.

As noted above, enteral feedings may result in increased fistula output; as a result, the patient's fluid and electrolyte balance may be jeopardized, and healing of the fistula tract may be delayed. When fistula output increases simultaneously as the rate of administration of enteral solutions is increased, the parenteral route is warranted. During the early phases of fistula management while the patient is being stabilized, the parenteral route for nutritional support is often preferred. Once the fistula tract is more clearly described, sepsis is controlled, and the patient's fluid and electrolyte balance is established, one can consider conversion to an enteral route.

Radiologic examination. The site and size of the fistula tract should be explored once the patient's fluid and electrolyte status has been stabilized and infection has been controlled. Contrast radiographic studies are used to visualize the tract to rule out underlying pathosis such as distal intestinal obstruction, diseased bowel, or an anastomotic separation. Water-soluble contrast agents (that is, Renografin, Hypaque or Gastrografin) are preferred to visualize the fistula tract.[13]

Spontaneous closure. Spontaneous fistula closure will occur in at least 50% of all enteric fistulas when the patient receives adequate nutritional support and infection is con-

Table 8-4   Signs and symptoms of fluid and electrolyte imbalance

	Normal values (mEq/L)	Causes for:		Signs and symptoms of:		Sources in diet
		Gains	Losses	Excess	Deficit	
Water		IV fluids Cirrhosis Stress Steroid treatment Nephrosis Cardiac insufficiency Protein depletion	Diarrhea Vomiting Gastrointestinal suction Diabetes insipidus Diuretics Intestinal obstruction Systemic infection Fistulas	↑ Venous pressure Edema Neck vein distention Bounding pulse Shortness of breath ↓ Hemoglobin ↓ Hematocrit	Dry skin Oliguria ↓ Body temperature Exhaustion Longitudinal wrinkling of tongue Lethargy Dry mucous membranes Atonic muscles Orthostatic hypertension ↑ Hemoglobin ↑ Hematocrit	All liquids Fruits Vegetables Meats
K^+	3.5–5.0	Renal disease Metabolic alkalosis Diabetic acidosis Adrenal insufficiency	Diarrhea Vomiting Anorexia Gastrointestinal suction Ulcerative colitis IV fluids Uncontrolled diabetes mellitus Trauma Diuretics Fistulas	Malaise Diarrhea Muscle weakness ↓ Respirations ↓ Pulse Arrhythmias Nausea Oliguria ECG changes	Muscle weakness Paresthesia Weak, irregular pulse ↓ Reflexes Speech changes ECG changes Anorexia ↓ Gastrointestinal motility Leg cramps Arrhythmias	Orange juice Strong tea Coke Dried fruit Gatorade Tomato juice Bananas

Table 8-4 cont'd

	Normal values (mEq/L)	Causes for:		Signs and symptoms of:		Sources in diet
		Gains	Losses	Excess	Deficit	
Na^+	136-145	Cushing's syndrome Renal disease Aldosteronism Tracheobronchitis Osmotic diuretics	Fever Vomiting Diarrhea Diuretics Gastrointestinal suction Addison's disease Starvation Fistulas Perspiration Excessive ingestion of water	Dry, sticky mucous membrane Flushed skin Thirst Rough, dry tongue Restlessness Fever Oliguria ↓ Reflexes	Weakness Anorexia, nausea Confusion and apprehension Abdominal cramps Syncope Hypotension Headaches ↓ Skin turgor Shock	Salt water Bouillon Gatorade Pepsi Preserved foods Dried fruits
Ca^{++}	4.5-5.5	Excessive administration of vitamin D Prolonged immobility Hyperparathyroidism Multiple myeloma	Excessive administration of citrated blood Recent correction of acidosis Acute pancreatitis Primary hypoparathyroidism	Lethargy Anorexia Nausea Vomiting Bone pain Dehydration Flank pain Constipation or diarrhea Polyuria	Twitching muscles Tetany Seizures Tingling and numbness of fingers Carpopedal spasm Arrhythmias Thirst	Milk Milk products Broccoli Shrimp
Cl^-	95-109	Dehydration Head injury Primary hyperparathyroidism Metabolic acidosis Respiratory alkalosis	Prolonged IV D5W Thiazide diuretics Gastric suction	Few clinical symptoms	Only after prolonged vomiting Few clinical symptoms	Salt Milk

From Irrgang S and Bryant R: J Enterstom Ther 11:214-215, 1984.

Box 8-1   GUIDELINES FOR ROUTE OF NUTRITIONAL SUPPORT IN PATIENTS WITH ENTERIC FISTULAS

ENTERAL NUTRITION
Oral route
   Colocutaneous fistula
   Low-output distal ileum fistula
Gastrostomy or jejunostomy route
   Esophageal fistula
   Gastric, duodenal, or jejunal fistula (access
     must be placed distal to fistula)

PARENTERAL NUTRITION
High-output fistula
Upper gastrointestinal fistulas when enteral
   access is not possible
Intolerance to enteral solutions
Distal bowel obstruction

---

trolled.[10,30,31] The time required to achieve spontaneous closure is reported to range from 4 to 7 weeks.[10,17,31] Many studies report that 90% of the enteric fistulas that close spontaneously will do so within 50 days.[3,11,21,31]

When it is anticipated that the fistula will heal spontaneously, the patient should receive aggressive medical management and nutritional support for 4 to 6 weeks.[31] At that time, if the fistula does not show a significant decrease in output and the patient is free of infection and in positive nitrogen balance, surgical closure may be indicated.[25]

Recently, octreotide acetate (Sandostatin) has been added to the medical management of fistulas to enhance the potential for spontaneous closure. Octreotide acetate (an analog of the naturally occurring somatostatin) exerts pronounced inhibitory effects at various sites in the central nervous system and gastrointestinal tract. These effects include inhibition of secretions from the stomach, pancreas, biliary tract, and small intestine.[22,27] Administration of this hormone to patients with a small bowel fistula has been reported to reduce fistula output. Ladefoged and colleagues[22] found that high doses of octreotide acetate divided into two or three daily subcutaneous injections significantly reduced fecal loss of water and sodium in high-output fecal diversions. Because pancreatic secretions are inhibited, the patient should be monitored for a decrease in insulin production and resultant hyperglycemia.

Surgical procedures. Several factors have been identified as impediments to spontaneous closure (Box 8-2). If these variables are present and closure of the fistula is the ultimate goal for the patient, a surgical approach is appropriate. Surgical procedures may also be indicated for palliation.

The exact timing for surgical intervention is variable, depending on the patient's status. Surgical intervention is emergent in the presence of bowel necrosis or abscess.[9] Otherwise, operative interventions to close the fistula tract should be delayed until the patient is in optimum condition (that is, has a positive nitrogen balance and control of infection).[13] In the presence of irradiated tissue it is important that definitive surgery be delayed until the patient is well nourished and tissues have returned to a normal soft pliable state.[32]

The surgical management of enterocutaneous fistulas usually involves either diversion or resection.[1] Factors such as location, size, and cause of the fistula, the patient's overall status, and the presence of irradiated tissue will determine the approach selected.[13,39]

Diversion techniques divert the fecal stream away from the fistula site; removal of the fistula is not accomplished. Resection of the fistula is not always appropriate or possible in

---

Box 8-2   FACTORS THAT DELAY SPONTANEOUS FISTULA CLOSURE

Complete disruption of bowel continuity	Cancer in site
Distal obstruction	Previous irradiation to site
Foreign body in fistula tract	Crohn's disease
Epithelium-lined tract contiguous with the skin	Presence of large abscess

---

the presence of extensive or recurrent malignancy or when there is inadequate tissue perfusion in the vicinity of the fistula (secondary to numerous surgical resections, scar formation, uncontrolled diabetes, or prior irradiation).

Diversion can be achieved by creation of a stoma proximal to the fistula or by the making of an anastomosis (end to end or side to side) of the two segments of bowel on both sides of the fistula (such as an ileotransverse anastomosis when the fistula communicates with the right colon). This latter procedure may be referred to as an intestinal bypass in which the segment of bowel containing the fistula is completely isolated and separated from the fecal stream.

When closure of the fistula is the goal, resection of the fistula will be necessary. The advantage of this technique is that the diseased tissue is removed. An end-to-end anastomosis of the intestine with resection of the fistula tract is performed. To protect the anastomosis, diversion of the fecal stream through a temporary stoma may be indicated. If the distal part of the rectum is not suitable for anastomosis or the anal sphincters are not competent, a permanent stoma with a Hartmann's pouch may be the safest procedure.[33]

Enteric fistulas communicating with the urinary tract will always require diversion of the fecal stream proximal to the fistula site to prevent urinary tract infections and pyelonephritis.

NURSING MANAGEMENT

The *nursing* management of patients with fistulas is complex and intense and demands critical thinking skills as well as technical skills. Critical thinking skills are needed by the nurse to assess the fistula, its characteristics, and the patient's status; to develop an individualized management plan based on this assessment; and to facilitate discharge planning. Competence in technical management implies knowledge of available products (advantages, disadvantages, effectiveness, and guidelines for use).

Goals

Effective nursing management of fistulas strives to achieve seven goals:
- Skin protection
- Containment of drainage
- Odor control
- Patient comfort
- Accurate measurement of effluent
- Patient mobility
- Cost containment

Optimally, all goals can be achieved simultaneously; at times, however, the nurse must prioritize among these objectives. For example, a pouching system may effectively contain output, contain odor, and provide significant skin protection. However, complete skin protection may not be feasible, and slight denudation may be inevitable immediately surrounding the fistula orifice.

Interventions to achieve the above goals of fistula management begin as soon as the patient presents with a fistula; they are not contingent upon medical management. To effectively care for a patient with a fistula, the nurse must proceed in an orderly fashion. The nursing process is a framework that can provide such an orderly process.

Assessment

The method selected to manage a fistula is guided by the assessment of four key fistula characteristics, as outlined in Box 8-3.

Source

When the nurse first encounters the patient with a fistula, little information may be available regarding the origin of the fistula or the involved organs (if diagnostic studies have not yet been conducted). However, the nurse can determine probable origin of the fistula based on assessment of fistula output (volume, consistency, odor, amount, and corrosive nature) (Table 8-3). This information provides insight into the patient's risk for altered skin integri-

---

Box 8-3 FISTULA ASSESSMENT GUIDE

BOWEL SOURCE
Diagnostic studies done
Odor
Color
Consistency of effluent
Corrosive nature

SKIN INTEGRITY
Intact
Denuded or eroded
Erythema
Ulceration
Maceration

ANATOMIC LOCALE OF ORIFICE
Proximity to bony prominence or
    protrusions
Irregular skin surfaces (scars)
Stability of perifistular skin
    Mobile
    Flaccid
    Stable

Level fistula orifice exits onto skin:
    Skin level
    Deep in wound
    Retracted
Number of fistular openings
    More than one
    Proximity of tracts to each other

CHARACTERISTICS OF EFFLUENT
Nature
    Activated enzymes
    Odor
Volume
    500 ml/24 hr or less
    1000 ml/24 hr or less
    1500 ml/24 hr or more
Consistency
    Liquid
    Particulate matter present
    Thick or pasty

Modified from Irrgang S and Bryant R: J Enterostom Ther 11:211-225, 1984.

ty and so is valuable when one is selecting products and fistula management method. For example, a fistula producing thick, odorous effluent is likely communicating with the descending colon and will be less corrosive than the liquid effluent typical of the ileum.

Skin Integrity. Denudation of perifistular skin is a common complication in fistula patients and is often present when the patient first presents with the fistula. The volume and enzymatic nature of the effluent impinges on the potential for altered skin integrity.

The constant presence of moisture can cause maceration, whereas effluent with enzymatic drainage will create erythema, erosion, and ultimately ulceration of perifistular skin. It is best to visually inspect the skin to assess the condition. However, data can also be obtained from the nursing staff and patient to aid assessment. For example, when frequent dressing changes (every 4 hours) are reported, the nurse can anticipate that the skin will deteriorate quickly and preventive strategies should be implemented. Patient reports of burning or stinging sensations around the fistula or wound commonly indicates denudation of the epidermis.

Patients with a fistula may also develop an infection in the perifistular skin as a result of entrapment of exudate against the skin. Origin of the infection is most commonly fungal and is characterized by an erythematous, papular rash with satellite lesions (Plate 24). Although less common, herpes zoster skin lesions may also occur. At times, it may be difficult to distinguish between the erythema caused by such an infection and the erythema caused by chemical irritation from contact with the effluent.

Anatomic Locale of Fistula Orifice. The actual cutaneous location of the fistula must be assessed so that it will guide product selection and management method. Several factors should be considered. Proximity to bony prominence or other protrusions (that is, retention sutures or stoma) will require products with a flexible adhesive surface that can be trimmed so as to avoid impinging on the prominence or protrusion.

With the patient in a supine and semi-Fowler's position, the patient should be evaluated for the presence of irregular skin surfaces that are created by scars or creases (Plates 24 and 25). Skin-barrier paste or strips of skin-barrier wafers will be needed to "level" the irregular surface for an effective pouching system (Plates 26 and 27).

The surrounding skin should also be assessed to determine if the skin appears mobile and flaccid or stable (Plate 24). Because the normal aging process can weaken muscular and subcutaneous tissue support, a more mobile abdominal skin surface is created. Additional adhesive support (that is, large adhesive surface or cement), convexity, or a belt may be necessary when the surrounding skin is mobile. Scar tissue or a lean muscular abdomen will create a more stable skin surface.

It is also important to notice the level at which the fistula orifice exits onto the skin. Fistulas emptying into deep open wounds often require more modifications and special techniques than fistulas emptying flush with intact skin.

Assessment of the number and proximity of cutaneous fistula exit sites is also necessary to determine appropriate management. When more than one fistula exits onto the skin in proximity, they can frequently be pouched within one pouching system. Separate pouching systems may be required when the cutaneous fistula sites are more widely spaced.

Characteristics of Effluent. Fistula output must be assessed in terms of enzymatic nature, volume, and consistency—key factors that guide the method selected for fistula management. Until radiographic studies are performed, the enzymatic nature of the effluent can be implied from the volume and consistency of the drainage[12] (Table 8-3). When the enzymatic nature of the effluent is known to be high in digestive enzymes, aggressive skin protection will be necessary; therefore skin barriers will be needed and the pouch may need to be changed more frequently.

Generally, the volume of effluent dictates whether pouches or dressings should be used; dressings are contraindicated when the volume exceeds 100 ml in a 24-hour period. The type of pouch outlet (fecal drainable versus urinary spout) will be determined by both the volume and consistency of the drainage.

Planning

When planning the management of a fistula or drain site, the nurse needs knowledge of available products, technical skills to effectively use these products, and knowledge of available resources. The plan should be agreed upon by the multidisciplinary team members (typically the nurse, surgeon, internist, social worker, dietician, patient, and family).

Fistulas can be managed with pouches, dressings or suction, or all three. When planning the management approach, the nurse must consider each of the nursing management goals and select appropriate interventions that will meet those goals.

Goal: Skin Protection. The potential for skin breakdown is always present when a fistula exists. The enzymatic nature of effluent is far more detrimental to skin integrity than the volume of effluent. Skin integrity can also be jeopardized by entrapment of fluid against the skin, which precipitates maceration (as with dressings).

Skin protection is a priority goal for all fistulas regardless of the management option selected. Pouching accomplishes skin protection by containing effluent. Dressings alone do not offer skin protection and require the concurrent use of a skin barrier to protect the skin.

It should be noted that skin-barrier pastes and wafers commonly need to be applied over an intact incision when one is managing a fistula. This is done to prevent contamination of the incision with effluent and to prevent leakage of effluent from the fistula along the incision.

Skin barriers are available in various forms. Box 8-4 summarizes the characteristics and indications of each type.

Skin-barrier powders are used only to absorb moisture from denuded surface and to create a dry surface. Adhesives or ointments can then be applied to the dry surface. Skin-barrier powders should not be confused with talc or cornstarch, which do not provide skin protection. Skin-barrier powders should be discontinued once the skin is intact.

Solid-wafer skin barriers are pectin-based wafers that have an adhesive surface and can be placed around the fistula to provide skin protection. Gauze dressings can then be applied over the skin-barrier wafer. These barriers are changed only when they loosen from the wound or fistula edges.

Skin sealants are used to protect the skin from adhesives, to enhance adhesion (particularly on oily or dry skin or over skin barrier powders), or to provide skin protection around low-output fistulas. However, because skin sealants contain alcohol, it is preferable to avoid their use over denuded skin. Skin sealants must be allowed to dry before additional products are applied (to permit solvents to dissipate, thus avoiding chemical skin damage). Skin sealants are available in various forms (wipes, spray, gel, and brush-on liquid).

Box 8-4   GUIDE TO THE USE OF SKIN BARRIERS IN FISTULA MANAGEMENT

SOLID WAFERS
Characteristics:
   Available as wafers or rings
   Have moist tack
   Have varied flexibility
   Have varied durability to effluent
Indications:
   Level irregular skin surfaces
   Protect perifistular skin from
      effluent when dressings are used or
      skin is exposed

PASTE
Characteristics:
   Commercial preparations contain
      alcohol, which can create burning
      sensation if skin is denuded
Indications:
   Level irregular skin surfaces
   Protect exposed skin from effluent (that
      is, with pouching)
   Extend duration of solid wafer barrier
      when pouching

POWDER
Characteristics:
   Must be used lightly
   Residual powder alters adhesion
Indications:
   Absorb moisture from superficial
      denudement before applying
      ointments or adhesives

SEALANTS
Characteristics:
   Contain alcohol
   Create pain when applied over
      denudement
   Must be allowed to dry
Indications:
   Under adhesives to protect fragile skin
   Improve adhesion to skin (such as oily
      skin)
   Protect perifistular skin from effluent
      when dressings are used

Petroleum-based or zinc-based ointments are another approach to providing skin protection from effluent. They are used with dressings and must be reapplied frequently to assure adequate protection. Ointments are contraindicated when adhesives are being used because adherence will not be possible. They are of greatest value in low-output fistulas or when the skin contours are not amenable to pouching; meticulous skin care is essential, however.

Goal: Containment of Effluent. Containment of effluent can be accomplished, to varying degrees, with dressings, pouches, suction, or a combination of these. The volume of effluent, patient's activity level, and abdominal contours influence which approach is most desirable and effective.

Gauze dressings. Gauze dressings are appropriate when the output is low (less than 100 ml per 24 hours) and odor is not offensive. If the output exceeds 100 ml per 24 hours, dressings become less effective and more time intensive. The application of additional dressings will not increase the absorbency of the dressing or lengthen the time between dressing changes. Furthermore, entrapment of effluent against the skin may cause maceration and breakdown. A good rule is that when dressings have to be changed more often than every 4 hours, a pouching system should be considered.

Although dressings are easy to use and readily available, dressings do not offer skin protection, odor control, or accurate output measurement. Skin protection must be provided by use of a skin barrier product. Odor can be controlled by application of a charcoal deodorant dressing over the gauze; however, particularly pungent fistulas may be best managed with odorproof pouches despite the low output.

Frequent dressing changes that require tape removal and reapplication can jeopardize skin integrity. The nurse should anticipate the potential for skin breakdown when using dressings, particularly on fragile, elderly skin or irradiated skin, and institute preventive measures. Many methods can be used to secure dressings over a fistula or drain site. Refer to Chapter 1 for more discussion on prevention of taping injuries.

Routine pouch techniques

GENERAL MEASURES. Effective pouching of a fistula will achieve all seven nursing management objectives. Numerous techniques have been reported in the literature.[1,6,14,20,36,37] The various ostomy pouches (fecal or urinary; adult or pediatric) can be used, as well as pouches specifically designed for wound management. Pouching offers a sense of control to the patient and nursing staff because effluent is contained and can be emptied at specific intervals and the pouch can be changed at convenient times.[40] By preventing the embarrassment of leaking dressings that loosen when the patient is ambulatory, the patient's dignity is also supported.

The frequency for changing a fistula pouch will vary. For complex, high-output fistulas, a 24-hour pouch setup may be considered successful. The pouch must be changed frequently enough to prevent the skin breakdown that occurs as the skin barriers dissolve because of exposure to fistula drainage.

FEATURES OF A FISTULA POUCH. Several features must be considered when one is selecting a pouch for fistula containment, as outlined in Box 8-5.[17] The decision tree in Fig 8-2 can be used to guide fistula pouch selection.

Box 8-5   FEATURES OF A FISTULA POUCH

ADHESIVE SURFACE
Size and shape of cutting surface
Sizable versus presized adhesive surface
Presence or absence of starter hole
Attached skin barrier preferred
Degree of flexibility of skin-barrier wafer

POUCH CAPACITY
Predetermined by size of adhesive surface
3 to 4 hours' capacity preferred

POUCH FILM
Odorproof or odor-resistant film
Rustle-free film
Transparent versus opaque film

POUCH OUTLET
Urinary outlet
Wide tubular outlet
Fecal outlet

WOUND ACCESS
Two-piece pouch
Access window
Open-end drain with wide outlet

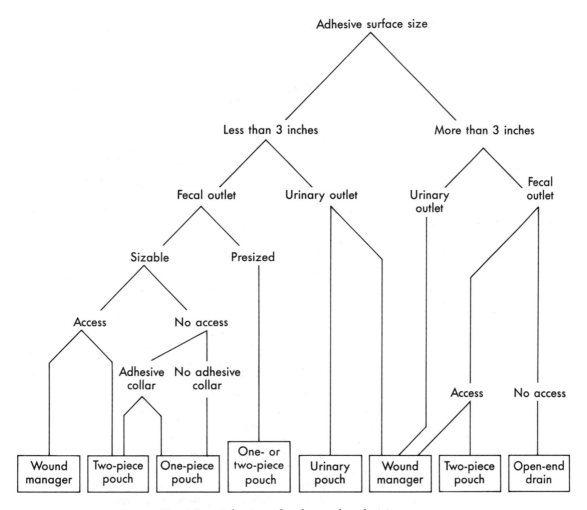

Fig. 8-2.   Selecting a fistula pouch: a decision tree.

Adhesive surface. An adhesive surface must be large enough to accommodate the fistula orifice and generally allow a minimum of 1-inch adhesive contact around the fistula. Although more adhesive surface is usually desirable, it may not be possible in the presence of obstacles such as retention sutures.

Sizable pouches are most appropriate for fistulas because they can be customized to irregular fistula contours. Adhesive surfaces often have a starter hole; although these may be convenient, at times, starter holes restrict the positioning of the pouch on the abdomen. Most pouches have an attached skin-barrier wafer, which is usually preferred because it simplifies the pouching procedure. However, a pouch *without* an attached skin barrier may be selected because other features (such as large capacity, type of outlet needed, desire to avoid a starter hole, or preference for a pouch without a floating collar) are determined to be a priority; in this case, a skin-barrier wafer is added to the pouch or applied directly to the skin before pouch application.

Pouch capacity. The capacity of the pouch is predetermined by the size of the adhesive surface; pouches with larger adhesive surfaces have larger pouch capacities. It is preferable to use a pouch with the capacity to contain 3 to 4 hours of drainage so that the risk of leakage is minimized. However, a smaller capacity pouch may be used if the staff or patient is willing to empty the pouch more frequently or if the pouch can be connected to bedside drainage.

Pouch film. Consideration may also be given to the odorproof qualities of the pouch film. Large pouches and urinary drainage equipment may be more odor-resistent than odorproof, hence requiring more frequent pouch changes to control the odor from permeating the pouch film. Some pouch films may be more "rustle free" than other pouch films. Finally, pouches are available with transparent, opaque, or beige-tone films. Most often, the fistula pouch should be transparent so that application can be closely observed.

Pouch outlet. An important consideration in selecting a fistula pouch is determining the most appropriate outlet needed. Generally, 24-hour volumes of less than 1000 ml are easily managed with a feces-drainable outlet, whereas volumes in excess of 1000 ml are more appropriately managed with a urinary outlet.

By using a urinary outlet, one can achieve continuous drainage. The antireflux present in most urinary pouches may need to be "popped," or removed so that fistula effluent can drain without clogging the pouch. Tubing is attached to the pouch so that drainage is facilitated to stay away from the skin and go into a larger receptacle such as a bedside drainage collector. Nursing care is therefore economized, and overfilling of the pouch is avoided.

Continuous drainage is still possible when particulate matter is present in the effluent by use of a wider tubular outlet, by attachment of latex drainage tubing to a fecal pouch, or by "rubber banding" of a urinary pouch adapter into a pouch spout (Box 8-6). An open-end drain or feces-drainable pouch is indicated for thick, mushy effluent.

WOUND ACCESS. At times access to the fistula site may be desirable so that tubes can be advanced, the fistula can be assessed easily, or skin-barrier pastes can be reinforced. Access to the site without disruption of the pouch adhesive can be achieved with a two-piece pouch or with a pouch that has an attached "access window" (Plate 28). When such access features are not available or have an inadequate adhesive surface size, wide open-end drains can be used. One can obtain limited access by cuffing the pouch film back to expose the site.

Pouch modifications

ADHESIVES. Additional adhesives are often needed when one is pouching fistulas. Although pouches and solid skin-barrier wafers already have an adhesive surface, additional adhesives may be needed to (1) attach two surfaces, (2) enhance the tack of an existing adhesive, or (3) extend the adhesive surface on a pouch. Adhesives are particularly beneficial on mobile, flaccid skin because they provide more support to the surrounding tissue. In some instances, by enhancement of the adhesive tack, the wearing time of the pouch may be extended. Adhesives may also be warranted to improve the tack when several applications of skin-barrier powder are required in the presence of severe denudation.

Adhesives are commercially available in a liquid, aerosol, or sheet form. Liquid and aerosol adhesives are applied lightly, and contain solvents that must evaporate before application of additional products. The directions that accompany these products should be followed closely.

Box 8-6   ADDITION OF CONTINUOUS DRAINAGE TUBE TO FECAL OUTLET POUCH

EQUIPMENT
Fecal pouch or open-end drain
10 in 1 connector
5 inches of latex tubing
Rubber band
Bedside drainage system

PROCEDURE
1. Attach latex tubing to connector.
2. Cut desired opening in fecal pouch or open-end drain.
3. Working at the adhesive surface, reach through the inside of the pouch and pull the tail of the pouch through the inside of the pouch out the adhesive surface opening.
4. Grasp the connector and tubing and insert the connector upward through the now "cuffed" end of the pouch, through the inside of the pouch, and

out the tail of the pouch (and adhesive surface).
5. Rubberband the tail of the pouch to the 10 in 1 connector.
6. Now pull on the latex tubing so that the tail of the pouch is no longer in the adhesive area. The tail of the pouch is now cuffed around the 10 in 1 connector on the inside the pouch.
7. Attach to bedside drainage system.
NOTE : When the pouch is removed, the latex tubing and connector can be cut off the pouch and reused or the entire system can be discarded.
NOTE : A urinary adapter can also be used by fanfolding of the tail of the open-end drain around the adapter. The pouch is secured to the adapter with a rubber band, and a beside drainage bag can then be easily attached to the adapter.

Although not an intended use, liquid adhesives have also been used in combination with skin-barrier powders to protect exposed skin from caustic effluent. In this procedure, several layers of skin-barrier powder and liquid adhesives (cement) are alternately applied to the skin. Principles for proper usage of skin-barrier powders and adhesives should be followed when one is using this technique.

Because fistulas vary in size and shape and abdominal contours can be dramatic, large and unusually shaped pouch apertures are often necessary (Fig. 8-3). Sheets of adhesives (or double-faced adhesive disks) can be used to either create or increase the adhesive surface on a pouch. Box 8-7 describes the procedure for adding an adhesive sheet to a pouch.

An adhesive surface can also be created or added to a pouch by use of cloth tape and cement. This procedure is outlined in Box 8-8 and may be quite useful in situations where resources are limited.

Another method that can be used to acquire a large adhesive surface is to attach two open-end drainable pouches (Fig. 8-4). Pouch features that facilitate saddlebagging include no attached solid-wafer skin barrier, no floating collar, and no starter hole. A large solid-wafer skin barrier is then attached to the new combined adhesive surface, and the pouch is prepared in the usual fashion. Box 8-9 describes the saddlebagging technique.

CATHETER PORTS. Occasionally, drainage will develop around a percutaneous tube (such as biliary tube or sump tube) that is attached to suction or dependent drainage. A catheter port is a nipple-shaped device that attaches to the external wall of a pouch. The percutaneous tube is disconnected, threaded through the fistula pouch opening and catheter port, and then reconnected to drainage. The pouch is then secured to the skin as detailed in Box

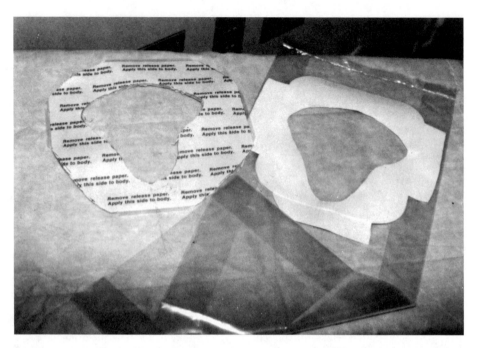

Fig. 8-3. Example of adding adhesive surface to large open-end drain to accommodate unusually shaped pouch opening needed. (Courtesy Abbott Northwestern Hospital, Minneapolis.)

7-4. In this way, drainage around the catheter is isolated and collected in the pouch while the catheter is connected to dependent drainage or suction.

Catheter ports may also be used with suction catheters that have been placed in or adjacent to the fistula opening. In these situations, the catheter port again serves to secure the catheter as it exits the wall of the pouch.

Box 8-7 PROCEDURE FOR ADDING ADHESIVE SHEETS TO ENLARGE POUCH ADHESIVE SURFACE

EQUIPMENT
Pouch without floating collar
Double-faced adhesive sheet or disk

PROCEDURE
1. Remove protective paper from one side of adhesive sheet.
2. Attach this adhesive sheet adjacent to existing adhesive on pouch (edges may overlap slightly).
3. Trace desired opening size on protective paper covering adhesive surface.
4. Cut to desired size.
5. Prepare solid skin-barrier wafer (usually 8 × 8 inches) and attach to adhesive surface on pouch and continue in usual fashion.

Box 8-8   PROCEDURE FOR CREATING A POUCH ADHESIVE SURFACE

EQUIPMENT
Pouch or plastic bag
1-inch cloth tape
Cement

PROCEDURE
1. Determine surface area on pouch to be enlarged or on plastic bag where adhesive surface is to be created.
2. Cut several strips of cloth tape.
3. Apply several strips of cloth tape on pouch or plastic bag side by side where adhesive surface is intended to be. Each strip should overlap slightly.
4. Apply more strips of cloth tape over the already placed tape but in a perpendicular fashion. Again, each strip should overlap slightly.
5. Trace the desired opening over the cloth tape and cut out.
6. Apply cement to tape to create tacky surface. Two or three coats of cement may be required because the tape absorbs some of the cement.
7. Prepare solid-barrier wafer, attach to cemented adhesive surface, and continue in usual fashion.

NOTE: Steps 2 to 5 can also be omitted; the desired opening is cut directly into the pouch film, cement is added, and the skin-barrier wafer is attached.

Complex pouch techniques

SILICONE MOLDS. A sophisticated and complicated pouching system using a dental mold material and presized pouch with a belt gasket is an option when the fistula orifice is recessed in an open wound or is surrounded by numerous irregular skin surfaces. Essentially, the mold fills the wound or surrounds the fistula and creates a smooth surface to which a pouch can be applied.[7,23,43]

A silicone mold is made from Silastic 382 Medical Grade Elastomer—a two-component silicone material that vulcanizes at room temperature without exotherming.[43] It is inherently nontoxic, nonirritating, and nonsensitizing. The elastomer is supplied as two separate liquids—an opaque viscous elastomer base and a catalyst. The elastomer base is composed of polydimethylsiloxane polymer and silica filler. The catalyst M is a specially tested grade of stannous octoate.

The elastomer is poured into the wound or onto the abdomen so that a mold of the fistula opening and wound is created as demonstrated in Plate 29; the fistula orifice is protected from the elastomer during the process. Once the mold dries it hardens and is then easily removed from the wound. The mold can be secured into the fistula opening with adhesives. Box 8-10 lists the directions for creating and applying a silicone mold. This technique is an intricate, complicated procedure that requires frequent revision of the mold as the wound contracts and changes.

Customized silicone faceplates can also be made by some ostomy suppliers or retailers. A Play-Doh impression of the fistula site serves as a template or model from which to make the faceplate.

TROUGH PROCEDURE. When fistulas are contained within the depressions of a wound such that a routine pouching system fails, this procedure may be useful. With the trough procedure, one or several strips of a transparent dressing are used to occlude the wound and trap effluent in the wound depression (Fig. 8-5). A small opening is made in the trans-

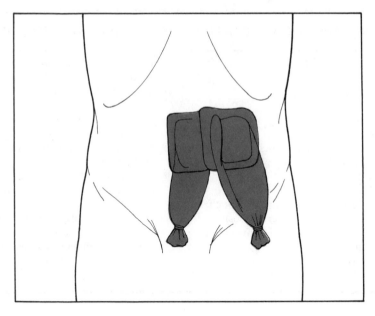

Fig. 8-4.   Sketch of saddlebagging technique where two open-end drainable pouches are connected along the adhesive surface to create a large adhesive surface.

parent dressing at the most dependent aspect of the wound, and an ostomy pouch is applied over this opening; no pattern is required.

To enhance adherence of the transparent dressing to the skin peripheral to the fistula or wound (and to protect perifistular skin), apply strips of a solid-wafer skin barrier. Directions for the trough procedure are listed in Box 8-11.

Box 8-9   SADDLEBAGGING TECHNIQUE

EQUIPMENT
Two open-end drains (without floating collar or attached skin barrier or starter hole)
Solid-wafer skin barrier (8 × 8 inches)
Skin-barrier paste

PROCEDURE
1. Align pouches as you intend final product to appear on abdomen.
2. Peel protective backing away from adhesive along common edges of pouches approximately $1/2$ to 1 inch.
3. Attach the two pouches along this $1/2$- to 1-inch margin *only*.
4. Trace pattern of wound onto new adhesive surface (combined pouch adhesive surfaces).
5. Cut out pouch opening; do not cut into "seam" created by combining pouches.
6. Trace pattern onto solid-wafer skin barrier and cut out.
7. Remove protective paper backing from pouch adhesive surface and attach to solid-wafer skin barrier.
8. Prepare skin as indicated by wound contours and continue pouching procedure.
NOTE: Both pouches will fill with drainage and require emptying.

Box 8-10   SILICONE MOLD

EQUIPMENT
Emesis basin
Tongue blade
Dow Corning Medical Grade Elastomer 382
Dow Corning Catalyst M and eye dropper
Red rubber catheter (optional)
Skin-barrier paste
Ostomy pouch with belt
Adhesives (silicone spray necessary to adhere
  to mold)

PREPARATION
1. Cleanse skin around the wound with water
   and pat dry.
2. Pour elastomer into dry emesis basin;
   usually 1 or 1 ¹/₂ ounces is enough for a
   moderate-sized cast.
3. Add 10 to 12 drops of Catalyst M for each
   ounce of elastomer.
4. Stir thoroughly with the tongue blade.
5. If necessary, place a suction catheter into
   fistula opening to contain drainage while
   the cast is setting.
6. When elastomer has slightly thickened,
   pour on patient's abdomen or in open

wound around fistula orifice to a one-
fourth inch thickness.
7. Allow mold to harden for 3 to 5 minutes in
   wound.
8. Gently lift mold out of wound.
9. Remove catheter from cast.
10. Trim edges of cast to form gently rounded
    surfaces.
11. Trim fistula opening in cast to be sure
    opening is adequate.

APPLICATION
1. Spread a smooth layer of skin-barrier paste
   on the back of the mold with a tongue
   blade, and allow it to set until it is firm to
   touch. NOTE: Silicone spray can be applied
   to this surface to increase adherence with
   or without the paste.
2. Place the mold into the wound. Seal the
   edges with the skin-barrier paste.
3. Apply tape on all edges of the mold.
4. Apply an ostomy pouch with belt tabs over
   the opening in the mold; attach belt.

CONDOM CATHETER FISTULA POUCH. At times, skin-surface contours or obstacles (such as retention sutures) may substantially reduce the surface that is available for attaching a pouch (Plate 30). A conduit for drainage can be made from a flexible skin-barrier washer and condom catheter as described in Box 8-12. This system has limited capacity but may make a significant contribution to keeping the patient dry.

BRIDGING TECHNIQUE. The bridging technique is a procedure that can be used to isolate one area of a wound from another part of the wound. It has two primary indications for use. (1) Wounds may present with two distinct areas of "needs": one area of the wound has drainage and requires containment, whereas another area needs moist wound healing or packing. (2) Very large wounds may be more manageable if the wound is "divided."

Solid-wafer skin barriers are cut into small pieces to fill the wound at the selected bridge location and layered into place (Fig. 8-6). A routine pouch or more complicated pouching system can then be applied over the bridge that now exists in the wound. Box 8-13 describes the steps involved in the bridging technique.

Suction catheters. Suction catheters attached to low, intermittent suction may be needed when routine pouching is ineffective or overwhelmed by the volume of output. Effluent must be liquid if suction is to be effective; thick or particulate drainage will occlude the catheter. Suction does not provide complete containment of effluent, and so dressings and different modes of skin protection must also be utilized.

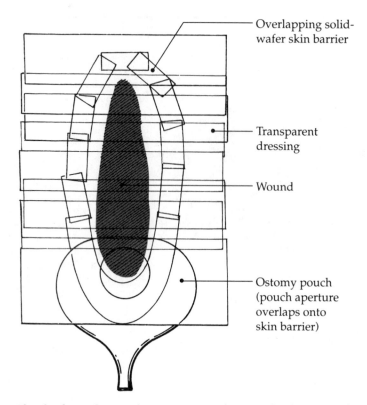

Overlapping solid-
wafer skin barrier

Transparent
dressing

Wound

Ostomy pouch
(pouch aperture
overlaps onto
skin barrier)

Fig. 8-5.   Sketch of trough procedure. Notice overlapping skin-barrier wafers and transparent dressing strips. Pouch opening must overlap onto the skin-barrier wafer at the inferior aspect of the wound.

Suction catheters can also be used in combination with routine and complex pouching techniques to enhance the effectiveness of the pouch. With this technique, the suction catheter is generally placed inside the pouch or laid on the surface of the abdominal wound or fistula versus placement within the fistula tract. It is more effective to insert the suction catheter through the wall of the pouch (with the use of a catheter port) as opposed to under the adhesive surface, a position that can result in leakage.

Suction catheters have also been used with a transparent dressing placed over the wound.[16,18,24] In this closed wound-drainage system, a multifenestrated suction catheter (such as Jackson Pratt) is laid in the wound and exits from the least dependent aspect of the wound (Plate 31). A transparent dressing is then used to cover the wound and the suction catheter. Skin-barrier paste is sometimes necessary to fill in irregular skin surfaces and to seal around the catheter as it exits from the transparent dressing. Suction tubing is then attached to the suction catheter and set at a low continuous suction level. A hemovac can provide the suction for short periods of time to increase the patient's mobility. To protect the wound edges and base from the suction catheter ports, the wound is lined with a thin layer of moist gauze or a commercially available wound liner. This dressing is commonly changed every other day.

Box 8-11   TROUGH PROCEDURE

1. Prepare skin and fill irregular skin surface as usual.
2. Apply overlapping strips of solid-wafer barrier along wound edges.
3. Apply skin-barrier paste to smooth "seams" (that is, between barrier edges and along skin edges). NOTE: Inferior aspect of wound should be bordered with a solid piece of barrier instead of overlapping strips to prevent leakage.
4. Cut strips of a transparent dressing so that they are wide enough to cover wound and skin-barrier strips. Calculate length of strips so that strips overlap intact skin with 1- to 2-inch margins.
5. Reserve one strip of transparent dressing to be applied to the most inferior aspect of the wound.
6. Attach a drainable pouch (can be urinary or fecal) to this one strip of transparent dressing.
7. Cut hole in pouch or transparent-dressing adhesive surface so that it is lower than the inferior wound margins (it should clear the wound edges to provide adequate drainage).
8. Beginning at top of wound, apply transparent dressing in overlapping strips.
9. Attach the final strip of the transparent dressing (with the attached pouch) so that the bottom of the pouch opening is secured onto the skin-barrier wafer.

A catheter that is inserted into the fistula tract will act as a foreign body and may therefore interfere with healing and even increase fistula output.[42] On the other hand, a catheter coiled in a defect above the orifice or in the open wound surrounding the fistulous orifice will not inhibit closure.

Box 8-12   CONDOM CATHETER FISTULA POUCH

EQUIPMENT

Solid skin-barrier wafer (flexible)
Condom catheter
Adhesive (spray or cement)
Skin-barrier paste
Microporous tape
Rubber tip (stopper) from laboratory blood tubes

PROCEDURE

1. Cut 4 × 4-inch solid-wafer skin barrier in half and then half again so that it is only one fourth of original size.
2. Round off corners.
3. Trim center opening to wound size needed.
4. Apply adhesive to top surface (nonadhesive) of skin-barrier wafer. Let dry.
5. Unroll condom catheter.
6. Working with larger opening end of condom catheter, attach condom to cemented skin-barrier wafer.
7. Prepare skin as warranted by contours and skin integrity.
8. Remove protective paper backing from solid-wafer skin barrier.
9. Attach adhesive surface of skin barrier (with condom attached) to skin.
10. Tape edges of condom catheter pouch to skin-barrier wafer and surrounding skin.
11. Cap tip of condom catheter with rubber tip of laboratory blood tubes.

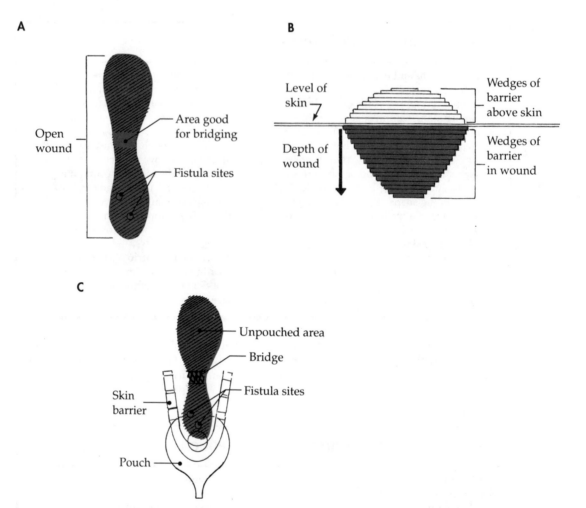

Fig. 8-6. **A,** Area of wound where fistula sites are located and identified can be separated from remainder of wound. **B,** Cross-section view of tapered skin-barrier wedges used to fill the wound defect and to extend slightly above the level of the skin. **C,** Sketch demonstrating how pouch is applied over bridge and fistula leaving the area of wound that is not draining available for more appropriate wound care.

Because firm tubes can injure fragile tissue, only soft, flexible suction catheters should be used with fistulas.[42] Suction catheters should be considered a short-term intervention because of the limitations placed on patient mobility and the time-intensive nature of the care.

Vaginal fistula drain device. Thus far, discussion of fistula management techniques has focused on cutaneous fistulas. Vaginal fistulas, which can occur in the female patient with a radiation-treated pelvic malignancy, create a challenging situation where the patient is essentially incontinent of feces through the vagina. The uncontrolled passage of fecal material vaginally results in severe perivaginal skin denudation and discomfort. Aggressive nursing care is essential to prevent these complications.

Box 8-13   BRIDGING TECHNIQUE

PROCEDURE

1. Assess wound and determine most appropriate location for "bridge." Be sure all sites from which drainage is produced are included in the side of wound to be pouched. For simplification of the bridging procedure, areas that are narrower or shallower should be selected.

2. Apply layered wedges of solid-wafer skin barrier and paste to create bridge. Wedges must be custom-cut to fit the dimensions of the wound at that level; usually the bottom wedge is narrowest because the deepest part of the wound is typically the narrowest area. Each successive wedge is a little wider until the skin-barrier wafer wedges reach skin level.

3. Continue to layer solid-wafer barrier wedges *above* skin level using progressively smaller and narrower wedges (to create a pressure-dressing effect).

4. Apply solid-wafer skin barrier to cover newly created bridge and extend onto intact skin. Paste may be needed to smooth "seams."

5. Continue with routine or complex pouching procedure as indicated.

NOTE: Skin barrier paste or adhesive spray or cement may be used between wedges but are not routinely necessary.

Skin protection can be achieved with ointments and pads; frequent dressing changes are necessary to avoid entrapment of caustic drainage contents against the skin. Unfortunately, ointments and pads for vaginal fistulas are less than optimal because they are labor intensive, do not promote patient mobility, do not adequately contain the fecal contents, and fail to control odor.

Various pouching techniques can be modified to adhere to the perivaginal surface (such as sizable one-piece fecal pouch or female urinary incontinence pouch).[7,26] However, the difficult location and moist surface surrounding the vaginal orifice make adhesive pouching systems very challenging.[4]

A vaginal fistula drain device is another method of managing a vaginal fistula and does not require adhesives. Such vaginal drain devices are available commercially. This type of system can also be improvised with an Evenflo nipple shield or vaginal diaphragm and a large Malecot catheter (Fig. 8-7).[4,28] A cruciate incision is made through the nipple shield or diaphragm through which the catheter is threaded. The shield or diaphragm serves to occlude the vagina so that the drainage is directed down the catheter.

The soft cone-shaped device, shield, or diaphragm is inserted a very short distance into the vagina. The discomfort such manipulation of the labia and vagina can create for the patient can be minimized by lubrication of the device with a lidocaine (Xylocaine) lubricant. Tubing is attached to the device to channel the fistula contents into a bedside collection bag. The drainage tubing can be anchored to the patient's inner thigh.

A vaginal fistula drain device will remain in place quite effectively while the patient is reclining. As the patient becomes more ambulatory, the device may have a tendency to become dislodged; however, because the procedure is so easy, the vaginal drain can be reinserted by the patient as needed. Gentle irrigation of the tubing may be indicated if the tubing becomes occluded by fistula material.

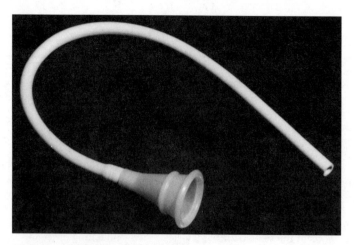

Fig. 8-7. Example of commercially available vaginal drain device. (Courtesy Abbott Northwestern Hospital, Minneapolis.)

A vaginal fistula drain device may be a temporary or permanent management technique depending on the patient's status.

Goal: Control Odor. Fistula effluent typically has a strong odor that can be offensive to the patient, family, and caregivers. The method of odor control will depend on whether dressings or pouches are being used. Gauze dressings will not control odor; therefore charcoal-impregnated dressings may be needed over the gauze dressings. However, because charcoal becomes inactivated with moisture, these dressings should not come into contact with drainage materials. Charcoal dressings are most cost effective with low-output fistulas where the charcoal dressing remains intact for 24- to 48-hour periods.

Odor is best controlled by use of a pouch to contain the effluent. In fact, a pouch may be the preferred management technique simply to contain the odor regardless of the volume of output. Although most pouches have an odorproof film, the quality of the film's ability to contain odor varies. For example, many urinary pouches and urinary drainable systems are not odorproof and so may become saturated with odor quickly.

To control odor the nurse should (1) dispose of soiled linens and dressings from the room promptly, (2) use care in emptying pouches to prevent splashing effluent on the patient or on linens, (3) cleanse the tail of drainable fecal pouches after emptying, and (4) use deodorants appropriately.

Deodorants can be taken internally (orally) or used externally (in the pouch or as a room spray). Internal deodorants are in a tablet form but are generally discouraged in the presence of pathologic condition such as a fistula. External deodorants are available in liquids, powders, and tablets and are placed in the pouch after each emptying. Room deodorants are particularly useful when the nurse is emptying the pouch, changing the pouch, or changing dressings. The room deodorant selected should be one that eliminates odor rather than masks odor. With the many types of deodorants now available, patients, families, and nurses should not have to tolerate the unfortunate odor that often accompanies fistulas.

Goal: Patient Comfort. The patient with a fistula is at risk for skin irritation, which can become a source of discomfort and exhausts the patient's morale. Factors contributing to skin irritation include damp dressings, presence of caustic effluent in contact with the skin, and frequent tape application and removal. When selecting and evaluating a management technique, the nurse should consider interventions appropriate to prevent unnecessary patient discomfort.

Goal: Accurate Measurement of Effluent. Accurate measurement of effluent from a fistula or drain site is critical to the success of fluid and electrolyte resuscitation and nutritional support. As the patient becomes stabilized, accurate measurement of the effluent is of less import. Seldom will the patient at home be required to monitor output volumes. Pouching offers the most objective method of monitoring output; suction is accurate only if the effluent does not leak around the catheters. Dressings can provide an estimate of volume if the dressings are weighed; however, this method is time consuming, messy, and inconsistent from caregiver to caregiver.

Goal: Patient Mobility. Consideration for optimizing the patient's activity should be of paramount importance when a fistula management method is being selected. Restrictions on physical activity predispose the patient to physical complications such as pneumonia, pressure ulcers, and thrombophlebitis as well as psychosocial complications such as depression and withdrawal. Because limitations on a patient's physical activity are sometimes necessary when suction or dressings are used to contain effluent, these interventions should be used only on a temporary basis. Pouches are less likely to restrict mobility.

Goal: Cost Containment. Accountable, appropriate fistula management also requires that the nurse select a treatment option that is cost effective. For example, a fistula pouch with a wound access window that is changed every other day is more costly than a sizable ostomy pouch, which would probably yield the same wear time. However, if use of a pouch with an access window prolongs wear time by providing access for wound care and paste application, it may be the most cost-effective option.

Cost containment implies attention not only to products and materials, but also to labor and time. Table 8-5 demonstrates the savings (cost and time) realized when pouching of a drain site is used instead of every-4-hour dressing changes.

Implementation

Preparation. After careful assessment of the wound or fistula and establishment of a care plan, it is time to implement the plan. Because fistula output can be unpredictable, it is best to be as organized as possible before beginning the procedure. A routine pouch change procedure is listed in Box 8-14. Water, gauze, towels, scissors, and the products that will be needed should all be set out before one starts. A receptacle for soiled linens and trash should be placed in proximity.

Preassemble as many items as possible. When using a pouch without an attached skin barrier, the pouch and barrier should be assembled so that it is applied to the patient as a complete unit. Doing so will be convenient and reduce application errors, which can result in leakage.

Fistula pouch changes can be complicated and time intensive. The procedure may be facilitated by scheduling a time that allows a fellow nurse to assist. The patient may also be

Table 8-5   Comparison of costs per management option (cost represents an average of the hospital's *acquisition* cost only)[*]

Management option	Frequency of change	Cost per week
OPTION 1: DRESSINGS: 2 pkg sterile gauze ($0.06) 1 pkg abdominal dressing ($0.10) Accessory items[†] ($1.02) TOTAL COST PER CHANGE: $1.18	6/day (42/week)	$49.56
OPTION 2: POUCHING: Medium pouch with access window and skin barrier attached ($13.00) ¼ tube skin-barrier paste[‡] ($1.50) Accessory items[†] ($1.02) TOTAL COST PER CHANGE: $15.52	3/week	$46.56
OPTION 3: POUCHING: Medium pouch; no access window; skin barrier attached ($2.30) ¼ tube skin-barrier paste[‡] ($1.50) Accessory times[†] ($1.02) TOTAL COST PER CHANGE: $4.82	3/week	$14.46
OPTION 4: POUCHING: Medium pouch; no skin barrier or access window ($1.25) 1 4×4 skin-barrier wafer ($2.15) ¼ tube skin-barrier paste[‡] ($1.50) Accessory items[†] ($1.02) TOTAL COST PER CHANGE: $5.92	3/week	$17.76

[*]Nursing labor is not quantified in this comparison because such is hospital specific. However, one can surmise that the dressing option requires substantially large nursing time, which could be reallocated to other nursing activities or, for some hospitals, could result in cost savings when pouching options are utilized appropriately.
[†]Accessory items include 2 pairs of nonsterile gloves, 4 nonsterile gauzes, one 35 ml syringe, and one 250 ml bottle of normal saline.
[‡]Assume that one tube would be used for 4 pouch changes.

willing to assist. One person could be responsible for removing soiled products, cleansing the skin, and wicking effluent while the second person prepares and applies the pouching system. Plates 25 to 27 demonstrate the steps used to pouch an enterocutaneous fistula.

Skin Cleansing. When preparing the skin for applying a pouch, it is essential that the skin be clean, dry, and greaseless. Small amounts of residual paste or cement may be left on the skin and should not hinder pouch adhesion; again, the surface of the residue should be clean and allowed to dry completely. Generally, tap water and soft gauze or cotton sponges are sufficient for cleansing perifistular skin. Many commercially prepared skin cleansers are also available to cleanse the skin; however, their use in fistula care should be quite limited. Soaps (cleansers) will emulsify fecal material and are primarily indicated when fistula

---

Box 8-14   SIZABLE POUCH-CHANGE PROCEDURE: FISTULA

1. Assemble equipment: pouch, skin-barrier wafer, pattern, skin-barrier paste, scissors, paper tape, closure clip, water, gauze or tissue.
2. Prepare pouch:
   a. Trace pattern onto skin-barrier wafer and pouch.
   b. Cut skin barrier to size of pattern.
   c. Cut pouch at least $^1/_{16}$-inch larger than skin-barrier wafer.
   d. Remove protective backing or backings from pouch.
   e. Apply nonadhesive side of skin-barrier wafer to pouch, matching center openings.
   f. Remove protective backing from skin-barrier wafer.
   g. Set assembled pouch aside.
3. Remove and apply pouch:
   a. Remove pouch, using one hand to gently push the skin away from the adhesive.
   b. Discard pouch and save closure clip.
   c. Control any discharge with gauze or tissue.
   d. Clean skin with water and dry thoroughly.
   e. Apply paste around fistula or stoma. Fill in any uneven skin surfaces with paste. Use a damp finger or tongue blade to apply paste.
   f. Apply new pouch, centering wound site in opening.
   g. Tape edges of adhesive surface in a picture-frame effect with paper tape.
   h. Close bottom of pouch with clip.
   NOTE: If pouch has attached skin barrier eliminate steps *2c* to *e*.

---

drainage is adherent to surrounding skin. Cleansers should be nongreasy and rinsed thoroughly; use on denuded skin is discouraged.

Adhesives are generally easily removed from the skin with only tap water and soft cloth or gauze. Solvents may be used to remove adhesive residue but must be cleansed thoroughly from the skin to avoid leaving a greasy film on the skin.

Sizing Pouch Aperture. A pouching system can succeed or fail by the size and shape of the opening cut in the pouch alone. Most commonly a $^1/_8$- to $^1/_4$-inch margin of skin is left exposed around the fistula to prevent leakage of effluent under the skin-barrier wafer. This exposed skin is then protected with another form of skin barrier, typically paste.

Apertures much larger than the actual fistula opening may be necessary with severe, deep depressions that create irregular skin surfaces. To prevent skin denudation, a skin barrier paste is applied to the exposed skin (Plate 32).

Skin-Barrier Paste. Skin-barrier pastes are used to level irregular skin surfaces before adhesives are applied, as shown in Plate 26, to extend the duration of solid-wafer skin barriers, to protect the perifistular skin that remains exposed to effluent, and to prevent leakage between the skin and pouch opening. Pastes should be applied in a thin bead, smoothed into place with a damp gloved finger or tongue blade, and allowed to dry briefly so that solvents can escape before other products are applied.

At times, when the pouch is being changed frequently, it is not possible to remove all residual skin-barrier paste. To avoid traumatizing the skin, residual paste can be dried and left on the skin, and new paste applied.

Because commercially prepared pastes contain alcohol, discomfort is experienced when applied to denuded skin. Occasionally, making up pastes is desirable. One can make such pastes by mixing skin-barrier powder with glycerin to achieve a toothpaste consistency. Because these products do not contain alcohol, the patient with denuded skin should not experience burning or stinging during the application process. These made-up pastes may be indicated when commercial pastes are not available, when large amounts are needed, or when the skin is severely denuded. However, because such pastes do not contain preservatives, they will not store well.

Routine Care. Drainage of effluent away from the fistula orifice should be facilitated to minimize the erosion of the skin barrier by corrosive effluent. This can be accomplished by interventions as simple as angling the pouch off to the reclining patient's side or by attaching tubing to enable continuous drainage into a larger receptacle. Patients should be encouraged to participate in monitoring the pouch and recognizing when it needs to be emptied.

The care of fistulas or drain sites is seldom a sterile procedure. Sterile products are an unnecessary expense and are not shown to control infection. Clean, aseptic technique should be followed.

Universal precautions are imperative when one is working with any body fluid, especially effluent from fistulas and drain sites because they are often contaminated with feces and blood. Gloves should be worn when one is emptying pouches, changing pouches, cleansing the skin, and changing dressings. One pair of gloves are worn to remove soiled dressings or pouches, and another pair of gloves are worn to apply new dressings or pouches.

Evaluation

Accomplishment of Goals. The nurse should take the time to reflect on the seven nursing management goals and evaluate how well these have been accomplished. If a pouch is being used, concerns focus primarily on the effectiveness of the pouching system at containing effluent, controlling odor, and protecting the skin. Dressings should also be evaluated in terms of effectiveness in containing effluent, protecting skin, and controlling odor. Efficient use of nursing time should not be overlooked.

Generally a pouching system should stay intact at least 24 hours, preferably 3 to 4 days. The length of time will be dependent on many variables such as abdominal contours, volume of effluent, and patient activities. It is advisable to begin conservatively and change the pouch 24 hours after initial application so that the condition of the perifistular skin and skin barrier can be assessed. If the skin barrier is intact and the skin is well protected, the wear time can gradually be extended a day at a time.

Making Changes. It is infrequent that the first fistula pouch applied will be effective. Generally, modifications are necessary in the pouch pattern, size of adhesive surface, and use of skin-barrier pastes or wafer strips. It is best to make one change at a time so that the effect of these changes can be accurately assessed.

Some modifications are quite simple but effective. The addition of a belt may be warranted to add security to the pouch system, particularly on obese patients, or when the perifistular skin is mobile. Frequency of pouch emptying and volume of effluent should also be evaluated. The pouch should be emptied whenever it is one third to one half full. Leakage can result just because the pouch overfills. Pouch overfilling can be a staffing-related problem or the result of passing large sudden volumes. Continuous drainage to keep the pouch from overfilling may provide an effective resolution to the problem.

One pouching system is seldom effective from the onset of the fistula until the closure of the fistula. Changes in the fistula output, patient activity, and abdominal contours will necessitate frequent reevaluation of the pouching pattern and procedure. As healing occurs, retraction of the fistula, scars, or wound develop and modifications in the pouching system will be necessary.

Discharge Planning. Once a pouching system is deemed effective, it is time to begin teaching the procedure to staff nurses and family members. Interested caregivers can be involved in the procedure before this time, and techniques can be explained. However, to avoid confusion, actual teaching of the procedure should be delayed until a clear, successful plan emerges. As the discharge date becomes clear, the home care nurse should be contacted and invited to participate in the pouch-change procedure before discharge. A complete discharge plan should contain the following elements legibly documented for the nurse or caregiver: step-by-step instructions on the pouch-application process, list of equipment and product numbers, list of retailers where supplies can be purchased, enough equipment for two or three pouch changes; phone number of ET nurse, home-care nurse referral, follow-up plan with physician, and follow-up plan with ET nurse. Follow-up observation and monitoring by a nurse who specializes in fistula management, such as the ET nurse, is necessary to anticipate contour changes, make necessary adjustments, monitor nutritional status, and identify complications.

SUMMARY

Patients with a fistula require complex, aggressive, and methodical care. State-of-the-art care mandates the utilization of a multidisciplinary team. Because the fistula may take weeks or months to close, the patient commonly requires acute care, home care, and outpatient care to monitor adequately the containment method and to make revisions as indicated. Successful containment methods challenge the nurse to be creative and patient.

Certainly, the nurse plays an extremely important role in the containment of effluent, skin protection, and emotional support. However, this is most effectively achieved when nursing management is complemented with an understanding of the medical and surgical fistula management plan.

SELF-EVALUATIONS

QUESTIONS AND PROBLEMS

1. List at least four factors that may contribute to fistula development after a surgical procedure.
2. Radiation-induced endarteritis may cause fistulas:
    a. only in the first month after irradiation.
    b. between 1 and 3 years after irradiation.
    c. from 3 to 5 years after irradiation.
    d. at any time after irradiation.
3. List three complications that contribute to death from fistulas.
4. Define the term "fistula."
5. A high-output fistula is defined as one that produces:
    a. more than 100 ml in 24 hours.
    b. more than 500 ml in 24 hours.
    c. more than 1000 ml in 24 hours.
    d. more than 750 ml in 24 hours.
6. Define the involved structures for the following:
    a. Enterocutaneous
    b. Colocutaneous
    c. Vesicovaginal
    d. Rectovaginal
    e. Colovesical
7. List the three phases of medical management for the patient with a fistula.
8. A high-output small bowel fistula is likely to cause which of the following?
    a. Fluid volume deficit; hyperkalemia
    b. Fluid volume excess; hyponatremia
    c. Fluid volume deficit; hypokalemia
    d. Fluid volume excess; hypernatremia
9. The major cause of death in the patient with a fistula is:
    a. malnutrition.
    b. sepsis.
    c. operative complications.
    d. hypovolemia.
10. Identify guidelines for nutritional support of the patient with a fistula to include the amount of calories and proteins needed and the route for nutritional support.
11. What percentage of fistulas will close spontaneously with nutritional support and infection control?
    a. 50%
    b. 90%
    c. 75%
    d. 25%
12. List at least four factors known to delay spontaneous closure of fistulas.
13. Surgical *closure* of fistulas commonly involves:
    a. fistula resection and end-to-end anastomosis.
    b. "oversewing" of fistula tract.

      c. creation of stomas proximal to the fistula.

      d. intestinal bypass procedure.

14. List seven goals for nursing management of the patient with a fistula.

15. Identify four factors that nurses should consider in assessing a fistula and establishing a management plan.

16. Which of the following is used to absorb moisture from irritated skin?

      a. Commercial skin-barrier pastes

      b. Adhesives

      c. Skin-barrier powders

      d. Skin sealants

17. Skin sealants are used for all of the following *except:*

      a. to protect skin from adhesives.

      b. to prevent maceration from low-output fistulas.

      c. to prevent erosion from caustic drainage.

      d. to enhance tack over oily skin.

18. Which of the following fistulas would be appropriately managed with gauze dressings?

      a. Volume of output 350 ml per 24 hours

      b. Output noncorrosive and odorous

      c. Volume of output 100 ml per 24 hours and noncorrosive

      d. Output with formed consistency and odorous

19. List features that should be considered in the selection of a fistula pouch.

20. Describe two methods for extending the adhesive area on a pouch.

21. Which of the following is appropriate for pouching a fistula located in an open wound and surrounded by irregular abdominal contours?

      a. Two-piece ostomy pouch

      b. Condom catheter fistula pouch

      c. One-piece ostomy pouch with convexity

      d. Trough procedure

22. Which of the following is the best option for managing a wound with very limited pouching surface?

      a. Bridging technique

      b. Saddlebagging technique

      c. Condom catheter fistula pouch

      d. Trough procedure

23. Explain when the bridging technique is indicated?

24. Describe the indications for using suction catheters in the management of draining wounds and fistulas.

25. Identify two approaches to management of vaginal fistulas.

26. Identify options for odor control in wounds managed with dressings and wounds managed with pouches.

27. Identify options for management and accurate measurement of high-volume output.

28. List five components critical to a discharge plan for the patient with a fistula.

29. What is a major drawback to the use of silicone molds for fistula containment?

      a. Mold material is quite expensive.

      b. New molds must be made as contours change.

       c. Adhesives must be used to adhere the mold.

       d. The mold is rigid and can traumatize skin.

30. Skin-barrier paste is used with fistulas to achieve which of the following objectives?

       a. Absorb moisture from denuded skin

       b. Increase tack of pouch adhesives

       c. Level irregular skin surfaces

       d. Protect the skin from adhesives

SELF-EVALUATION

ANSWERS

1. Presence of foreign body close to suture line
Tension on suture line
Improper suturing technique
Distal obstruction
Hematoma or abscess formation in mesentery at anastomotic site
Presence of tumor or disease in area of anastomosis
Inadequate blood supply to anastomosis

2. d

3. Fluid and electrolyte imbalances
Malnutrition
Sepsis

4. An abnormal passage between two or more structures or spaces.

5. b

6. a. Fistula between small bowel and skin
b. Fistula between colon and skin
c. Fistula between bladder and vagina
d. Fistula between rectum and vagina
e. Fistula between colon and bladder

7. Fluid and electrolyte stabilization
Evaluation and treatment of sepsis
Definitive therapy

8. c

9. b

10. Amount of calories and protein needs should be determined by a complete nutritional assessment. Calorie-intake guidelines suggest 37 to 45 calories/kg per 24 hours. Protein-intake guidelines suggest 1.5 to 1.75/kg per 24 hours.
Guidelines for selection of route:
    Enteral nutrition is appropriate orally for colocutaneous fistulas or low-output ileal fistulas. Enteral gastrostomy or jejunostomy nutrition is appropriate for esophageal fistulas and for gastric, duodenal, or jejunal fistulas.
    Parenteral nutrition is indicated for high-output fistulas, when enteral feedings are not possible because of the location of the fistula or intolerance of the solution and when the bowel is obstructed.

11. a

12. Complete disruption of bowel continuity
    Distal obstruction
    Foreign body in fistula tract
    Epithelium-lined tract contiguous with the skin
    Cancer in site
    Previous irradiation to site
    Crohn's disease in site
    Presence of large abscess
13. a
14. Skin protection
    Containment of drainage
    Odor control
    Patient comfort
    Accurate measurement of effluent
    Patient mobility
    Cost containment
15. Source of fistula drainage
    Skin condition
    Anatomic location and abdominal contours
    Characteristics of drainage (volume, consistency, presence or absence of enzymes, color)
16. c
17. c
18. c
19. Adhesive surface and cutting surface
    Pouch capacity
    Pouch film (odorproof versus odor-resistant)
    Pouch outlet
    Wound-access features
20. Use of double-faced adhesive disks or double-faced adhesive sheets
    Use of contact cement over cloth tape strips
    Use of saddlebagging technique
21. d
22. c
23. The bridging procedure should be used when it is helpful to isolate one area of a wound from another area of the wound. This may be needed for very large wounds or for wounds that have two distinct areas of "needs."
24. Suction catheters may be used as a supplement to routine pouching, to facilitate management of high-output fistulas, or to replace pouching when it is ineffective. If used to replace pouching, suction catheters are used with a closed wound-drainage system (as with use of transparent adhesive dressing).
25. Pouching
    Use of vaginal drain device (nipple shield and Malecot catheter)
    Ointments and pads
26. *Wounds managed with dressings:* charcoal dressings can be secured over wound dressings; charcoal dressings must be kept dry.

Wound managed with pouches: meticulous pouch hygiene, pouch deodorants, and room deodorants. Oral deodorants may be an option in either situation.

27. a. Use of pouching system with spout for attachment to bedside drainage.

b. Use of urinary adapter secured into drainable pouch with rubber band.

c. Use of 10 in 1 connector and latex tubing connected to pouch before pouch application.

28. Step-by-step instructions for pouch application

List of products and product numbers

List of retailers where products can be purchased

Home-care nurse referral

Follow-up appointment with physician and ET nurse

Phone number of ET nurse and physician

29. b

30. c

REFERENCES

1. Alexander-Williams J and Irving M: Intestinal fistulas, Boston, 1982, Wright-PSG.
2. Aguirre A, Fischer JE, and Welch C: The role of surgery and hyperalimentation in therapy of gastrointestinal-cutaneous fistulae, Ann Surg 180:393-400, 1974.
3. Allardyce DB: Management of small bowel fistulas, Am J Surg 145:593-595, 1983.
4. Boarini J, Bryant R, and Irrgang S: Fistula management, Semin Oncol Nurs 2:287-292, 1986.
5. Devereux DF, Sears HF, and Ketcham AS: Intestinal fistula following pelvix exenterative surgery: predisposing causes and treatment, J Surg Oncol 14:227-234, 1980.
6. Devlin HB and Elcoat C: Alimentary tract fistula: stomatherapy techniques of management, World J Surg 7:489-494, 1983.
7. Dunavant MK: Wound and fistula management. In Broadwell D and Jackson B, editors: Principle of ostomy care, St. Louis, 1982, Mosby–Year Book, Inc.
8. Everett WGL: Wound sinus or fistula? In Westaby S, editor: Wound care, St. Louis, 1986, Mosby–Year Book, Inc.
9. Fazio VW, Coutsoftides T, and Steiger E: Factors influencing the outcome of treatment of small bowel cutaneous fistula, World J Surg 7:481-488, 1983.
10. Fischer J: The pathophysiology of enterocutaneous fistulas, World J Surg 7:446-450, 1983.
11. Fischer JE: Enterocutaneous fistulas. In Najarian JS and Delaney JP, editors: Progress in gastrointestinal surgery, Chicago, 1989, Mosby–Year Book, Inc.
12. Given BA and Simmons SJ: Gastroenterology in clinical nursing, ed 4, St. Louis, 1984, Mosby–Year Book, Inc.
13. Goldberg SM, Gordon PH, and Nivatvongs S, editors: Essentials of anorectal surgery, Philadelphia, 1980, JB Lippincott, pp 316-332.
14. Gross E and Irving M: Protection of the skin around intestinal fistulas, Br J Surg 64:258-263, 1977.
15. Hollender LF, Meyer C, Avet AA, and Zeyer B: Postoperative fistulas of the small intestine: therapeutic principles, World J Surg 7:474-480, 1983.
16. Hollis HW Jr and Reyna TM: A practical approach to wound care in patients with complex enterocutaneous fistulas, Surg Gynecol Obstet 161:179-180, 1985.
17. Irrgang S and Bryant R: Management of the enterocutaneous fistula, J Enterostom Ther 11:211-225, 1984.
18. Jeter KF, Tintle TE, and Chariker M: Managing draining wounds and fistulae: new and established methods. In Krasner D, editor: Chronic wound care: a clinical source book for healthcare professionals, King of Prussia, Penn, 1990, Health Management Publications, Inc.
19. Jones CR, Woodhouse CR, and Hendry WF: Urological problems following treatment of carcinoma of the cervix, Br J Urol 56:509-613, 1984.

20. Krasner D: Managing draining wounds: fistulae, leaking tubes and drains. In Krasner D, editor: Chronic wound care: a clinical source book for healthcare professionals, King of Prussia, Penn, 1990, Health Management Publications, Inc.
21. Kurtz R, Heimann T, and Aufses A: The management of intestinal fistulas, Am J Gastroenterol 76:377-380, 1981.
22. Ladefoged K, Christensen KC, Hegnhøj J, and Jarnum S: Effect of a long acting somatostatin analogue SMS 201-995 on jejunostomy effluents in patients with severe short bowel syndrome, Gut 30:943-949, 1989.
23. Laing BJ: Making silicone casts for enterocutaneous fistulas, ET J, fall:11, 1977.
24. Lange MP, Thebo L, Tiede S, et al: Management of multiple enterocutaneous fistulas, Heart Lung 18:386-390, 1989.
25. Moran JR and Greene HL: Digestion and absorption. In Clinical nutrition: enteral and tube feeding, ed 2, Philadelphia, 1990, WB Saunders Co.
26. North AP: Management of an enterovaginal fistula. In Krasner D, editor: Chronic wound care: a clinical source book for healthcare professionals, King of Prussia, Penn, 1990, Health Management Publications, Inc.
27. Nubiola-Calonge P, Badía JM, Sancho J, et al: Blind evaluation of the effect of octreotide (SMS 201-995), a somatostatin analogue, on small-bowel fistula output, Lancet 2(8560):672-674, 1987.
28. O'Connor E: Vaginal fistulas: adaptation of management method for patients with radiation damage, J Enterostom Ther 10(6):229-230, 1983.
29. Reber H and Austin J: Abdominal abscesses and gastrointestinal fistulas. In Sleisenger M and Fortran J, editors: Gastrointestinal disease pathophysiology diagnosis management, vol 1, ed 4, Philadelphia, 1989, WB Saunders Co.
30. Rombeau J and Rolandelli R: Enteral and parenteral nutrition in patients with enteric fistulas and short bowel syndrome, Surg Clin North Am 67(3):551-568, 1987.
31. Rose D, Yarborough M, Canizaro P, and Lowry S: One hundred and fourteen fistulas of the gastrointestinal tract treated with total parenteral nutrition, Surg Gynecol Obstet 163:345-350, 1986.
32. Rothenberger DA and Goldberg SM: The management of rectovaginal fistulae, Surg Clin North Am 63(1):61-79, 1983.
33. Schmitz RL, Chao JH, and Bartolome JS Jr: Intestinal injuries incidental to irradiation of carcinoma of the cervix of the uterus, Surg Gynecol Obstet 138:29-32, 1974.
34. Schwartz S: Complications. In Schwartz S, Shires GT, Spencer R, and Storer E, editors: Principles of surgery, vol 1, ed 4, New York, 1984, McGraw-Hill Book Co.
35. Sitges-Serra A, Jaurrieta E, and Sitges-Creus A: Management of postoperative enterocutaneous fistulas: the roles of parenteral nutrition and surgery, Br J Surg 69:147-150, 1982.
36. Smith DB: Fistulas of the head and neck, J Enterostom Ther 9(5):20-24, 1982.
37. Smith DB: Multiple stomas, fistulas and draining wounds. In Smith DB and Johnson DR, editors: Ostomy care and the cancer patient: surgical and clinical considerations, New York, 1986, Grune & Stratton, Inc.
38. Smith DH, Pierce VK, and Lewis JL Jr: Enteric fistulas encountered on a gynecologic oncology service from 1969-1980, Surg Gynecol Obstet 158:71-75, 1984.
39. Smith ST, Seski JC, Copeland LJ, et al: Surgical management of irradiation-induced small bowel damage, Obstet Gynecol 65:563-567, 1985.
40. Thelan LA, Davie JK, and Urden LD: Textbook of critical care nursing: diagnosis and management, St. Louis, 1990, Mosby–Year Book, Inc.
41. Thomas RJS: The response of patients with fistulas of the gastrointestinal tract to parenteral nutrition, Surg Gynecol Obstet 153:77-80, 1981.
42. Welch JP: Duodenal, gastric, and biliary fistulas. In Schwartz SI and Ellis H, editors: Maingot's abdominal operations, vol 1, ed 8, East Norwalk, Ct, 1985, Appleton-Century-Crofts.
43. Watts R: Personal communication, 1982.

9 Principles of Nutritional Support

NANCY NUWER KONSTANTINIDES

OBJECTIVES

1. Define the term "malnutrition."
2. Describe the effects of malnutrition on the following systems or processes:
   Cardiorespiratory system
   Gastrointestinal system
   Wound healing
3. List some common causes of malnutrition.
4. Identify the three major components of a nutritional assessment.
5. Describe at least two approaches to obtaining an accurate dietary history.
6. Explain the significance of anthropometric measurements in a nutritional assessment.
7. Define the term "anergy" and explain its relevance to nutritional assessment.
8. Explain the significance of nitrogen balance studies in monitoring a patient's nutritional status.
9. Compare the following studies in terms of sensitivity to changes in nutritional status: serum albumin, transferrin, prealbumin.
10. List at least two conditions other than malnutrition that may cause low TLC (total lymphocyte count) levels.
11. Differentiate between the following formulas in terms of composition and indications for use:
    Milk based versus lactose free
    Protein intact versus chemically designed (elemental)
12. List at least two nursing measures for improving tolerance or reducing diarrhea in the patient receiving enteral feedings.
13. Identify indications for parenteral nutritional support.

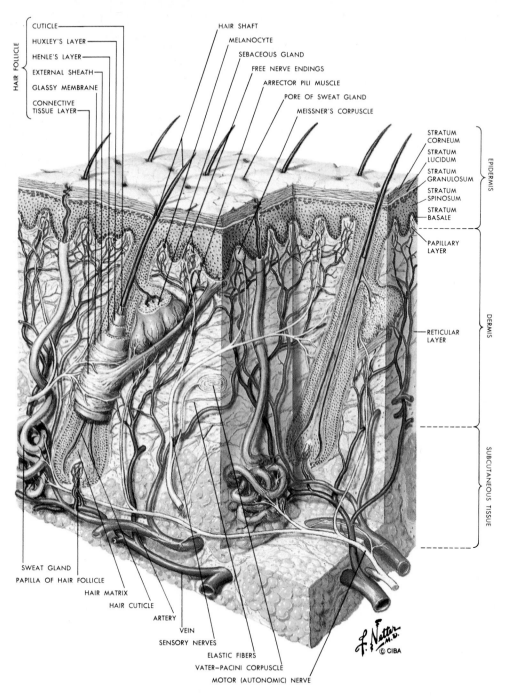

CUTICLE
HUXLEY'S LAYER
HENLE'S LAYER
EXTERNAL SHEATH
GLASSY MEMBRANE
CONNECTIVE TISSUE LAYER

HAIR FOLLICLE

HAIR SHAFT
MELANOCYTE
SEBACEOUS GLAND
FREE NERVE ENDINGS
ARRECTOR PILI MUSCLE
PORE OF SWEAT GLAND
MEISSNER'S CORPUSCLE

STRATUM CORNEUM
STRATUM LUCIDUM
STRATUM GRANULOSUM
STRATUM SPINOSUM
STRATUM BASALE

EPIDERMIS

PAPILLARY LAYER

RETICULAR LAYER

DERMIS

SUBCUTANEOUS TISSUE

SWEAT GLAND
PAPILLA OF HAIR FOLLICLE
HAIR MATRIX
HAIR CUTICLE
ARTERY
VEIN
SENSORY NERVES
ELASTIC FIBERS
VATER–PACINI CORPUSCLE
MOTOR (AUTONOMIC) NERVE

Plate 1 Schema of anatomy of skin and subcutaneous tissue. (From Habif TPL: Clinical dermatology: a color guide to diagnosis and therapy, ed 2, St. Louis, 1990, Mosby–Year Book, Inc.)

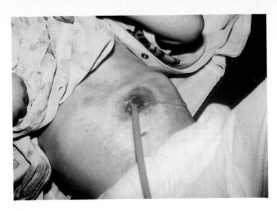

Plate 2 Erosion of epidermis because of chemical irritation from an unhealed gastrostomy site. (Courtesy Abbott Northwestern Hospital, Minneapolis.)

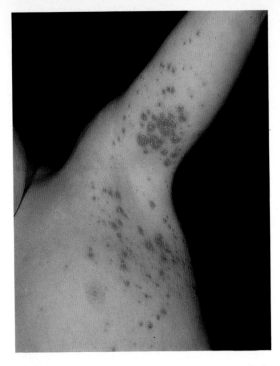

Plate 3 Bullous impetigo. Numerous unroofed bullae revealing shallow ulcerations. (From Habif TP: Clinical dermatology: a color guide to diagnosis and therapy, ed 2, St. Louis, 1990, Mosby–Year Book, Inc.)

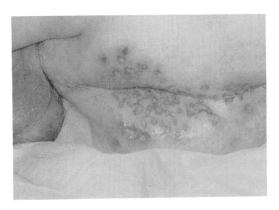

Plate 4 Herpes simplex on buttocks. Notice cluster of vesicles on erythematous base. (Courtesy Mary Brachman, Abbott Northwestern Hospital, Minneapolis.)

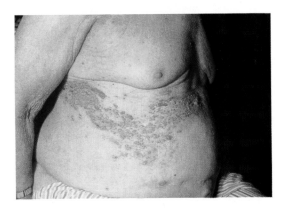

Plate 5 Herpes zoster involving single thoracic dermatome. Vesicles are clustered and erythematous. (Courtesy Mary Brachman, Abbott Northwestern Hospital, Minneapolis.)

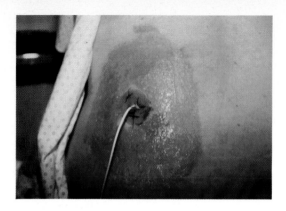

Plate 6   Moist desquamation after an allergic reaction in response to the second application of benzoin to a percutaneous nephrostomy site. (Courtesy Abbott Northwestern Hospital, Minneapolis.)

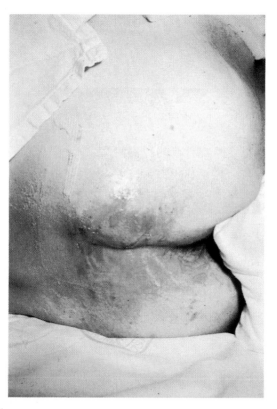

Plate 7   Partial-thickness lesion (extends into dermis) demonstrating islands of epidermal cells; stage 2 according to staging criteria of International Association for Enterostomal Therapy (IAET) and National Pressure Ulcer Advisory Panel (NPUAP). (Courtesy Emory University, Atlanta, Ga.)

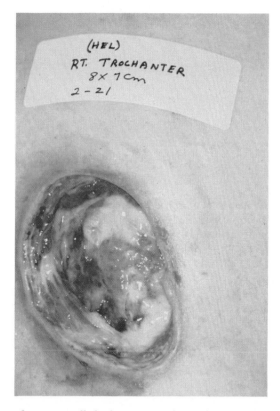

Plate 8   Full-thickness wound revealing muscle and the presence of yellow nonviable tissue; classified as a stage 4 ulcer according to the IAET and NPUAP staging criteria. (Courtesy Emory University, Atlanta, Ga.)

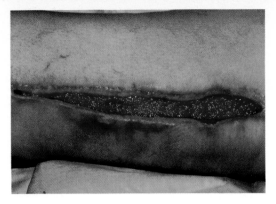

Plate 9 Surgical wound with granulation tissue present as evidenced by red, moist, grainy-appearing wound bed. (Courtesy Abbott Northwestern Hospital, Minneapolis.)

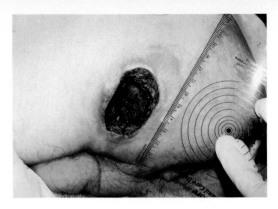

Plate 10 Eschar-covered pressure ulcer with evidence of infection in surrounding tissue. (Courtesy Emory University, Atlanta, Ga.)

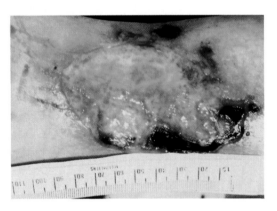

Plate 11 Full-thickness venous ulcer with necrotic tissue present (eschar and yellow nonviable) and exudate. (Courtesy Abbott Northwestern Hospital, Minneapolis.)

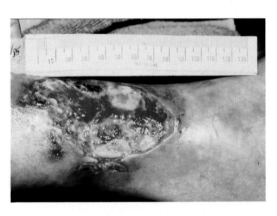

Plate 12 Stage 3 venous ulcer (same as in Plate 11) with evidence of healing: granulation tissue is now present in wound bed, and there is less nonviable tissue and poor drainage. (Courtesy Abbott Northwestern Hospital, Minneapolis.)

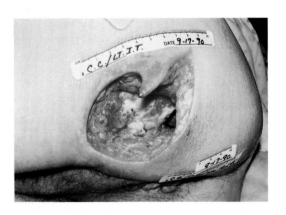

Plate 13 Full-thickness pressure ulcer with loss of tissue and with dead space. (Courtesy Emory University, Atlanta, Ga.)

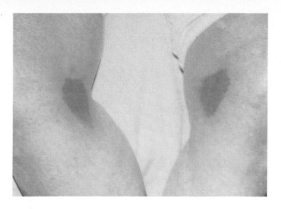

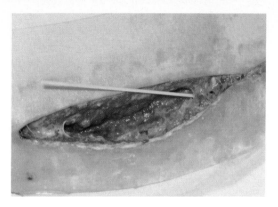

Plate 14 Stage 1 pressure ulcer according to IAET and NPUAP staging criteria. (Courtesy Abbott Northwestern Hospital, Minneapolis.)

Plate 15 Stage 3 dehisced surgical wound (according to IAET and NPUAP staging criteria) with undermining. (Courtesy Abbott Northwestern Hospital, Minneapolis.)

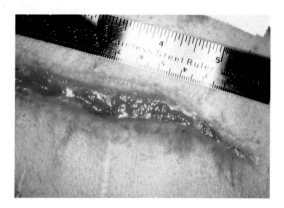

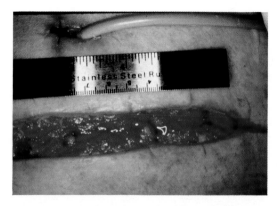

Plate 16 Surgical wound with epithelialization occurring; epithelial healing ridge apparent. (Courtesy Dr. Diane Cooper, San Francisco.)

Plate 17 Surgical wound lacking evidence of healing epithelial ridge. (Courtesy Dr. Diane Cooper, San Francisco.)

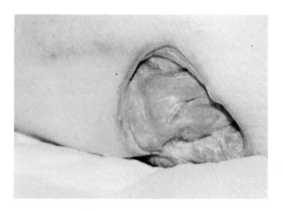

Plate 18 Stage 4 pressure ulcer with exposed muscle; notice the pale color of the muscle, which is suggestive of underlying suboptimal healing states such as anemia. Undermining of wound edges is also apparent. (Courtesy Abbott Northwestern Hospital, Minneapolis.)

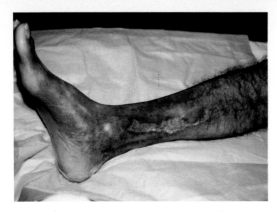

Plate 19 Classic appearance of lower extremity in patient with severe peripheral vascular disease. Notice shiny, taut epidermis and lack of subcutaneous tissue. (Courtesy Abbott Northwestern Hospital, Minneapolis.)

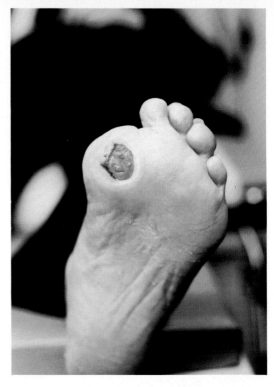

Plate 20 Classic neuropathic plantar ulcer on the first metatarsal head. Callus tissue has formed around the ulcer. Notice pale wound bed color. (Courtesy Dr. Jack Graber, Minneapolis.)

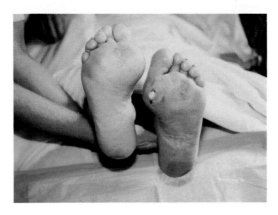

Plate 21 Neuropathic plantar ulcer on first metatarsal head after conservative débridement (packing is present in the ulcer). Notice foot and toe deformities and callus formation in this patient with diabetes mellitus. Stage 2 (blisters) pressure ulcers are also present on both heels. (Courtesy Abbott Northwestern Hospital, Minneapolis.)

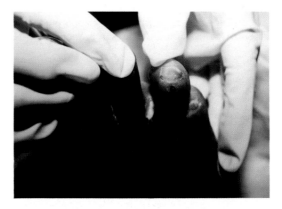

Plate 22 Insignificant-appearing interdigital ulcer in patient with diabetes, peripheral neuropathy, and peripheral vascular disease. (Courtesy Abbott Northwestern Hospital, Minneapolis.)

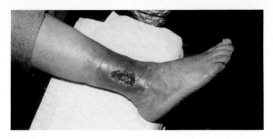

Plate 23 Typical appearance and location of a venous ulcer. Surrounding skin has been moisturized to eliminate the usual dry skin. (Courtesy Abbott Northwestern Hospital, Minneapolis.)

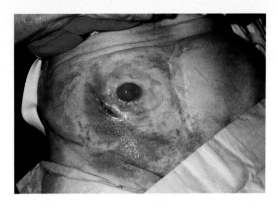

Plate 24 Patient with enterocutaneous fistula in proximity to previously established ileostomy and iliac crest. Perifistular skin is mobile and flaccid and has an erythematous rash typical of candidiasis infection. (Courtesy Abbott Northwestern Hospital, Minneapolis.)

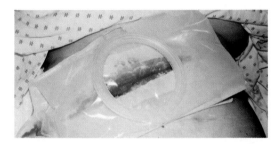

Plate 25 Enterocutaneous fistula with output of 1800 ml per 24 hours managed with sizable wound pouch with access window. Amount of skin exposed necessary to achieve adequate seal. Skin-barrier pastes dissolved quickly and could be reinforced daily to protect skin from effluent. (Courtesy Abbott Northwestern Hospital, Minneapolis.)

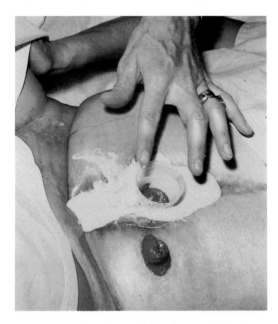

Plate 26 Medical-grade elastomer has been poured into abdominal wound to create a silicone mold. A medicine cup is in place to surround the fistula orifice and prevent contact with the mold. Elastomer dries to produce a firm mold. (Courtesy Mary Zink, Minneapolis.)

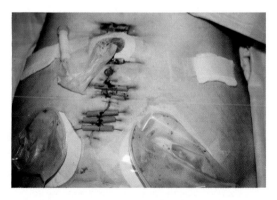

Plate 27 Condom catheter pouch technique used effectively in a fistula located in a midline incision with retention sutures present.

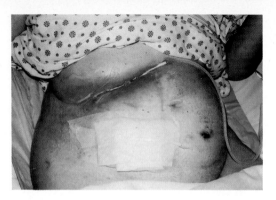

Plate 28   Closed wound drainage system with suction catheter laid in the wound and exiting from the transparent dressing covered wound. (Courtesy Abbott Northwestern Hospital, Minneapolis.)

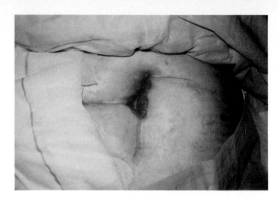

Plate 29   Patient with an enterocutaneous fistula with depressions in abdominal surface at upper left aspect. (Courtesy Abbott Northwestern Hospital, Minneapolis.)

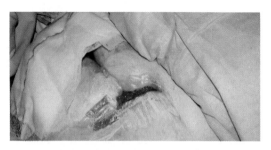

Plate 30   Tapered layers of solid-wafer skin barrier used to help level skin depression at inferior aspect. Skin-barrier paste has been applied to surrounding wound margins and in all three depressions (over skin-barrier wafer wedges) to level and protect the skin from effluent. Cement has been painted onto adhesive field (over paste and wedges) to increase adhesion. (Courtesy Abbott Northwestern Hospital, Minneapolis.)

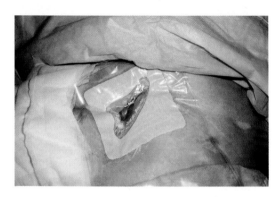

Plate 31   Open-end drain pouch is applied. A skin-barrier wafer had to be applied to the pouch and was selected because it provided a flexible adhesive surface that would conform to the skin contours and also had adequate cutting surface. (Courtesy Abbott Northwestern Hospital, Minneapolis.)

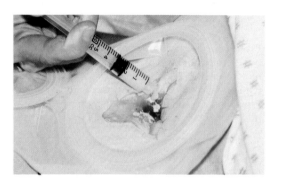

Plate 32   Additional skin-barrier paste being applied by a syringe after the pouch is applied to protect the perifistular skin and prevent leakage between skin and pouch opening. Notice radial slits that have been cut into pouch opening to facilitate conforming of adhesive to abdominal contours. (Courtesy Abbott Northwestern Hospital, Minneapolis.)

Proper wound healing can occur only with good nutrition. Unfortunately, although people are becoming more health and nutrition conscious, malnutrition remains a worldwide problem. Numerous adverse consequences such as increased morbidity (associated with decreased resistance to infections and impaired wound healing), increased mortality, and prolonged recovery from illness result from chronic malnutrition. This chapter reviews the causes and effects of malnutrition and the role of the health care professional in its prevention and treatment through nutritional assessment and intervention.

DEFINITION AND INCIDENCE OF MALNUTRITION

Malnutrition is a condition of inadequate nutrient intake or utilization (particularly calories and protein) relative to individual requirements. Malnutrition can also be defined as reduced lean body mass (or skeletal muscle mass).[1] Specific nutrient deficiencies (such as vitamins or minerals) can occur with or without malnutrition and are not discussed in this chapter. A general nutrition text should be consulted for more details on specific nutrient deficiencies.[4]

Malnutrition is a major health problem in hospitalized patients. Twenty-five percent to 50% of patients are malnourished upon hospital admission. Unfortunately, of those patients admitted in a well-nourished state, 25% to 30% develop malnutrition during hospitalization.[1]

EFFECTS OF MALNUTRITION

Malnutrition can affect all body systems. Without early identification and treatment many physiologic problems can develop. It is therefore critical to identify patients at risk for malnutrition; such identification is a multidisciplinary responsibility. Those patients identified as being at risk require appropriate nutritional intervention and present a unique challenge.

The effects of malnutrition are numerous. In acute malnutrition, organ system function is reduced, whereas in chronic malnutrition, both organ function and size are reduced. Malnutrition can impair cardiac and pulmonary efficiency leading to fatigue and shortness of breath. Absorption and metabolism of nutrients are also impaired in malnutrition because of effects on the gastrointestinal tract and the liver. The decreased white blood cell production and the efficiency of phagocytosis that occurs in malnutrition contribute to poor wound healing and increased wound infections. Protein deficiency impairs collagen synthesis, alters osmotic equilibrium, and contributes to edema formation, which further compromises tissue perfusion and metabolism.

CAUSES OF MALNUTRITION

Malnutrition can be caused by a variety of conditions including physiologic and psychosocial factors that lead to starvation. Sometimes malnutrition is caused by disease states that alter the normal metabolism of nutrients such as trauma. Hospitalized patients may also develop malnutrition as a result of iatrogenic factors. Table 9-1 details the causes of malnutrition.

TABLE 9-1   Causes of malnutrition

STARVATION
  Physiologic
    Disease induced
      Mucositis
      Esophageal stricture
      Head and neck surgery or radiation
      Reflux esophagitis
      Malabsorption
      Massive bowel resection
      Inflammatory bowel disease
    Drug-nutrient interactions
      Appetite suppressants
        Amphetamines
        Chemotherapy
      Drug-induced malabsorption
        Antibiotics
        Antacids
      Drug-induced altered metabolism
        Barbiturates decrease metabolism
        Steroids alter metabolism
    Age-related factors in the elderly
      Impaired taste
      Decreased salivation
      Impaired chewing from dental
        problems
      Impaired ability to prepare meals
  Psychosocial
    Poor dietary habits
      Fad diets
      Prolonged fasting
      Excess junk-food intake
      Drug or alcohol abuse

  Psychologic disorders
    Anorexia
    Bulimia
    Severe depression
  Psychologic stress
    Recent separation or divorce
    Anxiety-provoking events
    Work or family stress

ALTERED METABOLISM
  Hypermetabolism
    Severe trauma
    Overwhelming sepsis
    Major surgery
  Chronic disease
    Diabetes mellitus
    Cirrhosis
    Chronic obstructive pulmonary disease
      (COPD)

IATROGENIC FACTORS
  Lack of base-line nutritional assessment
  Lack of monitoring nutritional intake
  Frequent NPO (taking-nothing-by-
    mouth) status for diagnostic tests
  Inappropriate use of nutritional formulas
  Delay in initiating nutritional support
  Failure to recognize increased nutritional
    requirements

Modified from Konstantinides N: Malnutrition. In Kneisel C and Ames S: Adult health nursing, Menlo Park, Calif, 1986, Addison-Wesley Co.

NUTRITIONAL ASSESSMENT

An initial assessment provides base-line data regarding a person's nutritional status; subsequent assessments reflect changes in status and effects of interventions. The data derived should provide useful information for individualizing a nutritional plan. The assessment can help to identify the presence of or risk for malnutrition and nutrient deficiencies.

The nutritional assessment is best performed on a multidisciplinary basis. Depending on the institution, the responsibility for nutritional assessment can be shared among the dieticians, nurses, pharmacists, and doctors. Some institutions have a nutrition support team responsible for nutritional assessment and nutritional support therapies. The components of a nutritional assessment include the patient history, a physical examination, and laboratory data. Because subclinical malnutrition can be overlooked, the history, physical, and laboratory test data should be thoroughly evaluated.

Patient History

Much data relevant to nutritional status can be obtained by use of a careful patient history. The practitioner can utilize these data to identify nutritional problems, determine the need for further nutritional education, and plan realistic patient outcomes.

Information should be obtained regarding the current health status, previous illness, and dietary history, focusing on potential causes of malnutrition as described. Examples of specific information to obtain are listed in Table 9-2.

The diet history may include a dietary recall process.[2] These are most commonly used by dieticians when there is the need for more detailed information on nutritional intake. The *24-hour recall method* involves asking the patient to think of everything he or she ate or drank in the past 24 hours. The *dietary inventory method* involves asking the patient to record nutritional intake as it is consumed. This can include much detail such as the time of day, the specific amount consumed, and whether consumption was in response to hunger or other factors. The *food frequency form* has a list of foods from which the patient records intake. The *agency dietary history questionnaire* combines dietary intake with factors that affect food intake.

By obtaining this patient history information, the practitioner can identify patients at high risk for developing malnutrition. Box 9–1 lists the historical factors most relevant to

Table 9-2 Patient history for nutritional assessment

Current health	Recent change in dietary intake
	Recent stressful events
	Recent change in body weight
	Current medications
	Current medical problems
Previous illnesses	Major illnesses
	Trauma
	Past surgeries
	Dental problems
	Food allergies
	Eating disorders
	Weight loss program
Dietary history	Special dietary needs
	Intake from each food group
	Current versus past nutritional intake
	Daily eating patterns
	Food preparation habits
	Preferences and intolerances
	Weight history
	Use of alcohol and drugs
	Regular physical activity

Box 9-1   HIGH-RISK FACTORS FOR MALNUTRITION

1. Grossly underweight: weight-for-height below 80% of standard
2. Grossly overweight: weight-for-height above 120% of standard (The risk is attributable to the tendency to overlook protein and calorie requirements in the acutely ill obese patient.)
3. Experiencing recent loss of 10% or more of usual body weight
4. Alcoholism
5. Taking nothing by mouth for more than 5 days while being given simple intravenous solutions
6. Experiencing protracted nutrient losses
    a. Malabsorption syndromes
    b. Short-gut syndromes or fistulas
    c. Renal dialysis
    d. Draining abscesses, wounds
7. Experiencing increased metabolic needs
    a. Extensive burns, infection, trauma
    b. Protracted fever
8. Taking drugs with antinutrient or catabolic properties: steroids, immunosuppressants, antitumor agents

The presence of any one characteristic is a warning that a patient is at increased risk of malnutrition; the absence of these characteristics, however, does not mean that malnutrition does not exist or cannot occur.

---

identify high-risk patients. Some practitioners use this abbreviated history as a screening tool to determine the need for a more detailed history as described above.

Physical Examination

The physical examination for malnutrition is particularly challenging in early malnutrition because some signs do not appear until the malnutrition becomes advanced. Some physical changes associated with malnutrition also have nonnutritional causes (such as dermatitis). Obesity may mask the skeletal muscle wasting of malnutrition. No single physical finding is diagnostic of malnutrition; therefore the physical examination must be considered with the patient history and the laboratory data. The clinical signs of protein malnutrition are listed in Box 9-2.

One component of the physical examination is the determination of body measurements such as body weight and anthropometrics. Height and weight should be determined at base-line values with weights recorded at regular intervals. This base-line weight should be compared to the reported usual body weight and with the ideal body weight for height. Each institution should have a standard for determining ideal body weight.

Box 9-2   SIGNS OF PROTEIN MALNUTRITION

Thin, sparse and easily pluckable hair	Flaky dermatosis
Decreased muscle mass	Parotid enlargement
Decreased base-line body temperature	Hepatomegaly
Edema	Impaired wound healing
Lackluster nails	

Anthropometric measurements are used to indicate protein and fat stores in muscle and adipose tissue. Specific measurements include triceps skin fold, midarm circumference, and midarm muscle circumference. These measurements are most commonly obtained by the dietician and are compared to tables of standards that are available in most clinical nutrition texts.

Skin testing for delayed cutaneous hypersensitivity is another component of the physical examination and is used as an indicator to determine nutritional status. Skin testing, which is usually performed by the nurse, involves the intradermal introduction of various recall antigens. The patient's response to this antigenic challenge provides gross information about the patient's immune function, since the immune system is very sensitive to protein status. The site of injection of the antigens is palpated for induration at a given time period, usually between 24 and 48 hours. The malnourished person will have no induration and therefore negative skin testing, often referred to as "anergy." Unfortunately, there are many factors that can cause a false-negative response to skin testing such as surgery, cancer, recent radiation, or immunosuppressive drug therapy.

Laboratory data

Laboratory indices for nutritional assessment involve primarily tests related to protein metabolism. Protein status can be evaluated through a nitrogen-balance study, visceral protein blood levels, and gross tests of immune function, such as total lymphocyte counts.

The nitrogen-balance study is an important laboratory determination for nutritional status. The nitrogen balance is determined by an evaluation of a 24-hour intake of nitrogen (which is a proportion of the protein) relative to nitrogen output. Nitrogen output is determined from a 24-hour urine collection for urinary nitrogen collected during the same day as the intake. To calculate the nitrogen balance, the nitrogen output is subtracted from the nitrogen intake while one factors in nitrogen loses from other sites such as wounds or fistulas. Typically, this is calculated by a dietician. The goal in supporting nutritional status is to strive for a zero or positive nitrogen balance, which indicates that the patient is retaining more nitrogen than he or she is losing; retained nitrogen is therefore available for protein synthesis.

Visceral protein blood levels are another indicator of protein status and are also known as "transport proteins," or "plasma proteins." They are produced in the liver and include serum albumin, transferrin, and prealbumin. Each of these proteins have a different half-life (albumin, 21 days; transferrin, 7 days; prealbumin, 3 days). Because the proteins with the shorter half-life provide more current information on protein status, they are the preferred indicators for visceral protein status.

Normal levels of the visceral proteins vary slightly with the institution but are approximately 3.3 to 4.5 g/dl for albumin, 200 to 400 mg/dl for transferrin, and 20 to 40 mg/dl for prealbumin. Visceral protein levels are below normal in malnutrition. An important goal of nutritional support is to increase or normalize visceral protein levels because very low levels are associated with increased morbidity and mortality.

The immune system is very sensitive to protein status because protein is a major constituent of immune system components such as antibodies and lymphoctyes. Consequently, gross tests of immune function such as total lymphocyte count (TLC) also reflect protein status. Lymphocytes constitute a variable percentage of the circulating white blood cells and are reported in a white blood cell differential. The TLC is calculated when the percent of lymphocytes is multiplied by the white cell count. The normal level is 1500 to 3000 cells per mm^3. Below normal levels may be a reflection of malnutrition; however, TLC may also be depressed by chemotherapy, autoimmune diseases, stress, and infection (including HIV).

NUTRITIONAL SUPPORT

Optimal nutritional status is essential for optimal wound healing, thus it is essential that persons with wounds have their nutritional status and needs addressed. Some persons are able to maintain their nutritional status by oral intake of a balanced diet supplemented with multiple vitamins and minerals. Unfortunately, many patients with wounds have some degree of malnutrition. These are the persons who require special nutritional interventions. Having performed a nutritional assessment, the practitioner can devise an appropriate individualized nutritional plan for these patients. This usually involves collaboration with the dietician and possibly other nutritional professionals.

Nutritional support therapy should provide a balanced intake of necessary nutrients based on the person's energy and protein requirements. Because a person's nutritional needs are dependent on many variables (such as age, sex, height, weight, presence of severe wasting or obesity, current disease state and severity of illness, as well as the presence and severity of a wound), it may be an oversimplification to give a range of calories and protein that a patient with wounds will require. However, it is useful to remember that a healthy person requires approximately 0.8 g of protein per kilogram per 24 hours. Obviously, the presence of a wound will increase these protein requirements. In general, a patient with wounds needs adequate calories, increased amounts of protein (modified according to results of nitrogen-balance studies and visceral protein levels), increased vitamin C and zinc intake, and increased vitamin A if the patient is currently receiving corticosteroids. A clinical nutrition text can be referenced for more details on normal nutritional requirements.[3,4]

The route of nutritional support will depend on the patient's ability to eat adequately or the availability of the gastrointestinal tract for tube feedings. When the gastrointestinal tract cannot be used, parenteral nutrition should be the route of choice.

Oral Nutritional Support

The patient with a wound who needs nutritional interventions and is able to eat adequately can benefit from nutritional counseling. The nurse should collaborate with the dietician in devising a nutritional plan. The patient should receive information on foods necessary for balanced intake of the major food groups (bread and cereal, fruits, vegetables, meat and milk). Patients should be encouraged to eat foods high in protein (such as meats, milk products), vitamin C (as in orange juice) and zinc (as in seafood). The patient should also receive a multiple vitamin and mineral supplement by mouth. Frequent small meals with nutritious snacks are often warranted. A dietary inventory may be helpful to the patient and the dietician to ensure that intake is appropriate. If deficiencies are identified by means of this inventory, additional instruction may be necessary. To adequately meet their nutritional needs orally, some patients may benefit from supplements such as Meritene, Carnation Instant Breakfast, and Ensure.

Enteral Tube Feeding

Enteral tube feedings are provided to patients with a functional gastrointestinal tract when oral intake is inadequate or contraindicated (as with dysphagia from head and neck surgery or radiation, bowel obstruction, or enterocutaneous fistula.) Tube feedings may be administered through nasal feeding tubes or abdominal feeding tubes; the implications for care are related to the location of the feeding tube. The patient with a feeding tube in the small bowel (such as a nasoduodenal or jejunostomy tube) will benefit from slow administration of the tube feeding because of the lack of a reservoir to handle large volumes quickly. An enteral infusion pump may be necessary to enhance tolerance to these intestinal feedings.

Most enteral tube feeding formulas are nutritionally complete and are designed for a specific purpose. Several formulations are available, and each has specific nursing implications. The milk-based formulas (such as Meritene, Shake-up) are designed for oral consumption but are contraindicated for the patient who is lactose intolerant. The majority of enteral formulas are lactose-free formulas (such as Ensure, Osmolite, Resource) and are designed for intact gastrointestinal tracts. The chemically defined formulas (such as Citrotein, Isotein HN) are indicated when there is compromised gastrointestinal tract function (such as inflammatory bowel disease, radiation enteritis, malabsorption) because they are partially predigested. With these formulas the individual primarily needs to absorb the nutrients. Chemically defined formulas are sometimes referred to as "elemental formulas." "Elemental" implies that all major nutrients are predigested. Tolerex is one of the few enteral formulas that are truly elemental. Specialty formulas are formulas made for specific disease states including organ failure (such as Pulmocare for pulmonary disease) or hypermetabolism (such as Stresstein, Vivonex TEN). Many institutions have an enteral formulary where more information on enteral formulas can be found.

Certain measures are important to improve tolerance to enteral tube feeding formulas. Formulas are best tolerated when administered slowly, especially when being delivered directly into the small bowel. When formulas are initiated, they are often given at a dilute strength and low rate and then gradually increased to the goal rate and strength. The initiation and advancement should be individualized to optimize tolerance.

The nurse should implement measures to minimize and treat the potential gastrointestinal, mechanical, and metabolic complications. Because microbes grow quite readily in this room-temperature, nutrient-rich environment, formulas should be handled carefully so as to minimize contamination. Aspiration of the formula is of most concern and is prevented by ensuring that the feeding tube tip remains in the desired location and that the residual volume does not exceed a reasonable limit (50 to 150 ml).

Diarrhea is a common side effect of enteral tube feedings because tube feedings almost always change the stool consistency. However, diarrhea in the tube-fed patient may actually be induced by many variables: medications (such as antacids or antibiotics) disuse of the gut (which leads to villus atrophy), hypoalbuminemia (which precipitates mucosal edema), and the administration of a contaminated formula. Unfortunately because diarrhea has no universal definition, the timing of interventions is a subjective decision. Interventions for tube feeding–associated diarrhea is generally believed to be necessary after the patient has experienced greater than two stools per day for more than 2 days. When patients have liquid stools, 250 ml should be considered one stool. Diarrhea during tube feedings is best treated with liquid antidiarrheal medications after each stool or bulking agents. If the stooling pattern persists or worsens, it may be beneficial to decrease the concentration or volume of formula administered. Those with large amounts (greater than 1000 ml) of liquid stool require a stool culture and possibly bowel rest.

Feeding tube obstruction is prevented with frequent flushing and the avoidance of medications notorious for occluding the tube. Hyperglycemia can be minimized with careful monitoring of patients who are prone to glucose intolerance and by avoidance of the formulas high in carbohydrates.

When patients require tube feedings at home, the patient or a support person needs to learn procedures necessary to administer the formula and measures necessary to prevent complications. The patient and support person need to understand proper storage, preparation, and handling of formulas, proper care for the feeding tube, and how to monitor and record necessary parameters such as weight. Patients on tube feedings also need to be linked with the community resources, such as home health nurses.

Parenteral Nutrition

Parenteral nutrition is necessary in patients when enteral tube feeding is contraindicated, is insufficient to maintain nutritional status, or has led to serious complications (aspiration or excessive diarrhea). The components of the parenteral nutrition solution include dextrose, crystalline amino acids, eletrolytes, minerals, trace elements, and vitamins. Intravenous fat is usually administered in a separate container because of instability with certain combinations of other nutrients. The amount of parenteral nutrition administered will depend on the person's requirements.

The nurse is responsible for safe and effective delivery of the parenteral nutrition. The solution is administered into the peripheral veins or into a central vein. However, because the peripheral route is unable to handle the necessary high concentrations of amino acids and dextrose, it should be used as a short-term nutritional supplement. Central venous access is preferred when reliable and adequate parenteral nutrition is required for 1 week or more. Because of the high dextrose concentrations, the parenteral nutrition should be administered by means of an infusion pump to help regulate glucose homeostasis.

It is important to take measures to prevent solution contamination and infection at the catheter site. Fungi grow readily in the parenteral nutrition solution, whereas bacteria grow well in the intravenous fat. An in-line filter can be used to help trap any organisms that would be present in a contaminated solution and to trap tiny particles from the solutions. Special filters are necessary for fat emulsions because of their rather large globules.

Aseptic technique is used for the regular dressing changes at the catheter site. Gloves and masks for dressing changes are used by some nurses. The use of antiseptic solution and ointment and the type and frequency of dressing changes are specific to the institutional preferences.

The patient should be observed for potential complications such as catheter problems, infection, or metabolic abnormalities. Careful monitoring and early intervention should lead to few complications with parenteral nutrition therapy.

When parenteral nutrition is required at home, the patient and support person will need time to learn to safely handle the catheter and solution administration. In-home nursing visits are almost always beneficial in the transition from the hospital and in reinforcing teaching. Solution and equipment deliveries must be arranged with a home nutrition company.

SUMMARY

Nutritional status plays an important role in wound healing. Since malnutrition is so prevalent and is not always obvious, all patients with wounds should have their nutritional status evaluated. A thorough nutritional assessment should reveal the risk for or presence of malnutrition and provide the necessary information to develop an individualized nutrition-al plan. The nutritional status should be evaluated at base-line values and at regular inter-vals for determination of the effectiveness of the current nutritional plan.

CASE STUDY

K.W. is a 34-year-old female with a history of ovarian carcinoma that was resected 2 years previously followed by chemotherapy and radiation therapy. She came to the hospital with nausea and vomiting from bowel obstruction, which was relieved by surgical resection of the affected small bowel. Surgery was complicated with wound dehiscence and infection. K.W. continued to require hospitalization for intravenously administered antibiotics and wound management.

K.W.'s base-line nutritional assessment included her usual oral intake until 1 week before her admission. She had lost 30 pounds in 3 years, of which 10 pounds were lost in the preceding 6 months. Her usual body weight was 140 pounds, and her actual body weight was 110 pounds. Her height was 5 feet, 6 inches. Her laboratory data revealed sub-normal transferrin of 176 mg%, zinc of 50 mg%, and a magnesium of 1.1 mEq/L. The dieti-cian determined that her calorie needs were 1800 to 2000 calories and 75 to 90 g of protein. Parenteral nutrition was initiated on the second postoperative day during this hospitaliza-tion. The standard formula was supplemented with extra zinc and magnesium. This was administered through a central vein to ensure adequate intake during the necessary bowel rest. Several weeks postoperatively the wound infection was controlled, and K.W.'s bowel function returned. Oral intake was initiated and advanced as tolerated to a malabsorption diet with supplements of Citrotein and multiple vitamins and minerals. Her weight and transferrin levels improved, and she was discharged with an outpatient nutritional follow-up schedule.

SELF-EVALUATION

QUESTIONS AND PROBLEMS

1. Define the term "malnutrition."
2. Of the patients admitted in a well-nourished state, what percent develop malnutrition during hospitalization?
   a. 5%   **c.** 25%
   b. 15%   **d.** 40%
3. Explain why malnutrition is a major cause of increased morbidity and mortality.
4. Identify at least three categories of factors that may cause or contribute to malnutrition.
5. Outline the key components of a nutritional assessment.
6. Define each of the following:
   24-hour dietary recall
   Dietary inventory
   Food frequency form
7. Anthropometric measurements are used to evaluate:
   a. visceral protein stores.
   b. somatic protein and fat stores.
   c. immune system function.
   d. muscle tone and function.
8. Define "anergy" and explain the relationship between nutritional status and immunocompetence.
9. Which of the following most rapidly reflects changes in visceral protein stores and is therefore most useful in monitoring the response of a malnourished patient to nutritional intervention?
   a. Total lymphocyte count
   b. Serum albumin
   c. Transferrin
   d. Prealbumin
10. Identify at least two etiologic factors, other than malnutrition, for decreased total lymphocte count (TLC).
11. Explain what is meant by the term "positive nitrogen balance" and identify the method used to determine nitrogen balance.
12. Compare the following formulas in terms of composition and indications for use:
    Milk based
    Lactose free
    Protein intact
    Chemically designed (elemental)
13. Identify at least three etiologic factors for diarrhea in the patient receiving enteral feedings.
14. Identify at least three nursing measures to reduce diarrhea and promote tolerance of enteral feedings.
15. List three types of complications that may occur with total parenteral nutrition.

SELF-EVALUATION

ANSWERS

1. "Inadequate nutrient intake or utilization relative to individual requirements" or "reduced lean body mass (or skeletal muscle mass)"
2. c
3. Malnutrition compromises immune system function because of decreased production of white blood cells and antibodies; as a result, malnourished patients are at greater risk for infection.

   Malnutrition impairs wound healing because of depletion of the protein stores required for synthesis of repair substances.

   Malnutrition impairs cardiac and pulmonary function and reduces absorption of nutrients from the gastrointestinal tract.
4. Diseases that alter intake or absorption of nutrients

   Medications that suppress appetite, impair absorption, or alter metabolism

   Age-related factors in elderly patients affecting intake

   Psychosocial factors affecting nutrient intake

   Psychologic disorders or stress affecting nutrient intake

   Altered metabolic states

   Iatrogenic factors affecting intake
5. a. Historical data

      Current health status (such as current medical problems, current medications, recent stressors, recent changes in dietary intake or weight)

      Past history (such as major illnesses, trauma, surgeries, dental problems, eating disorders, food allergies, weight loss programs)

      Dietary history (such as weight history, current versus past nutritional intake, special dietary needs, daily eating patterns and food preparation, food preferences and intolerances, alcohol and drug use, usual physical activity)

   b. Physical assessment

      Overall physical appearance or signs of malnutrition (such as sparse, pluckable hair; edema; lethargy; flaky dermatosis)

      Body weight and height; comparison of actual weight to ideal body weight

      Anthropometric measurements (such as triceps skin fold, midarm circumference, midarm muscle circumference)

      Skin testing for delayed cutaneous hypersensitivity

   c. Laboratory data

      Nitrogen balance study

      Visceral protein studies (such as serum albumin, transferrin, prealbumin)

      Total lymphocyte count
6. *24-hour dietary recall:* Obtain diet history by asking the patient to think of everything he ate or drank in the past 24 hours.

   Dietary inventory: Obtain diet history by asking the patient to record nutrient intake as it is consumed (may include data on time, amounts, stimulus for eating)

   Food frequency form: List foods from which patient records intake.
7. b
8. Anergy refers to negative skin testing to common antigens, that is, loss of the normal cutaneous sensitivity response. A negative response to common antigens is

indicative of serious compromise of immune system function. Severe malnutrition may cause anergy because the immune system is very sensitive to protein status. However, anergy may also result from surgery, cancer, recent radiation, or immunosuppressive drug therapy.

9. d

10. Immunosuppressive disease states (such as HIV)
Chemotherapy
Stress

11. Positive nitrogen balance refers to a state in which the patient is retaining more nitrogen than he is losing. Determination of nitrogen balance usually involves a 24-hour urine test for urine urea nitrogen to determine nitrogen losses (and an estimate of nitrogen losses from other sources) compared to nitrogen intake (determined by the dietician or nutritional support expert).

12. *Milk-based:* Appropriate for patient who is "lactose tolerant"; patients who have had nothing by mouth for more than a week may be temporarily intolerant of lactose because of loss of the brush border containing lactase.
Lactose-free: Protein is derived from soybean or other nonmilk sources and so does not require lactase for digestion or absorption. Appropriate for patient who is lactose intolerant.
Protein intact: Formulas that require breakdown of proteins, complex carbohydrates, and fats before absorption can occur. Appropriate for patient who has intact gastrointestinal tract with normal function.
Chemically designed (elemental): Formulas that contain amino acids or peptides, simple sugars, and fatty acids ready for absorption. Appropriate for patient who has compromised gastrointestinal tract (reduced length or absorptive capacity).

13. Antibiotics
Edema of bowel wall because of malnutrition, resulting in decreased absorption
Atrophy of villi because of prolonged status of taking nothing by mouth, resulting in reduced absorption
Viral or bacterial gastroenteritis
Drug induced (such as magnesium-based antacids)
Hypertonic formula

14. Identify and address causative factors
Utilize bulking agent or fiber-based formula
Utilize antidiarrheal agent
Reduce rate of feeding

15. Catheter related
Infectious
Metabolic

REFERENCES

1. Cerra FB: Pocket manual of surgical nutrition, St. Louis, 1984, Mosby–Year Book, Inc.
2. Konstantinides NN: Nutritional care. In Illustrated Manual of Nursing Practice, Springhouse, Penn, 1991, Springhouse Corp.
3. Konstantinides N: Malnutrition. In Kneisel C and Ames S: Adult health nursing, Menlo Park, Calif, 1986, Addison-Wesley Co.
4. Weinsier RL, Heimburger DC, and Butterworth CE: Handbook of clinical nutrition, St. Louis, 1989, Mosby–Year Book, Inc.

10 Evolving Wound Care Modalities

DENNIS L. CONFER
RITA A. FRANTZ
PAUL M. NEMIROFF
ALISON JUNEN
SUSAN MITCHELL
JULANNE PALMER

OBJECTIVES

1. Describe the structural features of the protein that compose growth factors.
2. Identify three growth factors and at least two actions that relate to the wound repair process.
3. Distinguish between the three types of electrical stimulation that have been applied to wound repair.
4. Discuss four effects of electrotherapy on wound healing.
5. Define the phrase "galvanotaxic effects."
6. Define hyperbaric oxygenation.
7. Describe the steps necessary to prepare a patient for HBO (hyperbaric oxygenation).
8. State six positive systemic effects of HBO.
9. Describe three complications of HBO.
10. Describe the role of investigational wound care modalities in the treatment of chronic wounds.
11. Describe the importance of the following when one is evaluating clinical trials: blinding, randomization, study population, and outcomes.

Thus far this text has addressed the more established, "standard" wound care modalities: topical dressings and surgical procedures. These interventions are passive in that they are not known to stimulate the cellular components of the wound repair process or interact with the cellular components.

Currently, technology that is premised on wound repair physiology is being developed and investigated and is designed to interact actively with the wound, thereby optimizing desired cellular activities. Such advances are the result of an expanded understanding of wound pathophysiology, the mechanisms of tissue repair, and advanced biotechnology capabilities. Three such investigational therapies are molecular regulation, electrical stimulation, and hyperbaric oxygenation. Because these novel approaches to wound care are not as yet proved scientifically, they are available only through research centers. When a patient is enrolled in a study examining one of these modalities, data are collected and tabulated so that objective interpretation of the effectiveness of the therapy can be determined; thus one can eliminate the subjectivity of case reports and anecdotal results. The wound care nurse should be familiar with these investigational therapies and current research results. Each of these modalities are presented and described in this chapter.

Molecular Regulation

DENNIS L. CONFER

The cellular events in wound healing are well known. Platelets arrive first, deposited by bleeding capillaries of the fresh wound and stimulated to release their contents by the resulting activation of the hemostatic system. The spent platelets are promptly joined by neutrophils engaged in the first stages of cleansing the wound by removal of cellular debris, microorganisms, and foreign material. These are followed, in orderly progression, by monocytes and macrophages, fibroblasts, and, soon, vascular endothelial cells. Other cells, including lymphocytes, smooth muscle cells, nerve cells, and epithelial cells, are also found in wounds. All are engaged in the process of restoring, as much as possible, integrity and structure.

To the scientists who began microscopic examinations of wound healing, it was readily apparent that the entire process was carefully controlled and highly orchestrated. These scientists postulated the existence of regulatory molecules that were released by cells in the wound and that controlled wound healing. Few could have anticipated, however, the true, mind-boggling complexity of this system. Few could have anticipated the sheer number of distinct regulatory molecules involved, the myriad of actions and interactions they cause, or the critical roles these molecules play in other bodily processes.

The past 10 years have produced an explosion of information about growth factors and cytokines, an explosion fueled by remarkable advances in technology. Growth factors are typically found in only minute amounts, whether in a laboratory culture dish, an experimental wound, or a human patient. New techniques, however, have made it possible to isolate these minute quantities of growth factors in highly purified form. Once they are isolated, the powerful methods of molecular biology can be applied to obtain the parent gene directly, sequence it, and clone it into a vector that will produce large amounts of pure protein. Thus it is possible not only to compare individual growth factors in experimental systems, but also to obtain enough purified protein for therapeutic applications.

As the information on growth factors and cytokines has proliferated, it has become apparent that these regulatory molecules play pivotal roles in several bodily processes. Not only are they involved in wound healing directly, but they also control critical stages in fetal development and often appear to stimulate the proliferation of cancer cells. It is also clear that growth factors and cytokines are involved in the repair of internal organ injuries and probably regulate many day-to-day activities of the immune system and of the nervous system. Thus the importance of these molecules in sustaining life goes far beyond their crucial function in wound healing.

Growth Factors

The biologic properties and potential wound-healing functions of various growth factors are the subject of several reviews.[5,29,42,56] A general overview of growth factors is provided here.

Naming Conventions. There is no standard nomenclature for growth factors, and this is a source of confusion. Some growth factors are named for a cell of origin, such as platelet-derived growth factor (PDGF), others for a cell that is a target for their action, such as fibroblast growth factor (FGF), and epidermal growth factor (EGF), and still others for an action they cause, such as transforming growth factor-beta (TGF-β) and tumor necrosis factor-alpha (TNF-α). Furthermore, some growth factors have more than one name; TNF-α is also called cachectin, TNF-β is also called lymphotoxin, and PDGF is the c-*sis* gene product. Confusion can also arise because factors with similar names may be very dissimilar; for example, transforming growth factor-alpha (TGF-α) is more closely related to epidermal growth factor (EGF) than to TGF-β.

Structural Features. All of the growth factors considered here are proteins. They vary widely in size from only a few amino acids to several hundred. Among the three general classes of proteins—structural proteins (like collagen and fibronectin), enzyme proteins (like the digestive enzymes of the gastrointestinal tract), and hormones (like insulin)— growth factors are hormones. They tend to be paracrine or autocrine hormones. The former, paracrine hormones, are released by one cell and exert their action on another cell that is very close by; thus, in a wound, for example, one cell, such as a monocyte, releases a growth factor that affects a nearby neighbor, perhaps a fibroblast. Autocrine hormones are self-stimulating; that is, the cell that releases the hormone is also the one on which the hormone acts. Both of these are in contrast to the endocrine hormones, such as insulin, which are synthesized and released at one site and then travel by the bloodstream to exert an action at some distant locale.

Sources and Targets. The list of cell types that synthesize and release growth factors is ever expanding. Many growth factors were initially isolated from cultured cell lines, such as tumor cells and fibroblasts, whereas others were found in blood cells, such as platelets and monocytes. At least part of the reason for this is that these cell lines and blood cells are easily manipulated, readily available, and produce enough growth factor to be useful. As individual growth factors have become thoroughly characterized, however, it has been possible to examine numerous new cell types and catalog which ones are capable of synthesizing the growth factor and the conditions under which they do so. These results have been particularly enlightening because they show that most growth factors can be synthesized and released by several different cell types; for example, platelet-derived growth factor is made not only in platelets, but also in macrophages, endothelial cells, fibroblasts, smooth muscle cells, and, most likely, other cells as well.[39,42,52,56] Furthermore, the studies of growth factor production have revealed that some cells may continuously produce a given factor whereas others will do so only under certain conditions; thus monocytes continuously express

TGF-β genes, whereas blood lymphocytes will express the gene only when stimulated by other growth factors.[2,35] This last example hints at an important concept, which is expanded below, that is, that growth factors rarely act in isolation, rather they appear to act within a rich network of interacting growth factors. In this network, it is not the presence or absence of a single factor that determines a biologic response but, instead, the overall combination of factors, their relative concentrations, and the various cells in the milieu capable of responding.

A cell that can respond to an individual growth factor is termed a "target cell." Among the many different types of cells present in a healing wound, several may be targets for the same growth factor. However, the response of each cell type may differ; for example, in the presence of a single factor, the fibroblasts might synthesize and release collagen, whereas the monocytes are stimulated to release a protein-digesting enzyme, and the epithelial cells are caused to proliferate. Thus a single growth factor acting on multiple targets could have a variety of results. Furthermore, each cell being affected by a certain growth factor may have its response modified by the simultaneous presence of other growth factors.

Actions. Growth factors and cytokines affect their target cells through receptors found on the target. For the most part, an individual receptor is highly specific; that is, it can recognize only one growth factor molecule. An exception to this rule occurs for the cellular EGF receptor, which also "sees" transforming growth factor-alpha (TGF-α), even though EGF and TGF-α have clearly different structures.[40] Nevertheless, the existence of essentially specific receptors for each growth factor ensures that the cellular response will also be unique. Each receptor has an extracellular domain, which displays the correct structure to recognize a specific growth factor (termed its "ligand"), a membrane-spanning region, which anchors it to the cell, and a cytoplasmic domain, which transfers a message to the interior of the cell when the extracellular domain is occupied by a ligand.

Unfortunately, the details of what exactly occurs when a growth factor binds to its receptor are sketchy at best. Many growth factor receptors are known to express tyrosine kinase activity in the cytoplasmic domain, and this enzyme activity is stimulated when the extracellular domain undergoes binding by a ligand. The tyrosine kinase transfers phosphate molecules from adenosine triphosphate (ATP) to the tyrosine amino acids present within intracellular proteins, presumably proteins involved in the regulation of critical cell activities. This phosphorylation, too, occurs in a highly specific way, so that only certain intracellular proteins will be phosphorylated by a given receptor's tyrosine kinase. In general, the phosphorylation of any intracellular protein alters its activity: some proteins will become more active when phosphorylated; others will be less active. Thus, within a given cell, it is the pattern of phosphorylation on the multitude of regulatory proteins that will determine precisely what the cell is doing at any instant in time. This pattern will be controlled, at least in part, by the composition of growth factors in the extracellular fluid that bathes the cell's outside surface.

Types

TGF-β (transforming growth factor-beta). TGF-β, transforming growth factor-beta, was so named because it causes cultured cells in vitro to acquire malignant cell behaviors (transform). It has numerous other actions, however, and may be the most broadly reactive growth factor yet identified; essentially all nucleated cells appear to possess receptors for this molecule.[57] The molecule is constructed of two identical peptide chains, each with a molecular weight of 12,500 daltons, linked together by disulfide bonds.

TGF-β, at certain concentrations, causes migration of monocytes, macrophages, and fibroblasts. This may reflect a role for the growth factor in attracting inflammatory cells to wounded tissue. Under other conditions, it can also cause the proliferation of fibroblasts and other types of cells. It is interesting that in some circumstances TGF-β also inhibits cell proliferation. Fibroblasts, for example, exposed to the combination of TGF-β and PDGF will grow more rapidly than normal, but when EGF replaces PDGF in this experiment, growth is actually slower than normal.[49] Thus the TGF-β molecule exerts differing effects depending on the target cell type and the conditions under which exposure occurs.

TGF-β has also been shown to affect the differentiation of certain cells; in some instances it provokes cellular differentiation, in others, it prevents differentiation. Finally, TGF-β also stimulates the production and release of other growth factors and biologically active molecules. Monocytes, for example, treated with TGF-β synthesize interleukin-1 (IL-1), platelet-derived growth factor (PDGF), fibroblast growth factor (FGF), and tumor necrosis factor-alpha (TNF-α).[41,55]

PDGF (platelet-derived growth factor). Platelet-derived growth factor (PDGF) is a molecule made up of two dissimilar chains with a total molecular weight of 31,000 daltons. It was first identified in platelets but is also produced by monocytes, macrophages, endothelial cells, fibroblasts, and smooth muscle cells.[39,52] PDGF, too, can cause a variety of target cell responses including chemotaxis, proliferation, and secretion.[17] Fibroblasts, smooth muscle cells, and other mesenchymal cells are stimulated to grow by PDGF. This effect can be further enhanced by either TGF-β or EGF. Similarly, migration of monocytes, macrophages, fibroblasts, and smooth muscle cells is enhanced by PDGF, and monocyte secretion of enzymes and structural proteins is also stimulated. Since many of the same cells that produce PDGF are also targets, this growth factor is an example of those that may exhibit autocrine action.

FGF (fibroblast growth factor). Fibroblast growth factor (FGF), a product of macrophages and neural cells, appears to exist in several closely related forms. The two major structural forms, distinguished by their physicochemical properties, are acidic FGF and basic FGF. These share approximately 50% amino acid homology.

FGFs bind heparin, a property that facilitates their isolation and may also have a role in vivo. Heparan sulfates, molecules closely related to heparins, are richly arrayed along vascular endothelial cells, and these cells can both undergo chemotaxis and proliferate in response to FGFs. The heparan sulfates on the endothelial cell surface may work to concentrate FGFs near their target. Other cells responding to FGF include fibroblasts, smooth muscle cells, pericytes, and nerve cells. These target cells are stimulated either to proliferate or to synthesize and secrete new molecules in response to FGF.

EGF (epidermal growth factor) and TGF-α (transforming growth factor-alpha). Epidermal growth factor (EGF) is a small molecule (about 6000 daltons) that was first isolated from salivary glands.[58] This molecule is frequently detectable in saliva and in urine. Like many other growth factors, under the appropriate conditions, its target cells may be stimulated to migrate, to proliferate, or to secrete additional products. The target cells for EGF arise in many tissues and include epidermal cells, glial cells, fibroblasts, smooth muscle cells, and others.

Transforming growth factor-alpha (TGF-α) is a similarly small molecule that utilizes the EGF receptor but is otherwise distinct from EGF (and even more so from TGF-β). TGF-α has been found in platelets, macrophages, fibroblasts, keratinocytes, and fetal tissues. It too is a chemotaxin, a mitogen, and a stimulin for its various targets, which include epithelial cells, endothelial cells, and fibroblasts.

Interleukins. Interleukins are an expanding group of *leuko*cyte products that affect the activities of other leukocytes and, as recent investigations have shown, other cell types as well.[25] Interleukin 1 (IL-1) is a product of monocytes and macrophages that is also termed "endogenous pyrogen" because it reliably causes fever. IL-1 also stimulates the immune reactivity of T-lymphocytes and the proliferation of fibroblasts and other connective tissue cells. T-lymphocytes, stimulated by IL-1, release IL-2, a potent cytokine that further stimulates the T-cells directly and will also activate natural killer (NK) cells. Other interleukins stimulate the proliferation of bone marrow cells, either broadly, in some examples, or rather selectively. Because bone marrow–derived cells—platelets, granulocytes, monocyte and macrophages, and lymphocytes—are so critically involved in wound healing, the interleukins must also be considered as essential ingredients.

Therapeutic Use of Growth Factors in Wound Repair

Despite the obvious role of growth factors in wound healing, the utility of artificially applied growth factors is still being evaluated. Numerous studies have utilized animal models of wounding.[29,42] In most of these, experimental wounds are created in research animals and then treated with topical or implanted growth factors. In general, these studies show that, when compared to control treatments, growth factor therapy in healthy animals improves wound strength, enhances collagen deposition, and increases the cellular content of experimental wounds. Dosage is likely to be a critical factor, however, because at least one study has demonstrated that the beneficial effects of TGF-β are reversed as the dose is increased.[6] Combinations of growth factors are also being examined and show, not surprisingly, complex interactions.[20]

Examinations in diabetic animals may be particularly relevant to humans and have produced interesting results. In one study, parameters of wound healing improved in wounds of diabetic mice treated with either PDGF or FGF, though the combination was no better than either factor alone.[24] Another report found that EGF and insulin together in diabetic rats improved healing parameters, whereas neither alone was beneficial.[28] A study of TGF-β in diabetic rats showed that beneficial effects were dependent on the type of wound being tested; improved healing was seen in a wound model with subcutaneous implants, whereas no benefit of the growth factor was seen with an incisional wound model.[11] These same authors also examined FGF in the subcutaneous implant model and observed effects quite different from those of TGF-β; compared to control diabetic rats, FGF caused enhanced recruitment of cells into the wound but actually inhibited collagen formation and organization.[11]

Few human evaluations of growth factor therapy have been completed and published. One randomized, double-blinded study was conducted in burn patients to evaluate EGF for healing of skin graft-donor sites.[12] Each patient, who required a skin graft, had skin harvested from two similar donor sites, one of which was treated with vehicle alone (silver sulfadiazine cream) and the other with vehicle containing recombinant human EGF. In each of 12 cases, epidermal regeneration was more rapid on the EGF-treated wound. The time to 100% healing was shortened by about 1.5 days in the EGF-treated donor sites, and skin biopsy specimens showed improved dermal and epidermal regeneration.

A second randomized, double-blinded trial examined healing of chronic ulcers treated with a platelet-derived extract prepared from each subject's own blood.[38] Subjects had blood collected for preparation of "wound healing factor," but those randomized to the control arm were returned a salve that contained vehicle only. Wound-healing factor, or the placebo salve, was applied beneath a sterile dressing and left there for 12 hours. The wound was then covered for 12 hours with a dry sterile dressing, and then the application was repeated. Both groups were observed for 8 weeks, and then the blind was broken. Once unblinded, patients in the control arm were switched to wound-healing factor, whereas recipients of the authentic preparation, whose wounds had not healed, continued in the treatment arm. Thirteen patients with a total of 21 wounds were evaluable in the treatment arm, whereas 11 patients with 13 wounds were in the control arm. Both groups contained patients with wounds of diverse cause, and because the number of subjects was small, this is a potential drawback of the study. Additionally, the average surface area of wounds in the control group was almost double that of the treatment group, but because of the wide variation in wound size, this was not a statistically significant difference. At the 8-week unblinding point, 17 of the 21 wounds in the treatment group had healed completely, whereas only 2 of the 13 in the control group were healed. Once unblinded, with all remaining subjects receiving wound growth factor therapy, all wounds eventually healed completely. Probably the major drawback of this study was the provision for unblinding after only 8 weeks. This provision allowed the investigators to know the preliminary results of the trial while patients were continuing to enroll, which could, as discussed below, bias the study.

These studies will soon be supplemented by others in progress or planned. Thorough scientific evaluations of growth factor therapy are virtually assured because numerous factors are at work encouraging this new technology.

First, there is certainly a need for new approaches to wound care. As detailed elsewhere in this volume, the incentives for improved care of recalcitrant, nonhealing wounds are numerous and include issues that range from relief of suffering to control of health care costs. Furthermore, the notion that wounds occurring in normal persons, as a result either of an accident or of a surgical intervention, might be healed in a fraction of the usual time is highly attractive and no longer reserved for the realm of science fiction.

Second, growth factor therapy is innately attractive because it attempts to duplicate, or even enhance, natural processes of wound healing. These processes can be assumed to approach the ideal because they have been sustained and refined by thousands of years of evolutionary pressure.

Third, growth factor therapy represents new technology with potentially spectacular clinical efficacy. The proliferation of novel methods for characterizing new factors and for production of highly purified growth factor proteins has been an essential component of this new field; without the methodology, growth factor therapy would remain unrealized.

Finally, the push to make growth factors clinically useful is driven, in part, by economic forces. The biotechnology industry has invested heavily in growth factor research and development. For this investment to be returned, growth factor therapy must become a reality. Unfortunately, because of the remarkable technologies involved, growth factor therapy is not inexpensive. It is incumbent upon health care personnel to limit application of this therapy to situations where its benefit has been unambiguously demonstrated, or where its potential efficacy is under evaluation in a properly designed and controlled clinical investigation.

Potential Limitations of Growth Factor Technology

From a practical standpoint, growth factor therapy may suffer certain limitations. The first among these is the concept of "barren soil." If a growth factor or a mixture of growth factors is introduced into a wound and is expected to cause some positive result, living cells must be present, or recruitable, to respond to the stimulation. Thus a wound that is severely ischemic may be unable to supply sufficient oxygen to support the granulocytes, monocytes, fibroblasts, and numerous other cells necessary to cause healing. Similarly, some patients, such as those receiving high-dose cancer chemotherapy or radiation therapy, may have severe bone marrow suppression that renders them incapable of producing the cells required for a response to growth factor therapy.

A second potential limitation is that of adequately controlling the delivery of therapy. As detailed earlier in this section, the synthesis and release of various growth factors is normally under exquisite regulation at a microscopic level. Within a healing wound, the composition, concentration, and distribution of growth factors changes continuously. It is possible that one cannot easily replace this complex system with a simple concoction of one or two growth factors applied topically or injected into a wound. Still, the animal and human studies mentioned above are beginning to indicate that simple delivery systems may be entirely adequate in certain clinical situations. For the true potential of growth factor therapy to be realized, however, more sophisticated systems for the precise delivery and control of growth factors may be necessary.

A third consideration relates to the cost effectiveness of growth factor therapy. For this high-priced technology to find broad application, it must ultimately be shown to reduce the cost of health care. This requirement means that growth factor therapy should have a positive impact on factors such as the duration of confinement, the cost of supplemental therapies (such as nursing care, antibiotics, and dressings), or the length of disability.

The potential benefits of growth factor therapy are enormous. Transforming this potential into reality will require carefully conducted and properly designed clinical investigations. It is essential for nurses who practice wound care to remain apprised of this rapidly advancing technology, so that application of this therapy is certain to remain judicious and efficacious.

Electrical Stimulation
RITA A. FRANTZ

The effects of electrical currents on wound healing were first documented in the late 1600s when gold foil applied topically over cutaneous ulcerations was found to promote healing and prevent scarring.[50] However, serious study of the role of electrical current in the wound-recovery process did not occur until 1960 when Becker[7] discovered that after amputation the regenerating limb of the salamander produced a measurable current and that the polarity of that current varied in a specific way during the regeneration process. His hypothesis that the body maintains an electrical current within itself, which is responsible for healthy tissue, provided the impetus for basic and clinical research on its role in all phases of the wound-healing process. These studies provide a body of knowledge from which clinicians can develop guidelines for practice.

Types of Electrical Stimulation

A variety of electrotherapy modalites are cited in the literature. Although several terms are used to describe these therapies, only three types of electrical waveforms have been applied to wound healing: low-intensity direct current (LIDC), high-voltage pulsed current (HVPC), and pulsed electrical stimulation. These waveforms are distinguished by the pattern of the current being delivered. Low-intensity direct current, also called "galvanic current," is characterized as a continuous, monophasic waveform in which the voltage does not vary with time. High-voltage pulsed current, a form of transcutaneous electrical nerve stimulation (TENS), features a waveform of paired short-duration pulses with a long inter-pulse interval. When compared to sound waves, a low-intensity direct current would be represented by a continuous hum, whereas high-voltage pulsed current would be characterized by short staccato sounds. Because of the constancy of direct current, its current intensity is five to eight times higher than high-voltage pulsed current, increasing the risk of heat developing under the surface electrodes and of burns occurring. The third type of waveform, pulsed electrical stimulation, is similar to high-voltage pulsed current but is actually an interrupted direct current with a wide rectangular pulse width and a short interpulse interval. This is the newest form of electrical stimulation being applied to wound healing and is still undergoing clinical investigation.

Effects of Electrotherapy on Wound Healing

Underlying the physiologic effects of electrotherapy on wound healing is the influence of electrical charge, that is, positive or negative polarity. All three modalities of electrical stimulation (waveforms) have the capability of delivering current of the same charge to the active electrode. A synthesis of the research literature indicates that certain physiologic changes occur at the tissue and cellular level in a wound exposed to exogenous electrical stimulation. These changes provide the basis for stimulation of the wound-healing process.

Current of Injury. The concept of "current of injury" has evolved from experiments demonstrating that the surface of the human and animal skin is electronegative with respect to inside deeper skin layers.[3,4,15,21] As a result the skin has electrical potentials across it resembling the model of a battery. This biologic battery is driven by a sodium-ion pump.[32] Current can flow between parts of the skin if the current is completed, as when wounding occurs and ionic fluids are available to transmit electricity between the outer and inner layers.[9] This effect was demonstrated by Becker,[8] who found that after amputation the regenerating limb of the salamander produces a measurable current and that the polarity of this current varies in a specific way during the regeneration process. As healing is completed or arrested, these currents no longer flow. It is postulated that electrical stimulation may work by mimicking the natural currents of injury, thereby restarting or accelerating the wound-healing process.[21]

Galvanotaxic Effects. It has been demonstrated that cells move along the path of current, a phenomenon referred to as the "galvanotaxic effect." When applied to wounded tissue, electrical currents have influenced migration of cells essential to the inflammatory process. Fukushima[22] demonstrated a galvanotaxic effect on neutrophils that were attracted to both the anode and cathode but in the presence of inflammation were attracted to the cathode. Eberhardt[18] showed that electrical stimulation increased the relative number of neutrophilic granulocytes in human skin exudate. Orida and Feldman[48] found that macrophages migrate toward the cathode. Given the role of neutrophils and macrophages in the inflammatory phase of wound healing, the capability to enhance cell migration implies that electrotherapy can promote the initial phase of wound healing. Furthermore, Weiss[59] has suggested that mast cells, which are associated with diseases of abnormal fibrotic healing and keloid formation, may be inhibited from migrating into a wounded area when treated with electrical stimulation. His finding of decreased mast cells and reduced scar-tissue thickness in healing human wounds undergoing electrotherapy substantiates further the potential benefit of electrical stimulation on soft-tissue repair.

Stimulatory Effects on Cells. Electrical current has been shown to have a stimulatory effect on fibroblasts, a key cell in wound contraction and collagen synthesis. Cruz and colleagues,[14] using the pig model, demonstrated that there are significantly more fibroblasts in burn wounds treated with electrical stimulation than in controls. Alvarez and others,[1] also employing the pig model, documented more fibroblasts and increased collagen synthesis in partial-thickness wounds. The effect of electrical current on fibroblasts has been reported by Bourguignon and Bourguignon,[10] who found that fibroblasts in culture increase DNA and protein (including collagen) synthesis in response to electrical stimulation. This effect was most noticeable near the negative electrode.

Blood Flow. Several studies have documented improved blood flow as a result of electrical stimulation. Hecker and others[27] have shown in normal subjects that negative polarity increased blood flow in the upper extremity as measured by plethysmography. In 1982, Kaada[33] demonstrated that application of distant, low-frequency transcutaneous electrical nerve stimulation produced pronounced and prolonged cutaneous vasodilatation in patients diagnosed with Raynaud's disease and diabetic polyneuropathy. Using skin temperature as a measure of peripheral vasodilatation, he found a rise in the temperature of ischemic extremities from 22° to 24° C to 31° to 34° C. The latency from the stimulus onset to the abrupt rise in temperature averaged 15 to 30 minutes with a duration of response from 4 to 6 hours.

Antibacterial Effects. Preliminary evidence indicates that electrical stimulation has bacteriostatic and bactericidal effects on microorganisms that are known to infect chronic wounds. Rowley[51] demonstrated inhibition of *Pseudomonas aeruginosa* in infected ulcers of rabbit skin when negative polarity was used. He hypothesized that the inhibition was the result of electrochemical changes created by the current. In a study of 20 patients with burn wounds that had been unresponsive to conventional therapy for 3 months to 2 years, Fakhri and Amin[19] showed a quantitatively lower level of organisms after treatment with direct current stimulation for 10-minute intervals twice weekly. This decrease in bacterial count was accompanied by epithelialization of the wound margins within 3 days of beginning electrical stimulation. Karba[34] studied bacterial growth in decubitus ulcers and found that *Pseudomonas aeruginosa* vanished after 2 weeks of electrical stimulation and did not reappear.

In summary, the literature provides evidence that electrical stimulation is associated with enhanced cellular processes that normally accompany the restoration of injured soft tissue and with inhibition of certain types of bacteria. These studies provide indirect evidence of its potential to enhance wound healing. However, the reliance on small sample sizes and the variability in type and level of electrical stimulation tested supports the need for additional research to identify the optimum treatment protocol to support these wound-healing processes.

Clinical Application

At present, the use of electrical stimulation for wound healing continues to be investigational in nature. Its efficacy is being evaluated by use of different types of electrical-current waveforms on a variety of chronic wounds including diabetic ulcers, pressure ulcers, venous ulcers, accidental injuries, and ulcers associated with arteriosclerotic disease. Preliminary reports provide encouraging support for its potential to enhance the wound-healing process.

Wolcott and Wheeler[61] conducted one of the earliest clinical trials testing low-intensity direct current on human subjects with 75 ischemic skin ulcers previously resistant to healing. They reported complete healing of 34 of the lesions with treatment and the range of improvement in the remaining 41 ranged from 0% to 97%. Gault and Gatens[23] subsequently reported similiar results with the use of low-intensity direct current. Using six subjects with contralateral ulcerations as controls, their results showed a mean weekly healing ratio of 30% for the treated group as compared to 14.7% for the control group. Mean healing after 4 weeks was 74% in those treated with electrical stimulation and 27.3% in the controls. The beneficial effects of low-intensity direct current were further substantiated by Carley and Wainapel,[13] who studied 30 subjects with chronic ulcerations who were paired according to age, diagnosis, and ulcer cause, location, and size. One member of the pair received low-intensity direct current therapy, whereas the other acted as the control. Results showed a 1.5 to 2.5 times faster healing rate for the treated group as compared to the controls. More recently, the efficacy of high-voltage pulsed current was tested on 16 subjects with stage IV pressure ulcers.[37] Subjects were randomly assigned to receive either a high-voltage, monophasic, pulsed current or a sham treatment. The ulcers treated with the HVPC had a mean healing rate of 44.8% with 100% healing in a mean period of 8 weeks. Those in the sham treatment group showed an increase in ulcer size of 11.59% over a period of 7.42 weeks.

Preliminary experimental evidence indicates that application of electrical stimulation has the potential to enhance the healing of chronic, recalcitrant wounds. However, many questions remain regarding the optimum treatment protocols, timing of the treatments, and compatibility with various local wound care regimes. Before widespread clinical application of electrotherapy can be considered, additional controlled clinical trials are needed to delineate its efficacy as a treatment modality for chronic wound healing.

Hyperbaric Oxygen

PAUL M. NEMIROFF
ALISON JUNEN
SUSAN MITCHELL
JULANNE PALMER

Hyperbaric oxygenation (HBO) is the administration of 100% oxygen at pressures two to three times that of normal atmospheric pressure. The entire body must receive the pressure in order for the oxygen to be effective; research has shown that HBO is useful because of its systemic (not local) effects.[30,36] Thus topical oxygen pressure devices that are promoted as providing local hyperbaric oxygen are not included in this discussion.

Indications

The use of HBO was first implemented in the early 1930s to treat decompression sickness (also known as the "bends"). Since that time, the applications for HBO have expanded through the implementation of experimental and clinical studies.

In the early 1970s, the Undersea Hyperbaric Medical Society (UHMS) was established to ensure the efficacious and safe use of HBO. The UHMS has defined the acceptable indications for primary or adjunctive HBO therapy as listed in Box 10-1. Typically, these are the only indications for which Medicare and third-party carriers will reimburse.

Generally, HBO therapy is considered to be primary therapy for arterial gas embolism, carbon monoxide poisoning, and decompression sickness only. HBO therapy must be integrated with the appropriate clinical and surgical treatments for all other indications (such as chronic refractory osteomyelitis, or chronic nonhealing wounds).

Considerable research[43-46,62] has shown the efficacy of using adjunctive HBO to enhance flap and graft survival. To be maximally effective HBO treatments should be initiated as soon as there is any doubt as to the viability of the flap.[43,44,62]

Specific examples of problem wounds that may respond well to *adjunctive* HBO therapy are diabetic ulcers, venous ulcers, arterial ulcers, and pressure ulcers.

Method of Delivery

HBO can be provided by use of one of two types of hyperbaric chambers: multiplace and monoplace units. The multiplace unit can accommodate several patients along with one or two attendants. These patients may be rolled directly into the unit by gurney and may require direct "hands-on" care during the treatment. The monoplace unit accommodates only one patient at a time and is a clear acrylic cylinder. When using the monoplace unit, the attendant sits beside the chamber and communicates with the patient by microphone. Patients may be monitored in either type of chamber with all the standard life-support systems (such as ECG, IV therapy, arterial lines, and mechanical ventilation). During the treatment, the patient may participate in whatever activity he or she chooses: watching television, listening to the radio, or sleeping.

Patient Preparation

To reduce the risk of spark formation in the oxygen-enriched environment of the chambers, patients are asked to remove all cosmetics, paper and metal products, hearing aides, and synthetic materials. Dressings with a petroleum base are removed before treatment: Silvadene, Xeroform gauze, Vaseline gauze, Adaptic, and antibiotic ointments are contraindicated during treatments. These products may be reapplied after the treatment; how-

---

Box 10-1   INDICATIONS FOR HYPERBARIC OXYGENATION

Acute blood loss anemia	Radiation necrosis
Arterial gas embolism*	Refractory osteomyelitis
Carbon monoxide poisoning*	Smoke inhalation
Cyanide poisoning	Thermal wounds
Decompression sickness*	Compromised flaps and grafts
Gas gangrene	Problematic wounds
Necrotizing fasciitis	

*Considered primary indications for HBO therapy.

From Hyperbaric therapy: a committee report, publ. no 30, Bethesda, Md, 1986, Undersea and Hyperbaric Society, Inc.

ever, for the patient receiving many treatments, this frequent removal and reapplication may prove exhausting as well as painful. Alternative topical wound care therapy should be encouraged to prevent disruption of the wound.

A thorough medical history must be obtained before HBO treatment. For example, a chest roentgenogram is necessary to rule out neoplasms or an untreated pneumothorax. If left untreated, the pneumothorax would produce a tension pneumothorax because of the expansion of the chest during decompression.[16] Patients with COPD or emphysema must be identified. They may not be candidates for HBO because these patients depend on a lower level of oxygen to stimulate respiration. If placed in a 100% oxygen environment, they may not receive a stimulus to breathe.

A thorough cardiac history, including an ECG, must also be obtained. The patient with borderline cardiac failure may be pushed into acute pulmonary edema by the stresses of apprehension, heat, or confinement within the chamber. Additionally, hyperbaric oxygen–induced vasoconstriction in peripheral arteries may produce a central fluid shift, and patients with borderline cardiac decompensation may develop acute heart failure while in the chamber.[16]

Blood glucose levels should be obtained on all patients with diabetes before treatment. Because blood glucose levels tend to decrease during treatments, a snack or a meal should be provided.

Finally, various tests, such as tissue oxygen monitoring, arteriograms, and Doppler flow studies, may be indicated before one begins HBO. These base-line data will serve to determine the extent of perfusion to the affected area.

Effects of HBO

Several positive systemic effects result from HBO.[31] First, as stated in Boyle's law, the increased pressure reduces the volume of a gas, thus bubble reduction is one positive systemic effect. This effect is the basis for the treatment of the bends and arterial air embolism.

Second, hyperoxygenation occurs because of the administration of oxygen under pressure. Although the hemoglobin in the blood can carry a maximum of molecules of oxygen, with HBO, additional oxygen can be forced into the blood as well as into the plasma. Consequently, increased oxygenation of tissues results and may improve perfusion to areas with compromised blood flow. The volumetric levels of diffusion achieved with HBO are two to three times those obtained under normobaric conditions.[50,53] Hyperoxygenation may be a critical interim measure while one is awaiting angiogenesis after vascular surgery for reestablishment of adequate blood flow.

Third, HBO acts as a vasoconstrictor, reducing edema or swelling in compromised flaps, burns, and crush injuries.

Fourth, fibroblastic activity is stimulated when abnormally low tissue P_{O_2} values are increased. Fibroblasts are stimulated to synthesize collagen and form a matrix, which provides support for new capillary beds. The improved oxygenation also supports endothelial proliferation and neovascularization.[30,44,47,60]

A fifth systemic effect of HBO is enhanced antimicrobial activity. By stimulating the phagocytic activity of white blood cells and preventing certain bacteria from producing harmful toxins, HBO improves the ability of antibiotics to kill bacteria.[26] Necrotizing fasciitis, gas gangrene, and refractory osteomyelitis are just a few of the infections that respond well to adjunctive HBO therapy.

Sixth, HBO enhances the function of osteoclasts within the bone; these cells are responsible for the breakdown and removal of dead bone. This enhanced removal, in turn, enables the osteoblasts to produce new bone tissue.[54]

Complications

Although HBO is a safe and effective treatment, it is not without complications. When delivered at 100%, oxygen is considered to be a drug. Strict guidelines must be followed to prevent oxygen toxicity. These guidelines include frequency, duration, and depth of treatments. Most treatments are approximately 90 to 120 minutes long at 2 atmospheres absolute (ATA) with approximately 6 to 8 hours between treatments. Oxygen toxicity is typically manifested in the form of a grand mal seizure. The patient is watched carefully for signs of an impending seizure (such as facial twitching, increased anxiety, restlessness, visual disturbances, and diaphoresis). Certain conditions and medications that may predispose a patient to oxygen toxicity seizures are high fever, sepsis, steroids, amphetamines, and nicotine. To minimize the risk of an oxygen-induced seizure, the patient may be given prophylactic diazepam. The length of the treatment may also be decreased. In some instances, a 10-minute "air break" may be provided to reduce the exposure to 100% oxygen.

Another complication that may be encountered is that of ear or sinus squeeze. Before the treatment, the patient is counseled on performing the Valsalva maneuver, swallowing repeatedly, or yawning to facilitate pressure equilibration. In a few cases, small ventilation tubes are placed in the patient's eardrums if he is unable to perform the maneuvers.

Claustrophobia may be controlled with antianxiety medications such as diazepam. A professional and confident staff should be able to allay anxiety through education and reassurance, thus reducing the patient's reliance on medication.

Indications and effects of HBO are currently being explored. Under investigational status at this time is the use of HBO with spinal cord and head injuries as well as various military applications. NASA is currently designing a hyperbaric chamber for use aboard the space station.

Evaluating Clinical Trials

DENNIS L. CONFER

The usefulness of new interventions for wound healing will ultimately be shown only through the completion of carefully designed human trials. Several factors are important for evaluating such trials and deserve brief consideration.

Type of Therapy

The type of therapy being investigated should be carefully reviewed to evaluate such things as the source of the product (such as growth factors) and the technique used to apply the product or therapy.

For example, the source of the growth factor may be important. Some investigators have advocated partially purified, cellular extracts as a source of growth factors. These extracts are typically prepared from cells present in the patient's own bloodstream. A potential advantage of these extracts is that they are not pure; that is, in contrast to the application of a single factor in isolation, the extracts may contain a rich mixture of various factors that will work in concert to cause wound healing. On the other hand, the impurity is also the major disadvantage of cellular extracts. It is very difficult to ensure that extracts prepared from the same patient on more than one occasion are the same in their content, and it is virtually impossible to know that extracts prepared from different patients are comparable. Many patients have chronic illness, and so extracts prepared from their blood may produce inferior results. Extracts from other patients may contain growth factor inhibitors, which will render the extract ineffective. Similarly, even when a patient's extract appears to be highly efficacious, it is impossible to explain why it worked because the exact composition is unknown. Even if the extract is known to contain, say, PDGF, it is insufficient to conclude that PDGF caused the healing because the extract may also contain numerous other factors, unmeasured or unknown, that contributed to its efficacy. In general then, studies that employ manufactured, recombinant growth factors are more likely to give clear-cut results and will also ensure that each patient receives an identical therapy.

Similarly, it is important to use the therapy in a consistent fashion. Furthermore, controls must be applied to the type of topical wound care provided during the study. For example, when one is evaluating the effectiveness of HBO, it is important to have consistency in the duration and frequency of each treatment. However, the type of topical therapy utilized during each treatment and between each HBO treatment should also be consistent. Without a properly designed study that controls these variables it would be difficult to prove that enhanced wound repair was truly the result of the investigational therapy; it may also have occurred as a result of the topical wound dressings, for example.

Blinding and Randomization

The best clinical studies are prospective, randomized, and blinded. A prospective study is one where, in order, hypotheses are advanced, a study is designed, the subjects are enrolled, and the data are collected for analysis. In a retrospective study, by contrast, the subjects have all been treated, often without complete uniformity and without an appropriate control group, before the study is ever conceived. This latter approach is more likely to yield misleading results because of biases, often unintentional, that are introduced.

Randomization, the random assignment of patients between one or more novel therapies and the standard therapy, is a constant feature of good clinical research. By random assignment of the treatments, any urge to bias the study is avoided. For example, an investigator could be so absolutely convinced that a new treatment is superior, that he or she insists on giving the new treatment to all the highest-risk patients. As a result, all the low-risk patients get standard therapy, and because they are low risk, they do just fine. In the end, the standard therapy appears better than the new therapy. The investigator is left wondering whether this result is true or it occurred because the two treatments were given to fundamentally different groups of patients. The only way to settle the issue is to repeat the study, this time with randomization.

Randomized studies should always include a control arm. The control therapy, against which the new therapies are compared, should be the best available current treatment. The best available current treatment is usually equivalent to "standard therapy" because it would be very unusual for a "standard therapy" to persist in use if it were not also the "best therapy." If standard therapy is omitted from the study as a treatment option, it could be shown that "new treatment A" is better than "new treatment B," but it would remain unknown whether either or both were superior to standard treatment.

Finally, blinding a study will also help to eliminate bias. In a "single-blind" study, the subjects are not allowed to know which treatment they are receiving. In a "double-blind" study, not only are the subjects unknowing, but also the medical personnel are unaware of the particular treatment. For eliminating bias and ensuring that all subjects receive similar levels of medical care, double blinding is clearly preferred.

Many medical personnel do not like the notion of blinding because they would like to "know" the results of the study while it is still in progress. When a subject has a particularly gratifying response, for example, everyone involved in the study would like to know which treatment the patient received. Unfortunately, providing such information to the medical staff can hopelessly confound a study and prevent its successful completion. As a practical solution, most double-blinded studies include provisions for monitoring the results as they unfold. In this way, a treatment that is clearly inferior can be dropped, or if there is a treatment clearly superior to the rest, the study can be terminated early. For the blinded medical personnel, they can be reassured that so long as the study continues unaltered no dramatic differences exist between the treatment arms.

Study Population

The study population is of course important in evaluating the results of a clinical study. In general, the more homogeneous the patient population, the better it is. If the study contains subjects with widely varying age, severity of illness, or underlying diagnosis, each treatment group must be examined carefully to ensure that the randomization resulted in an even distribution of patient types. Because randomization is under the assumption that each patient is identical, a diabetic subject is not different from a postoperative subject. When small numbers of subjects are involved therefore, there is a risk that all patients with the same diagnosis will be assigned to the same treatment. If this occurs, the study conclusions may be suspect.

Similarly, even when the study population is relatively homogeneous, care must be taken not to make inappropriate extrapolations from the conclusions. For example, a properly designed study could be performed with burn patients suffering second- or third-degree burns over less than 10% of their skin surface. Even if the study demonstrated that growth factors accelerate healing in this patient population, little could be inferred about the potential beneficial effects of growth factor therapy for chronic diabetic ulcers.

Outcomes

What did the study measure? In a study of lower extremity skin ulcers, the investigators could choose to measure a variety of outcomes. These may be direct measures of the ulcer, such as the total surface area of ulceration versus the duration of treatment; the time to 50% reduction of initial surface area; or the time to complete healing. Each of these should be a direct reflection of possible treatment benefits. If one is trying simply to determine whether growth factors accelerate ulcer healing, these direct measures are most relevant. However, knowing that an ulcer was healed is not a complete story; a more critical question is, "Did healing of the ulcer have a positive effect on the overall health of the subject?" Indirect measures of the treatment, designed for assessment of the impact of therapy on the overall severity of the illness, might help answer this question. Such indirect measures could include the duration of parenteral antibiotic therapy, the duration of oral antibiotic therapy, the total cost of therapy, or the duration of hospitalization. Additionally, one could also measure long-term outcomes. These might include the rate of ulcer recurrence, the rate of recovery from partial or total disability, the rate of rehospitalization, and so forth. The indirect measures of outcome are more difficult to assess and may require long-term follow-up study. Still, these indirect measures will provide the proof that the new therapy is beneficial and cost effective.

SELF-EVALUATION

QUESTIONS AND PROBLEMS

1. True or false: Growth factors are enzymes.
2. Which growth factor is also known as cachectin?
   a. Epidermal growth factor
   b. Fibroblast growth factor
   c. Transforming growth factor beta
   d. Tumor necrosis factor alpha
3. For the following growth factors, state two effects on the wound repair process:
   Platelet-derived growth factor
   Fibroblast growth factor
   Epidermal growth factor
   Transforming growth factor-beta
4. Which of the following statements is true of high-voltage pulsed current (HVPC)?
   a. Currents of high voltage are delivered with a wide rectangular pulse width.
   b. Currents are continuous and have a monophasic waveform.
   c. Skin burns are at greater risk of occurring under the electrode with HVPC.
   d. HVPC features a waveform of paired short-duration pulses with a long pause between pulses.
5. Describe the effects of electrotherapy on each of the following:
   Cellular migration
   Cell stimulation
   Blood flow
   Bacterial counts
6. Define hyperbaric oxygenation.
7. Describe how to prepare a patient for a hyperbaric oxygen treatment.
8. State three positive effects of HBO and two complications of HBO.
9. Distinguish between the role and the use of conventional therapy and investigational therapy in wound care.
10. Distinguish between randomization and blinding.

SELF-EVALUATION

ANSWERS

1. False
2. d
3. *Platelet-derived growth factor* (PDGF) is produced by monocytes, macrophages, endothelial cells, fibroblasts, and smooth muscle cells. PDGF causes a variety of responses including chemotaxis of monocytes, macrophages, fibroblasts, and smooth muscle cells; stimulation of the secretion of enzymes and structural proteins by monocytes; and proliferation of fibroblasts and smooth muscle cells.
   Fibroblast growth factor (FGF) is produced by macrophages and stimulates fibroblasts, smooth muscle cells, and other cells either to proliferate or to synthesize and secrete new molecules.
   Epidermal growth factor (EGF) stimulates target cells (epidermal cells, fibroblasts,

smooth muscle cells, and others) to migrate, proliferate, or secrete additional products.

Transforming growth factor-beta (TGF-β) causes migration of monocytes, macrophages, and fibroblasts; under certain circumstances TGF-β will also cause stimulation or inhibition of fibroblast proliferation.

4. d

5. *Cellular migration:* Cells move along the path of current; this phenomenon is referred to as the "galvanotaxic effect." Electrical currents influence neutrophil and macrophage migration.

Cell stimulation: Electrical current has been shown to stimulate fibroblasts to increase DNA and protein synthesis in the pig model.

Blood flow: Electrical stimulation has been shown to increase blood flow (cutaneous vasodilatation).

Bacterial counts: Electrical stimulation has shown, in some early studies, to exert bacteriostatic and bactericidal effects on microorganisms such as *Pseudomonas aeruginosa*.

6. Hyperbaric oxygen is the administration of 100% oxygen at pressures two to three times that of normal atmospheric pressure.

7. Rule out chest neoplasms or pneumothorax, COPD or emphysema.

Obtain ECG to rule out borderline cardiac failure.

Obtain blood glucose level before treatment.

Remove all cosmetics, paper and metal products, hearing aids, and synthetic materials.

Remove wound dressings with petroleum base.

8. *Positive effects of HBO:*
   a. Hyperoxygenation, which may increase tissue perfusion.
   b. Vasoconstriction, which reduces edema in compromised flaps or burns.
   c. Stimulation of fibroblasts by increasing abnormally low Po_2 values.
   d. Enhanced antimicrobial activity by stimulating the phagocytic activity of white blood cells.
   e. Enhanced function of osteoclasts within the bone to produce new bone tissue.

Complications of HBO:
   a. Oxygen toxicity
   b. Ear or sinus squeeze
   c. Claustrophobia

9. Conventional therapy is considered standard therapy and is widely accepted; investigational therapy consists in a treatment regimen that is under investigation. It is believed, either intuitively or anecdotally, to have beneficial results; however, this has yet to be proved scientifically. Investigational therapy should be conducted in research environments where specific types of data are being monitored and recorded so that results can be published as formal research.

10. Randomization is the random assignment of patients between one or more novel therapies and the standard therapy and serves to eliminate the urge to bias the study.

Blinding can be single or double. Single blinding is achieved when the subjects are not allowed to know which treatment they are receiving; in a double-blind study, both the subjects and the medical personnel are unaware of the particular treatment. Blinding further reduces the introduction of bias into the study.

REFERENCES

1. Alvarez OM, Mertz P, Smerbeck R, and Eaglstein W: The healing of partial thickness wounds is stimulated by external electrical current, Clin Res 30:574A, 1982 [Abstract].
2. Assoian RK, Fleurdelys BE, Stevenson HC, et al: Expression and secretion of type β transforming growth factor by activated human macrophages, Proc Natl Acad Sci USA 84:6020-6024, 1987.
3. Barker AT: Measurement of direct current in biological fluids, Med Biol Eng Comput 19:507, 1981.
4. Barker AT, Jaffe LF, and Vanable JW: The glabrous epidermis of cavies contains a powerful battery, Am J Physiol: Regulatory, Integrative and Comparative Physiology 11:R358, 1982.
5. Barnes D: Growth factors involved in repair processes: an overview, Methods Enzymol 163: 707-715, 1988.
6. Beck LS, Chen TL, Hirabayashi SE, et al: Accelerated healing of ulcer wounds in the rabbit ear by recombinant human transforming growth factor-beta 1, Growth Factors 2:273-282, 1990.
7. Becker RO: The bioelectric factors in amphibian limb regeneration, J Bone Joint Surg 43:643, 1961.
8. Becker RO: The electrical control system regulating facture healing in amphibians, Clin Orthop Rel Res 73:169, 1970.
9. Black J: Tissue response to exogenous electromagnetic signals, Orthop Clin North Am 15(1):15, 1984.
10. Bourguignon GJ and Bourguignon LYW: Electric stimulation of protein and DNA synthesis in human fibroblasts, FASEB J 1(5):398-402, 1987.
11. Broadly KN, Aquino AM, Hicks B, et al: Growth factors bFGF and TGFβ accelerate the rate of wound repair in normal and in diabetic rats, Int J Tissue React 10:345-353, 1988.
12. Brown GL, Nanney LB, Griffen J, et al: Enhancement of wound healing by topical treatment with epidermal growth factor, N Engl J Med 321:76-79, 1989.
13. Carley PJ and Wainapel SF: Electrotherapy for acceleration of wound healing: low intensity direct current, Arch Phys Med Rehabil 66:443, 1985.
14. Cruz NI, Bayron FE, and Suarez AF: Accelerated healing of full-thickness burns by the use of high-voltage pulsed galvanic stimulation in the pig, Ann Plast Surg 23:49, 1989.
15. Cunliffe-Barnes T: Healing rate of human skin determined by measurement of electric potential of experimental abrasions: study of treatment with petrolatum and with petrolatum containing yeast and liver extracts, Am J Surg 69:82, 1945.
16. Davis JC et al: Hyperbaric medicine: patient selection, treatment procedures, and side-effects. In Davis JC and Hunt TK, editors: Problem wounds—the role of oxygen, New York, 1988, Elsevier Science Publishing Co.
17. Deuel TF and Huang JS: Platelet-derived growth factor: structure, function, and roles in normal and transformed cells, J Clin Invest 74:669-675, 1984.
18. Eberhardt A, Szczypiorski P, and Korytowski G: Effect of transcutaneous electrostimulation on the cell composition of skin exudate, Acta Physiol Pol 37:41-46, 1986.
19. Fakhri O and Amin M: The effect of low-voltage electric therapy on the healing of resistant skin burns, J Burn Care Res 8:15, 1987.
20. Finesmith TH, Broadley KN, and Davidson JM: Fibroblasts from wounds of different stages of repair vary in their ability to contract collagen gel in response to growth factors, J Cell Physiol 144:99-107, 1990.
21. Foulds IS and Barker AT: Human skin battery potentials and their possible role in wound healing, Br J Dermatol 109:515, 1983.
22. Fukushima K et al: Studies of galvanotaxis of leukocytes, Med J Osaka Univ 4:195, 1953.
23. Gault WR and Gatens P: Use of low intensity direct current in management of ischemic skin ulcers, Phys Ther 56:265, 1976.
24. Greenhalgh DG, Sprugel KH, Murray MJ, et al: PDGF and FGF stimulate wound healing in the genetically diabetic mouse, Am J Pathol 136:1235-1246, 1990.
25. Hamblin AS: Lymphokines and interleukins, Immunology, suppl 1:39-41, 1988.
26. Hart GB, Lamb RC, and Strauss MB: Gas gangrene: a collective review, J Trauma 23:911-925, 1983.

27. Hecker B, Carron H, and Schwartz D: Pulsed galvanic stimulation: effects of current frequency and polarity on blood flow in healthy subjects, Arch Phys Med Rehabil 66:369, 1985.

28. Hennessey PJ, Black CT, and Andrassy RJ: Epidermal growth factor and insulin act synergistically during diabetic healing, Arch Surg 125:926-929, 1990.

29. Hudson-Goodman P, Girard N, and Jones MB: Wound repair and the potential use of growth factors, Heart Lung 19:379-384, 1990.

30. Hunt TK and Pai MP: The effect of varying ambient oxygen tensions on wound metabolism and collagen synthesis, Surg Gynecol Obstet 135:561-567, 1972.

31. Hyperbaric oxygen therapy: a committee report, Bethesda, Md, 1986, Undersea Medical Society, pp 2-3.

32. Jaffe LF and Vanable JW: Electric fields and wound healing, Clin Dermatol 2:34, 1984.

33. Kaada B: Vasodilation induced by transcutaneous nerve stimulation in peripheral ischemia (Raynaud's phenomenon and diabetic polyneuropathy), Eur Heart J 3:303, 1982.

34. Karba R et al: Effects of electrical current on healing and bacteria growth in decubitus ulcers, Abstract, 3rd International Symposium on Tissue Repair, Miami, Florida, 1990.

35. Kehrl JH, Wakefield LM, Roberts AB, et al: Production of transforming growth factor β by human T lymphocytes and its potential role in the regulation of T cell growth, J Exp Med 163:1037-1050, 1986.

36. Kivisaari J and Niinikoski J: Effects of hyperbaric oxygenation and prolonged hypoxia on the healing of open wounds, Acta Chir Scand 141:14-19, 1975.

37. Kloth L and Feedar J: Acceleration of wound healing with high voltage, monophasic, pulsed current, Phys Ther 68:503, 1988.

38. Knighton DR, Ciresi K, Fiegel VD, et al: Stimulation of wound repair in chronic, nonhealing, cutaneous ulcers using platelet-derived wound healing formula, Surg Gynecol Obstet 170:56-60, 1990.

39. Martinett Y, Bitterman PB, Mornex JF, et al: Activated human monocytes express the c-*sis* proto-oncogene and release a mediator showing PDGF-like activity, Nature 319:158-160, 1986.

40. Massagué J: Epidermal growth factor–like transforming growth factor. II. Interaction with epidermal growth factor receptors in human placenta membranes and A431 cells, J Biol Chem 258:13614-13620, 1983.

41. McCartney-Francis N, Mizel D, Wong H, et al: TGF-β regulates production of growth factors and TGF-β by human peripheral blood monocytes, Growth Factors 4:27-35, 1990.

42. McGrath MH: Peptide growth factors in wound healing, Clin Plast Surg 17:421-432, 1990.

43. Nemiroff PM, Merwin GE, Brant T, and Cassisi NJ: Effects of hyperbaric oxygen and irradiation on experimental flaps in rats, Otolaryngol Head Neck Surg 93:485-491, 1985.

44. Nemiroff PM and Lungu AL: The influence of hyperbaric oxygen and irradiation on vascularity in skin flaps: a controlled study, Surg Forum 38:565-567, 1987.

45. Nemiroff PM: Synergistic effects of pentoxifylline and hyperbaric oxygen on skin flaps, Arch Otolarygnol Head Neck Surg 114:977-981, 1988.

46. Nemiroff PM and Rybak LP: Applications of hyperbaric oxygen for the otolaryngologist-head and neck surgeon, Am J Otolaryngol 9:52-57, 1988.

47. Niinikoski J and Hunt TK: Oxygen tension in human wounds, J Surg Res 12:77-82, 1972.

48. Orida N and Feldman JD: Directional protrusive pseudopodial activity and motility in macrophages induced by extracellular electric fields, Cell Motility 2:243, 1982.

49. Roberts AB, Anzano MA, Wakefield LM, et al: Type β transforming growth factor: a bifunctional regulator of cellular growth, Proc Natl Acad Sci USA 82:119-123, 1985.

50. Robertson WGA: Digby's receipts, Ann Med History 7(3): 216, 1925.

51. Rowley BA, McKenna J, and Chase G: The influence of electrical current on an infecting microorganism in wounds, Ann NY Acad Sci 238:543, 1974.

52. Shimokado K, Raines EW, Madtes DK, et al: A significant part of macrophage-derived growth factor consists of at least two forms of PDGF, Cell 43:277-286, 1985.

53. Strauss MB: Chronic refractory osteomyelitis: review and role of hyperbaric oxygen, HBO Rev 1:231-255, 1980.

54. Strauss MB, Malludhe MM, Faugere MC, et al: Effect of HBO on bone resorption in rabbits, Presented at Seventh Annual Conference on Clinical Applications of HBO, Anaheim, Calif, 1982.

55. Wahl SM, Hunt DA, Wakefield L, et al: Transforming growth factor type β induces monocyte chemotaxis and growth factor production, Proc Natl Acad Sci USA 84:5788-5792, 1987.
56. Wahl SM, Wong H, and McCartney-Francis N: Role of growth factors in inflammation and repair, J Cell Biochem 40:193-199, 1989.
57. Wakefield LM, Smith DM, Masui T, et al: Distribution and modulation of the cellular receptor for transforming growth factor-beta, J Cell Biol 105:965-975, 1987.
58. Waterfield MD: Epidermal growth factor and related molecules, Lancet 1:1243-1246, 1989.
59. Weiss DS, Eaglstein WH, and Falanga V: Pulsed electrical stimulation decreases scar thickness at split-thickness graft donor sites, Invest Dermatol 92(3):539, 1989.
60. Winter GD and Penins DJD: Effects of HBO on epidermal regeneration. In Wada J and Iwa T, editors: Proc Fourth International Congress on Hyperbaric Medicine, Baltimore, Md, 1970, Williams & Wilkins Co., p 363.
61. Wolcott LE et al: Accelerated healing of skin ulcers by electrotherapy: preliminary clinical results, South Med J 62:795, 1969.
62. Zamboni WA, Roth AC, Russel RC, et al: The effect of acute hyperbaric oxygen therapy on axial pattern skin flap survival when administered during and after total ischemia, J Reconstr Microsurg 5(4):343-347, 1989.

Glossary

abscess	Localized collection of pus in any part of the body.
aerobe	Microorganism that lives and grows in the presence of free oxygen.
altered tissue perfusion	Condition when oxygenated blood does not flow freely through the vessels to the tissue.
anaerobe	Microorganism that grows in the absence of free oxygen.
antibacterial	Agent that inhibits the growth of bacteria.
antimicrobial	Agent that inhibits the growth of microbes.
arterial	Pertaining to one or more arteries, which are vessels that carry oxygenated blood to the tissue.
arteriosclerosis	Term applied to several pathologic conditions in which there is thickening, hardening, and loss of elasticity of the walls of blood vessels, especially arteries.
autolysis	Disintegration or liquefaction of tissue or of cells by the body's own mechanisms, such as leukocytes and enzymes.
bactericidal	Agent that destroys bacteria.
bacteriostatic	Agent that is capable of inhibiting the growth or multiplication of bacteria.
blanching	Becoming white; maximum pallor.
cell migration	Movement of cells in the repair process.
cellulitis	Inflammation of tissue around a lesion, characterized by redness, swelling, and tenderness. Signifies a spreading infectious process.
claudication	Inadequate blood supply that produces severe pain in calf muscles occurring during walking; subsides with rest.
collagen	Main supportive protein of skin, tendon, bone, cartilage, and connective tissue.

Modified from *Standards of care: dermal wounds: leg ulcers* and *Standards of care: dermal wounds: pressure sores*, Irvine, CA, 1987, International Association of Enterostomal Therapy.

colonized	Presence of bacteria that cause no local or systemic signs or symptoms.
contamination	The soiling by contact or introduction of organisms into a wound.
contraction	The pulling together of wound edges in the healing process.
crater	Tissue defect extending at least to the subcutaneous layer.
crusted	Dried secretions.
débridement	Removal of devitalized tissue.
debris	Remains of broken down or damaged cells or tissue.
decubitus	A Latin word referring to the reclining position; a misnomer for a pressure sore; its plural is "decubitus ulcers."
demarcation	Line of separation between viable and nonviable tissue.
denude	Loss of epidermis.
dependent pain	Pain occurring when extremity is lower than the heart.
dermal	Related to skin or derma; synonym "integumentary."
dermal wound	Loss of skin integrity, which may be superficial or deep.
dermis	Inner layer of skin in which hair follicles and sweat glands originate; involved in grade II to IV pressure sores.
edema	Presence of abnormally large amounts of fluid in the interstitial space.
enzymes	Biochemical substances that are capable of breaking down necrotic tissue.
epidermis	Outer cellular layer of skin.
epithelialization	Regeneration of the epidermis across wound surface.
erythema	Redness of the skin surface produced by vasodilatation.
eschar	Thick, leathery necrotic tissue; devitalized tissue.
excoriation	Linear scratches on skin.
exudate	Accumulation of fluids in wound; may contain serum, cellular debris, bacteria, and leukocytes.
fibroblast	Any cell or corpuscle from which connective tissue is developed.
friction	Surface damage caused by skin rubbing against another surface.
full-thickness	Tissue destruction extending through the dermis to involve the subcutaneous layer and possibly muscle and bone.
granulation	Formation or growth of small blood vessels and connective tissue in a full-thickness wound.
hydrophilic	Attracting moisture.
hydrophobic	Repelling moisture.
hyperemia	Presence of excess blood in the vessels; engorgement.
induration	Abnormal firmness of tissue with a definite margin.
infection	Overgrowth of microorganisms capable of tissue destruction and invasion, accompanied by local or systemic symptoms.
inflammation	Defensive reaction to tissue injury; involves increased blood flow and capillary permeability and facilitates physiologic cleanup of wound. Accompanied by increased heat, redness, swelling, and pain in the affected area.
insulation	Maintenance of wound temperature close to body temperature.
ischemia	Deficiency of blood caused by functional constriction or obstruction of a blood vessel to a part.

lesion	A broad term referring to wounds or sores.
leukocytosis	Increase in the number of leukocytes (above 10,000 per cubic millimeter) in the blood.
maceration	Softening of tissue by soaking in fluids.
macrophage	Cells that have the ability to destroy bacteria and devitalized tissue.
necrotic	Dead; avascular.
partial-thickness	Loss of epidermis and possible partial loss of dermis.
pathogen	Any disease-producing agent or microorganism.
phlebitis	Inflammation of a vein.
pliable	Supple, flexible.
pressure sore	Area of localized tissue damage caused by ischemia because of pressure.
pus	Thick fluid indicative of infection containing leukocytes, bacteria, and cellular debris.
pyogenic	Producing pus.
reactive, hyperemia	Extra blood in vessels in response to a period of blocked blood flow.
scab	Dried exudate covering superficial wounds.
shear	Trauma caused by tissue layers sliding against each other; results in disruption or angulation of blood vessels.
sinus tract	Course or pathway that can extend in any direction from the wound surface; results in dead space with potential for abscess formation.
slough	Loose, stringy necrotic tissue.
stasis	Stagnation of blood caused by venous congestion.
strip	Remove epidermis by mechanical means; denude.
trophic	Changes that occur as a result of inadequate circulation, such as loss of hair, thinning of skin, and ridging of nails.
ulcer	Open sore.
undermine	Tissue destruction underlying intact skin along wound margins.
varicosities	Dilated tortuous superficial veins.
vasoconstriction	Constriction of the blood vessels.
vasodilatation	Dilatation of blood vessels, especially small arteries and arterioles; preferred spelling rather than "vasodilation."
venous	Pertaining to the veins.
wound base	Uppermost viable tissue layer of wound; may be covered with slough or eschar.
wound margin	Rim or border of wound.
wound repair	Healing process. Partial-thickness healing involves epithelialization; full-thickness healing involves contraction granulation and epithelialization.

A Risk Assessment Scales

GOSNELL SCALE*

PRESSURE SORE RISK ASSESSMENT

I.D. _____   Medical Diagnosis:
Age _____ Sex _____   Primary _____
Height _____ Weight _____   Secondary _____
Date of Admission _____   Nursing Diagnosis:
Date of Discharge _____   _____

Instructions: Complete all categories within 24 hours of admission and every other day thereafter. Refer to the accompanying guidelines for specific rating details.

DATE	Mental Status:	Continence:	Mobility:	Activity:	Nutrition:	TOTAL SCORE
	1. Alert 2. Apathetic 3. Confused 4. Stuporous 5. Unconscious	1. Fully controlled 2. Usually controlled 3. Minimally controlled 4. Absence of control	1. Full 2. Slightly limited 3. Very limited 4. Immobile	1. Ambulatory 2. Walks with assistance 3. Chairfast 4. Bedfast	1. Good 2. Fair 3. Poor	

Date	Vital Signs				Diet	24-Hour Fluid Balance		COLOR	GENERAL SKIN APPEARANCE				Interventions		
	T	P	R	BP		Intake	Output	1. Pallor 2. Mottled 3. Pink 4. Ashen 5. Ruddy 6. Cyanotic 7. Jaundice 8. Other	**Moisture** 1. Dry 2. Damp 3. Oily 4. Other	**Temperature** 1. Cold 2. Cool 3. Warm 4. Hot	**Texture** 1. Smooth 2. Rough 3. Thin/Transp 4. Scaly 5. Crusty 6. Other		No	Yes	Describe

PRESSURE SORE RISK ASSESSMENT
MEDICATION PROFILE

Medication	Dosage	*Frequency	Route	Date Begun	Date Discon.

© 1988 Davina Gosnell

*Suggested flow sheets for monitoring data.

GOSNELL SCALE

GUIDELINES FOR NUMERICAL RATING OF THE DEFINED CATEGORIES

Rating	1	2	3	4	5
Mental Status: An assessment of one's level of response to his environment.	**Alert:** Oriented to time, place, and person. Responsive to all stimuli, and understands explanations.	**Apathetic:** Lethargic, forgetful, drowsy, passive and dull. Sluggish, depressed. Able to obey simple commands. Possibly disoriented to time.	**Confused:** Partial and/or intermittent disorientation to transpulmonary pressure. Purposeless response to stimuli. Restless, aggressive, irritable, anxious and may require tranqualizers or sedatives.	**Stuporous:** Total disorientation. Does not respond to name, simple commands, or verbal stimuli.	**Unconscious:** Nonresponsive to painful stimuli
Continence: The amount of bodily control of urination and defecation.	**Fully Controlled:** Total control of urine and feces.	**Usually Controlled:** Incontinent of urine and/or of feces not more often than once. q 48 hrs. OR has Foley catheter and is incontinent of feces.	**Minimally Controlled:** Incontinent of urine or feces at least once q 24 hrs.	**Absence of Control:** Consistently incontinent of both urine and feces.	
Mobility: The amount and control of movement of one's body.	**Full:** Able to control and move all extremities at will. May require the use of a device but turns, lifts, pulls, balances, and attains sitting position at will.	**Slightly Limited:** Able to control and move all extremities but a degree of limitation is present. Requires assistance of another person to turn, pull, balance, and/or attain a sitting position at will but self-initiates movement or request for help to move.	**Very Limited:** Can assist another person who must initiate movement via turning, lifting, pulling, balancing, and/or attaining a sitting position (contractures, paralysis may be present.)	**Immobile:** Does not assist self in any way to change position. Is unable to change position without assistance. Is completely dependent on others for movement.	
Activity: The ability of an individual to ambulate.	**Ambulatory:** Is able to walk unassisted. Rises from bed unassisted. With the use of a device such as cane or walker is able to ambulate without the assistance of another person.	**Walks with Help:** Able to ambulate with assistance of another person, braces, or crutches. May have limitation of stairs.	**Chairfast** Ambulates only to a chair, requires assistance to do so OR is confined to a wheelchair.	**Bedfast:** Is confined to bed during entire 24 hours of the day.	
Nutrition The process of food intake.	Eats some food from each basic food category every day and the majority of each meal served OR is on tube feeding.	Occasionally refuses a meal or frequently leaves at least half of a meal.	Seldom eats a complete meal and only a few bites of food at a meal.		

Vital Signs:	The temperature, pulse, respiration, and blood pressure to be taken and recorded at the time of every assessment rating.
Skin appearance:	A description of observed skin characteristics: color, moisture, temperature, and texture.
Diet:	Record the specific diet order.
24-hour fluid balance:	The amount of fluid intake and output during the previous 24-hour period should be recorded.
Interventions:	List all devices, measures and/or nursing care activity being used for the purpose of pressure sore prevention.
Medications:	List name, dosage, frequency, and route for all prescribed medications. If a PRN order, list the pattern for the period since last assessment.
Comments:	Use this space to add explanation or further detail regarding any of the previously recorded data, patient condition, etc. OR
© 1988 by Davina Gosnell	Describe anything which you believe to be of importance but not accounted for previously.

BRADEN SCALE FOR PREDICTING PRESSURE SORE RISK

Patient's Name _____ Evaluator's Name _____ Date of Assessment

SENSORY PERCEPTION
Ability to respond meaningfully to pressure-related discomfort

1. Completely limited:
Unresponsive (does not moan, flinch, or grasp) to painful stimuli, due to diminished level of consciousness or sedation,
OR
limited ability to feel pain over most of body surface.

2. Very Limited:
Responds only to painful stimuli. Cannot communicate discomfort except by moaning or restlessness,
OR
has a sensory impairment which limits the ability to feel pain or discomfort over 1/2 of body.

3. Slightly Limited:
Responds to verbal commands but cannot always communicate discomfort or need to be turned,
OR
has some sensory impairment which limits ability to feel pain or discomfort in 1 or 2 extremities.

4. No Impairment:
Responds to verbal commands. Has no sensory deficit which would limit ability to feel or voice pain or discomfort.

MOISTURE
Degree to which skin is exposed to moisture

1. Constantly Moist:
Skin is kept moist almost constantly by perspiration, urine, etc. Dampness is detected every time patient is moved or turned.

2. Moist:
Skin is often but not always moist. Linen must be changed at least once a shift.

3. Occasionally Moist:
Skin is occasionally moist, requiring an extra linen change approximately once a day.

4. Rarely Moist:
Skin is usually dry; linen requires changing only at routine intervals.

ACTIVITY
Degree of physical activity

1. Bedfast:
Confined to bed

2. Chairfast:
Ability to walk severely limited or nonexistent. Cannot bear own weight and/or must be assisted into chair or wheelchair.

3. Walks Occasionally:
Walks occasionally during day but for very short distances, with or without assistance. Spends majority of each shift in bed or chair.

4. Walks Frequently:
Walks outside the room at least twice a day and inside room at least once every 2 hours during waking hours.

MOBILITY
Ability to change and control body position

1. Completely Immobile:
Does not make even slight changes in body or extremity position without assistance.

2. Very Limited:
Makes occasional slight changes in body or extremity position but unable to make frequent or significant changes independently.

3. Slightly Limited:
Makes frequent though slight changes in body or extremity position independently.

4. No Limitations:
Makes major and frequent changes in position without assistance.

NUTRITION
Usual food intake pattern

1. Very Poor:
Never eats a complete meal. Rarely eats more than 1/3 of any food offered. Eats 2 servings or less of protein (meat or dairy products) per day. Takes fluids poorly. Does not take a liquid dietary supplement,
OR
is NPO and/or maintained on clear liquids or IV's for more than 5 days.

2. Probably Inadequate:
Rarely eats a complete meal and generally eats only about 1/2 of any food offered. Protein intake includes only 3 servings of meat or dairy products per day. Occasionally will take a dietary supplement,
OR
receives less than optimum amount of liquid diet or tube feeding.

3. Adequate:
Eats over half of most meals. Eats a total of 4 servings of protein (meat, dairy products) each day. Occasionally will refuse a meal, but will usually take a supplement if offered,
OR
is on a tube feeding or TPN regimen, which probably meets most of nutritional needs.

4. Excellent:
Eats most of every meal. Never refuses a meal. Usually eats a total of 4 or more servings of meat and dairy products. Occasionally eats between meals. Does not require supplementation.

FRICTION AND SHEAR

1. Problem:
Requires moderate to maximum assistance in moving. Complete lifting without sliding against sheets is impossible. Frequently slides down in bed or chair, requiring frequent repositioning with maximum assistance. Spasticity, contractures, or agitation leads to almost constant friction.

2. Potential Problem:
Moves feebly or requires minimum assistance. During a move skin probably slides to some extent against sheets, chair, restraints, or other devices. Maintains relatively good position in chair or bed most of the time but occasionally slides down.

3. No Apparent Problem:
Moves in bed and in chair independently and has sufficient muscle strength to lift up completely during move. Maintains good position in bed or chair at all times.

Total Score _____

NORTON SCALE

NORTON RISK ASSESSMENT SCALE

		Physical Condition		Mental Condition		Activity		Mobility		Incontinent		TOTAL SCORE
		Good	4	Alert	4	Ambulant	4	Full	4	Not	4	
		Fair	3	Apathetic	3	Walk/help	3	Sl. limited	3	Occasional	3	
		Poor	2	Confused	2	Chairbound	2	V. limited	2	Usually/Urine	2	
		Very Bad	1	Stupor	1	Bed	1	Immobile	1	Doubly	1	
Name	Date											

Reprinted with permission, Norton D, McLaren R, and Exton-Smith AN: An investigation of geriatric nursing problems in hospital, 1962, reissue 1975, Churchill Livingstone, Edinburgh.

B Topical Wound Care Products
A Partial List

Category	Example	Manufacturer
ABSORPTION DRESSINGS		
Dextranomer beads	Debrisan®	Johnson & Johnson, New Brunswick, NJ 08903
Copolymer starch dressings	Bard® Absorption Dressing	Bard Home Health Division, Murray Hill, NJ 07974
	Comfeel® Paste	Coloplast, Inc., Tampa, FL 33634
	Comfeel® Powder	Coloplast, Inc.
	DuoDERM® Paste	ConvaTec, Inc., Princeton, NJ 08543
	DuoDERM® Granules	ConvaTec, Inc.
Calcium alginates	Kaltostat™	Calgon Vestal Laboratories, St. Louis, MO 63133
	Sorbsan™	Dow B. Hickam, Inc., Sugar Land, TX 77487
CARBON-IMPREGNATED DRESSINGS	LYOfoam® "C"	Acme United Corp., Fairfield, CT 06430
	Odor–Absorbent Dressing	Hollister Incorporated, Libertyville, IL 60048
CLEANSERS	Biolex™ Wound Cleanser	Catalina Biomedical Corp., Duarte, CA 91010
	Cara–Klenz™	Carrington Laboratories (Avacare), Dallas, TX 75247
	Dey-Wash	Dey Laboratories, Inc., Napa, CA 94558
	Dermal Wound Cleanser	Smith & Nephew United, Inc., Columbus, SC 29205
	Puri–Clens™	Sween Corp., Lake Crystal, MN 56055
	Saf–Clens®	Calgon Vestal Laboratories, St. Louis, Mo 63133
	Shur Clens®	Calgon Vestal Laboratories
COMBINATION DRESSINGS	Airstrip®	Smith & Nephew United, Inc., Columbia, SC 29205
	Viasorb®	Sherwood Medical Co., St. Louis, MO 63146
	Polymem	Ferris Manufacturing Co., Burr Ridge, IL 60521
	Mitraflex™	Calgon Vestal Laboratories, St. Louis, MO 63133

Modified from Krasner D: Wound care products, Ostomy/Wound Management 33:47, 1991.

Category	Example	Manufacturer
ENZYMATIC DEBRIDING AGENTS	Biozyme–C®	Armour Pharmaceutical Co., Blue Bell, PA 19422
	Elase®	Parke–Davis (Professional Medical Products), Greenwood, SC 29648
	Panafil® Ointment	Rystan Company, Inc., Little Falls, NJ 07424
	Panafil® White Ointment	Rystan Company, Inc.
	Santyl®	Knoll Pharmaceuticals, Whippany, NJ 07981
	Travase®	Flint, Division of Travenol Laboratories, Inc., Deerfield, IL 60015
GAUZE DRESSINGS		
Cotton mesh	Multiple	Multiple
Synthetic (nonwoven)	Multiple	Multiple
Hypertonic absorbing	Mesalt®	Scott Health Care, Philadelphia, PA 19113
HYDROCOLLOID WAFER DRESSINGS	Comfeel®	Coloplast, Inc., Tampa, FL 33634
	Comfeel® Pressure Relief Dressing	Coloplast, Inc.
	Comfeel® Transparent Hydrocolloid	Coloplast, Inc.
	Cuttinova–Hydro	Biersdorf, Inc., Norwalk, CT 06856-5529
	DuoDERM®	ConvaTec, Inc., Princeton, NJ 08543
	DuoDERM® CGF	ConvaTec, Inc.
	DuoDERM® Extra–Thin™	ConvaTec, Inc.
	Hydrapad™	Baxter Healthcare Corp., Deerfield, IL 60015
	Intact™	Bard Home Health Division, Murray Hill, NJ 07974
	IntraSite®	Smith & Nephew United, Inc., Columbia, SC 29205
	J & J Ulcer Dressing™	Johnson & Johnson, New Brunswick, NJ 08903
	Restore™	Hollister Incorporated, Libertyville, IL 60048
	Restore CX™	Hollister Incorporated
	3M Tegasorb™	3M Company, St. Paul, MN 55144
	ULTEC™	Sherwood Medical Co., St. Louis, MO 63146
	Sween A–Peel	Sween Corp., Lake Crystal, MN 56055
HYDROGELS	Elasto–Gel™	Southwest Technologies, Kansas City, MO 64108
	Geliperm® Wet/Granulate	E. Fougera, Melville, NY 11747
	Hydragran™	Pharmaseal Div. (Baxter Healthcare Corp.), Valencia, CA 91355
	IntraSite Gel®	Smith & Nephew United, Inc., Columbia, SC 29205
	Second Skin®	Spenco Medical Corp., Waco, TX 76702
	Vigilon®	Bard Home Health Division, Murray Hill, NJ 07974
NONADHERENT DRESSINGS		
Nonimpregnated	Adaptic™	Johnson & Johnson, New Brunswick, NJ 08903
	ETE® Sterile Protective Dressing	Scott Health Care Products, Philadelphia, PA 19113
	EXU–DRY®	Frastec Wound Care Products, Bronx, NY 10475
	Metalline®	Selomas Inc. (Carapace Inc., Lohmann Products Div.), Wilmington, DE 19810
	Release®	Johnson & Johnson, New Brunswick, NJ 08903
	Telfa®	Kendall Healthcare Products Co., Mansfield, MA 02048

Category	Example	Manufacturer
NONADHERENT DRESSINGS—cont'd		
Impregnated	Scarlet Red®	Sherwood Medical Co., St. Louis, MO 63146
	Vaseline® Gauze	Sherwood Medical Co.
	Xeroflo®	Sherwood Medical Co.
	Xeroform	Sherwood Medical Co.
SEMIPERMEABLE POLYURETHANE FOAM DRESSINGS	Allevyn® Cavity Wound Dressing	Smith & Nephew United, Inc., Columbia, SC 29205
	Allevyn®	Smith & Nephew United, Inc.
	Epi–Lock™	Calgon Vestal Laboraories, St. Louis, MO 63133
	LYOfoam®	Acme United Corp., Medical Div., Fairfield, CT 06430
	LYOfoam® "A"	Acme United Corp.
	LYOfoam® "C"	Acme United Corp.
	LYOfoam® Tracheostomy Dressing	Acme United Corp.
SYNTHETIC BARRIER DRESSING	Hydron Wound Dressing®	Bioderm Sciences Inc., Plainsboro, NJ 08536
TOPICAL EMOLLIENTS AND GELS	Biolex™ Wound Gel	Catalina Biomedical Corp., Duarte, CA 91010
	Carrington Dermal Wound Gel™	Carrington Laboratories (Avacare), Dallas, TX 75247
	Chloresium® Ointment/Solution	Rystan Company, Inc., Little Falls, NJ 07424
	Dermagran® Spray	Derma Sciences, Inc., Old Forge, PA 18518
	Dermagran® Ointment	
	Granulex™	Dow B. Hickam, Inc., Sugar Land, TX 77487
	Proderm™	Dow B. Hickam, Inc., Sugar Land, TX 77487
TRANSPARENT ADHESIVE DRESSINGS	ACU–Derm®	Acme United Corp., Medical Div., Fairfield, CT 06430
	Bioclusive™	Johnson & Johnson, New Brunswick, NJ 08903
	BlisterFilm®	Sherwood Medical Co., St. Louis, MO 63146
	Ensure–it™	Deseret Medical, Sandy, VT 84070
	Hi/moist™	Catalina Biomedical Corp., Duarte, CA 91010
	Omiderm™	DR Labs
	OpraFlex®	Professional Medical Products, Inc., Greenwood, SC 29648
	OpSite®	Smith & Nephew United, Inc., Columbia, SC 29205
	Polyskin® II	Kendall Healthcare Products Co., Mansfield, MA 02048
	Tegaderm®	3M Company, St. Paul, MN 55144
	Tegaderm® Pouch	3M Company
	TranSite® Exudate Transfer Film	Smith & Nephew United, Inc., Columbia, SC 29205
	UniFlex®	Smith & Nephew United, Inc.
	Vari/moist™	Catalina Biomedical Corp., Duarte, CA 91010
	Visi Derm II	Medline Industries, Inc., Mundelein, IL 60060

C Support Surfaces

Category	Example	Manufacturer
OVERLAYS		
Foam	Bio Gard	Bio Clinic Co., Rancho Cucamonga, CA 91730
	Geo-Matt	Span-America Medical Systems, Inc., Greenville, SC 29606
	HighFloat	Pre-Foam, Inc., Anaheim, CA 92807
	Iris	E.R. Carpenter Co., Richmond, VA 23261
	UltraForm	American Health Systems, Inc., Greenville, SC 29616-1688
Static air	K-Soft	Kinetic Concepts, Inc., San Antonio, TX 78208
	KoalaKair	Baxter Healthcare Corp., Deerfield, IL 60015
	Original Waffle Pads	EHOB, Inc., Indianapolis, IN 46220
	Roho	Roho, Inc., Belleville, IL 62222
	Sof Care	Gaymar Industries, Inc., Orchard Park, NY 14127
	Tenderair	Health & Medical Techniques Inc., Westport, CT 06880
Alternating air (some with air flow, some without)	AIRFLO/AIRFLO PLUS	Gaymar Industries, Inc., Orchard Park, NY 14127
	AlphaCare	Huntleigh Technology Inc., Manalapan, NJ 07726
	Bio Flote	Bio Clinic Co., Rancho Cucamonga, CA 91730
	DoubleBubble	Huntleigh Technology Inc., Manalapan, NJ 07726
	Dyna-CARE	Grant Airmass Corp., Stamford, CT 06905
	Lapidus	Baxter Healthcare Corp., Deerfield, IL 60015
	PCA Systems	Grant Airmass Corp., Stamford, CT 06905
Gel	Action Mattress Pads	Action Products, Inc., Hagerstown, MD 21740
	TenderGEL (gel)	Health & Medical Techniques Inc., Westport, CT 06880
	Jay	

Modified from: Krasner D: Patient Support Surfaces, Ostomy/Wound Management 33:57, 1991.

Category	Example	Manufacturer
Water	Rochester Modular Waterbeds	Flotation Systems, Inc., Syracuse, NY 13220
	TenderFLO (water)	Health & Medical Techniques Inc., Rathway, NJ 07065
	WaterFlotation Mattresses and System	Lotus Health Care Products, Naugatuck, CT 06770
Low air loss	Acucair	Support Systems International, Inc., Charleston, SC 29405
	Bio Therapy	Bio Clinic Co., Rancho Cucamonga, CA 91730
	CLINI-CARE	Clinicare Systems, Inc., Orchard Park, NY 14127
	CRS 4000 (Alamo)	National Patient Care Systems, Inc., East Rutherford, NJ 07073
	Bio Med X	Bio Clinic Co., Rancho Cucamonga, CA 91730
	First Step Plus	Kinetic Concepts, Inc., San Antonio, TX 78208
REPLACEMENT MATTRESSES	Akros Gel and Foam	Lumex, Inc., Bay Shore, NY 11706
	Bio Gard PLUS	Bio Clinic Co., Rancho Cucamonga, CA 91730
	Century 2000	Hill-Rom Co., Inc., Batesville, IN 47006
	Clinisert	Support Systems International, Inc., Charleston, SC 29405
	CPS (Controlled Pressure Sites)	Medline Industries, Inc., Mundelein, IL 60060
	Decube/Genesis	Comfortex, Inc., Winonà, MN 55987
	GravityI/Gravity II	Health & Medical Techniques Inc., Rathway, NJ 07065
	HighFloat	Pre-Foam, Inc., Anaheim, CA 92807
	Iris Pressure Reduction Mattress	E.R. Carpenter Co., Richmond, VA 23261
	MaxiFloat	Baxter Healthcare Corp., Deerfield, IL 60015
	TheraRest	Kinetic Concepts, Inc., San Antonio, TX 78208
	Top-Gard	Gaymar Industries, Inc., Orchard Park, NY 14127
	UltraForm	American Health Systems, Inc., Greenville, SC 29616-1688
SPECIALTY BEDS		
High air loss	Clinitron	Support Systems International, Inc., Charleston, SC 29405
	FluidAir Plus	Kinetic Concepts, Inc., San Antonio, TX 78208
	Skytron	Mediscus Group, Trevose, PA 19053
Low air loss	Flexicair	Support Systems International, Inc., Charleston, SC 29405
	KinAir	Kinetic Concepts, Inc., San Antonio, TX 78208
	Mediscus Low Air Loss System	Mediscus Group, Trevose, PA 19053
	Orthoderm Therapy Bed	Health Products, Inc., South Haven, MI 49090
Kinetic with low air loss	BioDyne	Kinetic Concepts, Inc., San Antonio, TX 78208
	Restcue	Support Systems International, Inc., Charleston, SC 29405
Kinetic without low air loss	Keane Mobility	Mediscus Group, Trevose, PA 19053
	RotoRest	Kinetic Concepts, Inc., San Antonio, TX 78208
Obese patient accommodation	Burke Bariatric Bed	Kinetic Concepts, Inc., San Antonio, TX 78208
	Magnum 800 System	Mediscus Group, Trevose, PA 19053
	Mediscus HD System	Mediscus Group

ETIOLOGIC (CAUSAL) MODEL OF PRESSURE SORE PRODUCTION (see Fig. 5-2, p. 112)

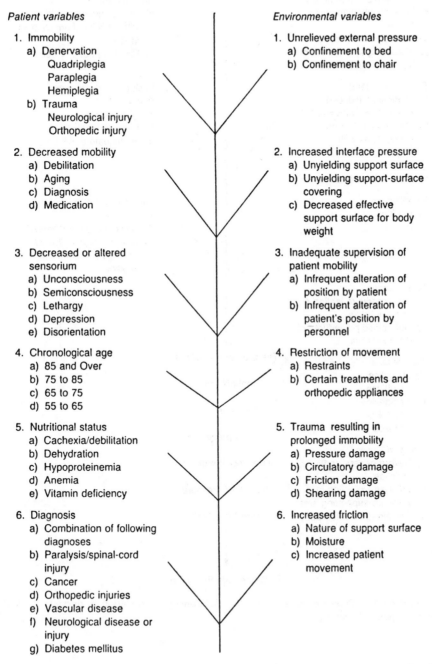

Patient variables

1. Immobility
   a) Denervation
      Quadriplegia
      Paraplegia
      Hemiplegia
   b) Trauma
      Neurological injury
      Orthopedic injury

2. Decreased mobility
   a) Debilitation
   b) Aging
   c) Diagnosis
   d) Medication

3. Decreased or altered sensorium
   a) Unconsciousness
   b) Semiconsciousness
   c) Lethargy
   d) Depression
   e) Disorientation

4. Chronological age
   a) 85 and Over
   b) 75 to 85
   c) 65 to 75
   d) 55 to 65

5. Nutritional status
   a) Cachexia/debilitation
   b) Dehydration
   c) Hypoproteinemia
   d) Anemia
   e) Vitamin deficiency

6. Diagnosis
   a) Combination of following diagnoses
   b) Paralysis/spinal-cord injury
   c) Cancer
   d) Orthopedic injuries
   e) Vascular disease
   f) Neurological disease or injury
   g) Diabetes mellitus

Environmental variables

1. Unrelieved external pressure
   a) Confinement to bed
   b) Confinement to chair

2. Increased interface pressure
   a) Unyielding support surface
   b) Unyielding support-surface covering
   c) Decreased effective support surface for body weight

3. Inadequate supervision of patient mobility
   a) Infrequent alteration of position by patient
   b) Infrequent alteration of patient's position by personnel

4. Restriction of movement
   a) Restraints
   b) Certain treatments and orthopedic appliances

5. Trauma resulting in prolonged immobility
   a) Pressure damage
   b) Circulatory damage
   c) Friction damage
   d) Shearing damage

6. Increased friction
   a) Nature of support surface
   b) Moisture
   c) Increased patient movement

Continued on p. 336.

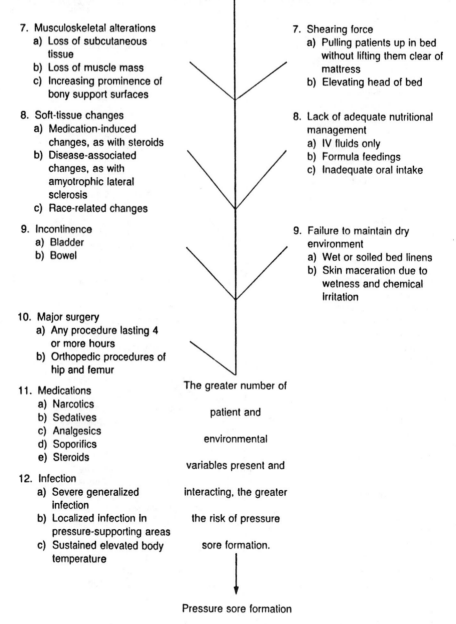

7. Musculoskeletal alterations
   a) Loss of subcutaneous tissue
   b) Loss of muscle mass
   c) Increasing prominence of bony support surfaces

8. Soft-tissue changes
   a) Medication-induced changes, as with steroids
   b) Disease-associated changes, as with amyotrophic lateral sclerosis
   c) Race-related changes

9. Incontinence
   a) Bladder
   b) Bowel

10. Major surgery
    a) Any procedure lasting 4 or more hours
    b) Orthopedic procedures of hip and femur

11. Medications
    a) Narcotics
    b) Sedatives
    c) Analgesics
    d) Soporifics
    e) Steroids

12. Infection
    a) Severe generalized infection
    b) Localized infection in pressure-supporting areas
    c) Sustained elevated body temperature

7. Shearing force
   a) Pulling patients up in bed without lifting them clear of mattress
   b) Elevating head of bed

8. Lack of adequate nutritional management
   a) IV fluids only
   b) Formula feedings
   c) Inadequate oral intake

9. Failure to maintain dry environment
   a) Wet or soiled bed linens
   b) Skin maceration due to wetness and chemical irritation

The greater number of patient and environmental variables present and interacting, the greater the risk of pressure sore formation.

Pressure sore formation

From Shannon ML: Pressure sores. In Norris CM: Concept clarification in nursing, Rockville, Md, 1982, Aspen Publications.

Index

A

ABI; *see* Ankle-brachial index
Absorption dressings, 52t, 53
  clinical features of, 56
Acetic acid, 51t
Acyclovir, herpes simplex infections
    treated with, 22
Adhesives, addition of, to fistula pouch,
    266-267, 268, 269
Advancement flaps, 143
Age
  advanced, pressure ulcer formation and,
    116
  skin characteristics altered by, 8
Aging, wound healing impaired by, 46
Air-filled overlays, 132
  alternating, 132-133
Air-loss beds
  high, 134-135
    advantages and disadvantages of, 136
  low, 135
    advantages and disadvantages of,137
Allergy, skin integrity affected by, 23-24
Allografts, cultured, venous ulcers treated
    with, 204
Anastomosis, inadequate blood supply to,
    fistula formation and, 250
Anergy, 293
Angiography, 179
  digital subtraction, 179-180
Angioplasty
  laser thermal, 184
  percutaneous transluminal, 183-184

Ankle-brachial index, 199
Ankle flare sign, 198
Antibacterials
  arterial ulcers treated with, 188
  venous ulcers treated with, 203
Antibiotics, topical, 48, 55
  venous ulcers treated with, 203
Anticoagulants, 185
Antiplatelet drugs, 186
Antiseptics, 51t
  wound care using, 50
Apocrine glands, 7
Arteriogram, 179
Arteriography, 179
Arteriosclerosis, 167
Arthritis, management of, venous ulcers
    and, 200
ASEPSIS, 78, 98, 99t
Atherosclerosis, 167
  diabetes mellitus and, 168
  hypertension and, 169
  smoking and, 168
Autolysis, 57, 59
Autonomic neuropathy, 192
Axial flaps, 143

B

B complex vitamins, wound healing and, 43
Baby nipple, tube stabilization with, 227,
    229
Bacteria
  interference with, 6
  types of, found in human skin, 6

Page numbers followed by *t* indicate tables.

Bacteroides, 48
Balloon inflow occlusion, 179
Basal cells, 3
Basement membrane zone, 3-4
Beds
   kinetic therapy provided by, 135-136
   speciality, 134-136
Bedsore, 109; *see also* Pressure ulcers
Bile, characteristics of, 254t
Biliary catheters
   irrigation of, 243
   percutaneous, 240
      complications with, 242t, 243
      nursing management of, 243
      placement procedures for, 241
Biliary drainage, percutaneous
   transhepatic, 240
Biologic dressings, 55
Blanching erythema, 117
Blinding a study, 315-316
Blood, stasis of, venous ulcers caused by,
   196
Blood flow
   dynamics of, 167
   effect of electrical stimulation on, 310
Blood glucose, control of, 200
Blood pressure, low, pressure ulcers and,
   116
Body temperature, elevated, pressure ulcer
   formation and, 116
Boot, Unna, venous ulcers treated with,
   201-202
Braden scale, 328
   features of, 124
   reliability and validity of, 123t
Bulla, definition of, *11*
Bullous impetigo, 21
Button, gastrostomy, 223-224
Bypass, procedures for, 183

C

Cachectin; *see* Tumor necrosis factor-alpha
Calories, wound healing and, 43
Candida albicans, 20
Candidiasis, 20-21
Capillaries, proliferation of, in wound
   healing, 39
Capillary closing pressure, 110, 112
   effectiveness of support surfaces
      measured with, 127
Capillary filling time, 171
Capillary pressure, 110
Carotene, 3

Carotenoids, 3
Casting, total contact, for neuropathic
   ulcers, 193-195
Catheter ports, 267-268
Catheters
   biliary, percutaneous, 240-243
   suction, fistulas managed with, 271-274
Cellulitis, periulcer, treatment of, 203
Chemicals, skin damaged by, 17-18
Chest tubes; *see* Empyema tubes
Cicatrization, index of, 74
Circulation
   impaired, 170-171
   as thermoregulatory mechanism, 6-7
Claudication, intermittent, 170
Cleansing, wound; *see* Wound cleansing
Clinical study
   blinding and randomization of, 315-316
   outcomes of, 316
   population for, 316
Collagen, 4, 5
   impaired synthesis of, hypoxia and,
      42
   synthesis of, in granulation process, 39-
      40
Colon, secretions from, characteristics of,
   254t
Color, wound, assessment of, 81-82
Communication, skin as organ of, 7-8
Compression stockings, graduated, 201
Congestive heart failure, management of,
   venous ulcers and, 200
Contact cast, total, for neuropathic ulcers,
   193-195
Contact dermatitis
   allergic, 23-24
   irritant, 17
Contraction, wound, 40
Contrast venography, 200
Copper, wound healing and, 43
Corium; *see* Dermis
Corneocytes, 2
Corticosteroids
   antiinflammatory effect of, 45
   effect of, on skin, 10
   venous ulcers and, 200
   wound healing impaired by, 45
Cortisol, pressure ulcer formation and, 116
Critical closing pressure, 110, 112
Crusts, definition of, *12*
Cultures, arterial ulcer, 187-188
Current of injury, 309
Cytokines, 302-303

D

Dead space
    full-thickness wounds with, topical
        therapy for, 59-60
    obliteration of, 48-49
Débridement, 81
    arterial ulcer, 186
    conservative instrumental, 59
    full-thickness wounds with necrosis
        managed by, 56-57, 59
Decubitus ulcers, 109; *see also* Pressure
    ulcers
Dehiscence, wound, 97
    definition of, 250
Deodorants, fistula, 276
Dermal papillae, 4
Dermatitis
    chemical, 17-18
    contact
        allergic, 23-24
        differentiated from candidiasis, 20
        irritant, 17-18
    stasis, 198
    venous, management of, 203
Dermatoheliosis, 9
Dermis, 4
    repair of, 35
Dermoepidermal junction, 3; *see also*
    Basement membrane zone
Diabetes
    regulation of, arterial ulcers and, 189-
        190
    vascular surgery in patient with, criteria
        for, 182-183
Diabetes mellitus
    care of feet in, 193, 194
    peripheral vascular disease and, 168
    surgical wound healing affected by,
        94
    wound healing impaired by, 44-45
Diarrhea, tube feeding and, 295
Dicloxacillin, impetigo treated with, 21
Diet, wound management and, 294
Diet history, 291
Digital subtraction angiography, 179-180
Diuretics, venous insufficiency and, 201
Documentation, guidelines for, 83-84
Doppler ultrasonography, 199
Dorsalis pedis pulses, 171
Drain sites; *see also* Fistulas
    definition of, 250
Drainage, biliary, percutaneous
    transhepatic, 240

Drainage system, nephrostomy, routine
    care of, 239-240
Draining, wound, definition of, 250-251
Dressings
    calcium alginate, venous ulcers treated
        with, 204
    gauze, effluent containment with, 263-
        264
    hydrocolloid, venous ulcers treated with,
        203
    over biliary tube insertion sites, 243
    topical, arterial ulcers treated with,
        187t, 188-189
    venous ulcers treated with, 203-204
    wound; *see* Wound dressings
Dry eschar, 48
Duodenum, secretions from,
    characteristics of, 254t
Duplex scanning with color-flow imaging,
    199

E

Eccrine glands, 7
Edema
    control of, arterial ulcers and, 189
    elimination of, venous ulcers and, 201
    grading of pulses and, 170
Education, patient; *see* Patient education
Effluent
    containment of, 263-276
    fistula
        characteristics of, 260, 261-262
        measurement of, 277
        refeeding of, 253
EGF; *see* Epidermal growth factor
Elastin, 4, 5
Elastic wraps, venous ulcers treated with,
    200
Elderly, prevalence of pressure ulcers in,
    108
Electrical current
    galvanotaxic effects of, 309-310
    stimulatory effect of, on cells, 310
Electrical stimulation
    antibacterial effects of, 310
    blood flow affected by, 310
    clinical application of, 310-311
    effects of, 309-310
    types of, 308-309
Electrolytes
    imbalance of, signs and symptoms of,
        256t-257t

Electrolytes—cont'd
  stabilization of, in fistula management, 253
Electrotherapy; *see* Electrical stimulation
Empyema, 230-231
Empyema tubes, 230-231
  nursing management of, 234
  placement of, 233-234
  pouching procedure for leakage around, 233-234
Endarteritis, radiation-induced, 250
Enteral nutrition, 255, 258
Enteral tube feeding, 294-296
Enterostomies, tube feeding; *see*
      Gastrostomy; Jejunostomy
Epidermal cells, migration of, 34
Epidermal growth factor, 303, 305
Epidermis, 2-33
  assessment of, with arterial ulcers, 174
  repair of, 34
  stripping of, 16-17
Epithelialization, 40
Erosions, definition of, *12*
Erythema, blanching, 117
Erythromycin, impetigo treated with, 21
Eschar, dry, 48
Exercise, limitations on, in peripheral vascular disease, 190-191
Extravasation, effect of, on skin, 25
Exudate
  assessment of, 82
  excess, 49
  full-thickness wounds with, topical therapy for, 59-60

F

Fascia, superficial; *see* Hypodermis
Fasciocutaneous flaps, 143
Feeding, enteral tube, 294-296
Feet, diabetic, care of, 193, 194
Femoroperoneal bypass, 183
Femorotibial bypass, 183
Fetal tissue, scarless healing of, 8
FGF; *see* Fibroblast growth factor
Fibrin cuffs, 197
Fibrinolysis, stimulation of, venous ulcers treated by, 202
Fibroblast growth factor, 303, 305
Fibroblasts, 39
Fibronectin, 4
Fissure, definition of, *12*
Fistula effluent, refeeding of, 253

Fistula pouch
  adhesive surface on, 265-266
    addition of, 268, 269
    modification of, 266-267
  capacity of, 266
  cleansing skin for, 278
  complex techniques for, 269-276
  condom catheter, 271, 273
  discharge planning for patient with, 280-281
  features of, 264-266
  odor control provided by, 276
  outlet for, 266
  procedure for changing, 277-278, 279
  routine care of, 279-280
  saddlebagging technique for, 267, 270
  silicone mold used for, 269, 271
  sizing aperature for, 278
  trough procedure for, 269-270, 273
  wound access and, 266
Fistulas
  assessment of, 260-262
  bridging technique for, 271, 275
  classification of, 251, 252t
  controlling odor of, 276
  definition of, 250
  definitive treatment of, 253, 255, 258-259
  enteral, route of nutritional support for patients with, 258
  etiology of, 250
  external, definition of, 251
  fluid and electrolyte stabilization of, 253
  high-output, definition of, 251
  implementation of care plan for, 277-280
  incidence of, 249-250
  internal, definition of, 251
  irradiation-induced, 250
  management of
    cost containment and, 277
    patient comfort in, 277
    patient mobility and, 277
    planning for, 262-277
    suction catheters for, 271-274
    surgical, 258-259
  manifestations of, 251-252
  medical management of
    goal of, 252-253
    phases of, 253-259
  nursing management of, 259-281
    goals of, 259-260

Fistulas —cont'd
  nutritional support for patients with, 253, 255
  orifice of, anatomic locale of, 260, 261
  pouching of, routine, 264-266
  radiologic examination of, 255
  skin-barriers for management of, 262-263
  source of, 260-261
  spontaneous closure of, 255, 258
    delay of, 259
  terminology for, 251, 252t
  vaginal, drain device for, 274-276
Flaps
  mycutaneous, 145, 147
  tissue, pressure ulcers treated with, 143
Fluids
  imbalance of, signs and symptoms of, 256t-257t
  interstitial, effect of pressure on, 120
  loss of, in burn patients, 5
  stabilization of, in fistula management, 253
  wound volume measured using, 77
Foam overlays, 130
  advantages and disadvantages of, 131
Foam wound dressings, 77
Folliculitis, differentiated from candidiasis, 20
Foreign bodies, presence of, in wounds, 83
Free flaps, 143
Friction
  pressure ulcer formation and, 115
  skin injured by, 16
Furacin; see Nitrofurazone

G

Gangrene, 171
Gastric juice, characteristics of, 254t
Gastrostomy
  definition of, 215
  endoscopic approach to, 221
  Janeway, 215
    summary of procedure for, 218t
  percutaneous endoscopic, 221
    summary of procedure for, 217t
  placement procedures for, 215-222
  Spivak, summary of procedure for, 219t
  Stamm, 215
    summary of procedure for, 216t
  surgical versus nonsurgical placement of, complications of, 223t
Gastrostomy button, 223-224

Gastrostomy tubes; see also Percutaneous tubes
  leakage around, 226, 229-230
  nursing management of, 224, 226-230
  site selection for, 224, 226
  stabilization of, 226-229
    external, 230t
  triple-lumen, 223
  types of, 222-224
    advantages and disadvantages of, 225t
Gauze, 96
Gauze dressings, 52t, 53
  clinical features of, 57
Gel dressings, 52t, 53
  clinical features of, 58
Gel-filled overlays, 131
  advantages and disadvantages of, 132
Glucose, blood, control of, 200
Gluteus maximus muscle flap, ischial ulcer closure with, 145
Goose bumps, 7
Gosnell scale, 326-327
  features of, 124
  reliability and validity of, 123t
Grading system, wound assessment using, 99
Graduated compression stockings, 201
Grafting, skin; see Skin grafting
Granulation, 39
Greater trochanteric ulcers, closure of, 147
Growth factors, 302-304
  actions of, 304
  naming conventions for, 303
  sources and targets of, 303-304
  structural features of, 303
  types of, 304-306
  venous ulcers treated with, 204
  wound repair stimulated by, 189
    potential limitations of, 307-308
    therapuetic use of, 306-307

H

Hamstring V-Y myocutaneous flap, ischial ulcer closure with, 145
HBO; see Hyperbaric oxygenation
Healing, wound; see Wound healing
Healing ridge, 97-98
Heart failure, congestive, venous ulcers and, 200
Hemostasis, 36
Heparan sulfate proteoglycan, 4
Herpes simplex virus, skin infections caused by, 21-22

Herpes zoster, 22
High-voltage pulsed current, 308-309
HSV; *see* Herpes simplex virus
HVPC; *see* High-voltage pulsed current
Hyaluronic acid, reduction in scar
    formation in postnatal wounds
    associated with, 8
Hydration, skin, 9
Hydrocolloid wafer dressings, 52t, 53, 54
Hydrocortisone, venous dermatitis treated
    with, 203
Hydrogen peroxide, 51t
Hyperbaric oxygenation, 311-314
    complications of, 314
    delivery of, 312
    effects of, 313-314
    indications for, 311-312
    patient preparation for, 312-313
Hyperemia, reactive, 117
Hyperlipidemia, peripheral vascular
    disease and, 168-169
Hypertension
    peripheral vascular disease and, 169
    venous, ulcerations of lower legs and,
    19
Hypoalbuminemia, venous ulcers and, 198
Hypochlorite solutions, 51t
Hypodermis, 4
Hypoxia; *see* Ischemia

I

ILD; *see* Indentation load deflection
Ileum, secretions from, characteristics of,
    254t
Immobility, venous ulcers and, 198
Immune system
    function of, nutritional status evaluated
        by, 293-294
    skin, 6
Immunosuppression, wound healing
    impaired by, 46
Impedance plethysmography, 199
Impetigo, 21
In situ saphenous bypass, 183
Incidence, definition of, 108
Incision, surgical, assessment of, 96-98
Incontinence, pressure ulcer formation
    and, 115
Indentation load deflection, foam overlays
    and, 130
Index of cicatrization, 74
Infection
    assessment of wounds for, 48
    eradication of, in arterial ulcers, 186-188

Infection—cont'd
    presence or absence of, wound healing
        and, 44
    pressure ulcers and, 140
    reduced resistance to, hypoxia and, 42
    reduction of, with percutaneous tubes,
        214-215
    skin; *see* Skin infections
Inflammation, 37-38
Injury, current of, 309
Instruments
    for evaluation of wound healing, 78-79
    schema of, for clinical evaluation of
        wound status and healing, 71t
Interleukins, 306
Interstitial fluid, effect of pressure on,
    120
IPG; *see* Impedance plethysmography
Iron, wound healing and, 43
Irrigation, wound, 50
Ischemia, 117
    duration and intensity of pressure and,
        113
    educating patients about, 190-191
    environmental factors in, 190
    evaluation of, 171
    nonblanching erythema and, 117
    redistribution of blood supply in, 119-
        120
Ischial ulcer, closure of, 144-147

J

Janeway gastrostomy, 215
    summary of procedure for, 218t
Jejunostomy
    definition of, 215
    needle catheter, summary of procedure
        for, 220t
    percutaneous endoscopic, summary of
        procedure for, 219t
    placement procedures for, 215-222
    Witzel, summary of procedure for, 219t
Jejunostomy tubes; *see also* Percutaneous
        tubes
    leakage around, 226, 229-230
    nursing management of, 224, 226-230
    site selection for, 224, 226
    stabilization of, 226-229
        external, 230t
    types of, 222-224
        advantages and disadvantages of, 225t
Jejunum, secretions from, characteristics
        of, 254t

K

Keloids, formation of, 41
Keratin, 3
Keratinocytes, 3
    basal, 3
Keratohyalin granules, 3
Kinetic therapy, provision of, by speciality
        beds, 135-136
Kundin wound gauge, 76-77

L

Lamina densa, 4
Lamina lucida, 4
Langerhans cells, 6
Laser thermal angioplasty, 184
Legs, elevation of, venous ulcers and, 199,
        200
Leukocytes, role of, in wound healing, 37
LIDC; see Low-intensity direct current
Lipodermatosclerosis, 198
Low air-loss overlays, 132
    advantages and disadvantages of, 133
Low-intensity direct current, 308-309
Lower extremity
    with arterial insufficiency, skin care for,
        191
    vascular perfusion of, assessment of,
        171-180
Lumbar sympathectomy, 184
Lymphotoxin, 303

M

Macrophages, role of, in wound healing,
        37-38
Macrophages, tissue, 6
Macule, definition of, *11*
Mafenide acetate, 188
Malnutrition
    causes of, 289, 290t
    definition of, 289
    fistulas and, 255
    high-risk factors for, 292
    incidence of, 289
    physical examination for, 292-293
    protein, signs of, 292
    venous ulceration and, 197-198
Malnutriton, effects of, 289
Mattresses
    overlay, 129-133
    replacement, 133-134
Medication, skin characteristics altered by,
        10
Meissner corpuscles, 7
Melanin, 6

Melanocytes, 3
Melanosomes, 3
Metabolism, function of skin in, 7
Moisture
    pressure ulcer formation and, 115
    preventing buildup of, 21
Molds, wound, 77
Motor neuropathy, 192
Muscles, damage to, pressure ulcers and,
        117-119
Myocutaneous flaps, 143
    ischial ulcer closure with, 145, 147
Myofibroblasts, 40

N

Necrosis, full-thickness wounds with,
        topical therapy for, 56, 59
Needle catheter jejunostomy, summary of
        procedure for, 220t
Neoangiogenesis, 39
Nephrostomy drainage systems, routine
        care of, 239-240
Nephrostomy tubes, percutaneous; see
        Percutaneous nephrostomy tubes
Neuropathy, motor, 192
Neuropathy, peripheral, 192-195
    management of, 192-195
    pathogenesis of, 192
    types of, 192
Nitrofurazone, 203
Nitrogen-balance study, nutritional status
        evaluated with, 293
Nocturnal pain, 170
Nodule, definition of, *11*
Nonadhesive semipermeable polyurethane
        foam dressings, 52t, 53
    clinical features of, 55
Nonocclusive dressings, venous ulcers
        treated with, 203
Nonsteroidal antiinflammatory agents,
        venous ulcers and, 200
Norton scale, 329
    features of, 124
    reliability and validity of, 123t
NSAID; see Nonsteroidal antiinflammatory
        agents
Nutrition
    assessment of, 290-294
        laboratory data for, 293-294
        patient history for, 291-292
        physical examination in, 292-293
    enteral, 255, 258, 294-296
    oral, 294
    parenteral, 255, 258, 296

Nutrition—cont'd
  for patients with arterial ulcers, 189
  poor, pressure ulcer formation and, 115
  pressure ulcers and, 140
  skin characteristics altered by, 10
  support of, 294-296
    in patients with fistulas, 253, 255
  surgical wound healing and, 95-96
  wound healing and, 43-44

O

Obesity, management of, venous ulcers
    and, 200
Obstructive biliary disease, 240
Occlusive dressings, venous ulcers treated
    with, 203
Orthotics, 193
Osteomyelitis, 188
  pressure ulcers and, 140
Overlays, 129-133
  dynamic, 132-133
  static, 130-132
Oxygen
  hyperbaric; *see* Hyperbaric oxygenation
  requirements for, in surgical wound
    healing, 94-95
Oxygen tension, transcutaneous, 177-179
Oxygen toxicity, 314
Oxygenation, hyperbaric; *see* Hyperbaric
    oxygenation
Oxygenaton, tissue perfusion and, 42

P

Pacinian corpuscles, 7
Pain
  nocturnal, 170
  peripheral arterial insufficiency and,
    169-170
  rest, 170
Pancreatic juice, characteristics of, 254t
Papillae, dermal, 4
Papillary dermis, 4
Papule, definition of, *11*
Parenteral nutrition, 255, 258
Patch tests, 24
  scale for interpretation of results of, 25
Pathogens, protection against, role of skin
    in, 6
Patient, optimizing, before surgical
    treatment of pressure ulcers, 141
Patient education
  about biliary catheters, 243
  about percutaneous tubes, 214

Patient education—cont'd
  about peripheral vascular disease, 190-
    191
  pressure ulcer prevention and, 141
PDGF; *see* Platelet-derived growth factor
PEG; *see* Percutaneous endoscopic
    gastrostomy
Pentoxifylline, microcirculation facilitated
    by, 185
Percutaneous endoscopic gastrostomy, 221
  summary of procedure for, 217t
Percutaneous endoscopic jejunostomy,
    summary of procedure for, 219t
Percutaneous nephrostomy tubes, 234-235
  nursing management of, 236-240
  obstruction of, 239
  patency of, 239
  placement procedures for, 235-236
  stabilization of, 237-239
Percutaneous transhepatic biliary
    drainage, 240
Percutaneous transluminal angioplasty,
    183-184
Percutaneous tubes; *see also* Gastrostomy
    tubes; Jejunostomy tubes
  patient education about, 214
  reduction of infection with, 214-215
Percutaneous gastrostomy, radiographic
    approach to, 221-222
Perfusion
  arterial, enhancement of, 182-186
  tissue, oxygenaton and, 42
  vascular
    assessment of, 171-180
    pharmacotherapy agents for, 185-186
Peripheral neuropathy, 192-195
Peripheral vascular disease
  assessment of, 171-180
  chronicity of, 191
  contributing factors in, 168-169
  diabetic and nondiabetic, 167-168
  exercise and activity limitations in, 190-
    191
  pathophysiology of, 166-168
  patient education about, 190-191
  pharmacotherapy agents used to treat,
    185-186
  positioning patient with, 190
  signs and symptoms of, 169-171
Phosphorylation, 304
Photoaging, 9
Photography, wound, 75
Photoplethysmography, 199
Planimetry, 75

Plaque, definition of, *11*
Platelet-derived growth factor, 303, 305
Popliteal pulses, 170-171
Positioning, patient, pressure ulcer formation and, 126
Posterior tibial pulse, 171
Pouch
  fecal outlet, addition of continuous drainage tube to, 266, 267
  fistula; *see* Fistula pouch
  rectal, 17
    procedures for, 18
Pouch film, 266
Pouching, fistula, 261, 264-274; *see also* Fistula pouch
  evaluation of system for, 280-281
Pouching, for leakage around empyema tubes, 233-234
Povidone-iodine, venous ulcers and, 202-203
Povidone-iodine preparations, 51t
PPG; *see* Photoplethysmography
Predictive value, screening tools measured by, 122t
Prednisone, venous ulcers and, 200
Pressure
  capillary closing; *see* Capillary closing pressure
  cellular response to, 117
  duration of, pressure ulcer formation and, 113
  intensity of, pressure ulcer formation and, 110, 112
  pressure ulcer formation caused by, 110-114
  segmental, 174-175
  tissue interface; *see* Tissue interface pressure
  tissue tolerance to, pressure ulcer formation and, 113-114
  toe, 175-176
Pressure-reducing devices, definition of, 129
Pressure-relieving devices, definition of, 128
Pressure sore; *see* Pressure ulcers
Pressure ulcers, 13-14
  advanced age and, 116
  clinical presentation of, 117
  closure of
    principles of, 144-145
    tissue expansion for, 144
  cortisol and, 116

Pressure ulcers—cont'd
  definitions of, 109-110
  economic impact of, 107
  elevated body temperature and, 116
  etiologic model for production of, 112, 335-336
  etiology of, 110-116
  extent of tissue damage caused by, 119-120
  friction and, 115
  as health threat, 106
  identifying patients at risk for, 120-124
  implementation of risk assessment program for, 124-125
  incidence of, 109
  incontinence and, 115
  interventions for, 126-127
  locations for, 110, *111*
  low blood pressure and, 116
  management of, 139-141
  miscellaneous factors in formation of, 116
  moisture and, 115
  mortality associated with, 106
  muscle damage related to, 117-119
  nutritional debilitation and, 115
  optimizing the microenvironment for, 140
  pathophysiologic changes occurring with, 117-120
  patient nutrition and, 140
  pressure and, 110-114
  prevalence of, 107-108
  prevention of, 120-141, 126-127
    patient education and, 141
    support surfaces used for, 127-139
  psychosocial status and, 116
  risk-assessment tools for, 121-122
  risk factors for
    assessment of patient for, 125
    minimizing negative effects of, 125-127
  scope of problem with, 107-109
  shear and, 114-115
  skin grafts used to treat, 142-143
  smoking and, 116
  staging of, 141-142
  surgical interventions for, 141-152
  surgical options for, 142-144
  tissue flaps used to treat, 143
  topical therapy for, 140
Prevalence, incidence of, 108
Prostacyclin, 186

Protein
  deficiency in, pressure ulcer formation
    and, 115
  dermal, 4
  metabolism of, laboratory studies used
    to evaluate, 293-294
  wound healing and, 43
Pseudomonas aeruginosa, 48
PTA; *see* Percutaneous transluminal
  angioplasty
PTBD; *see* Percutaneous transhepatic
  biliary drainage
Pulse volume recording, 177
Pulsed electrical stimulation, 308, 309
Pulses
  dorsalis pedis, 171
  grading of, edema and, 170
  lower extremity, palpation of, 170
  popliteal, 170-171
  posterior tibial, 171
Pustule, definition of, *11*
PVD; *see* Peripheral vascular disease
PVR; *see* Pulse volume recording
Pyelonephritis, 239-240

R

Radiation
  effect of, on skin, 24-25
  ultraviolet, protection against, 6
Radionuclide venography, 199-200
Random flaps, 143
Randomization, 315
Rating scales, identifying patients at risk
  for pressure ulcers with, 121, 122
Reactive hyperemia, 117
Rectal pouches, 17
  procedure for, 18
Red, Yellow, Black color system
  wound classification by, 73
  wound healing evaluated using, 78, 79
Remodeling, wound, 40-41
Rest pain, 170
Rete ridges, 3
Reticular dermis, 4
Revascularization surgery, 183-184
  indications for, 182
Risk assessment scales, 325-329
Risk-assessment tools for pressure-
  prevention program
  features of, 121-122
  implementation of, 124-125
  measures of predictive validity for, 122t
Rotation flaps, 143
Roux-en-Y, summary of procedure for,
  220t

RV; *see* Radionuclide venography
RYB; *see* Red, Yellow, Black color concept

S

Sacral ulcer, closure of, 147
Saliva, characteristics of, 254t
Scales, definition of, *12*
Scar tissue
  composition of, 39
  tensile strength of, 41
Scarring, hypertrophic, 41
Scar(s)
  definition of, *12*
  formation of, reduction in, 8
SCD; *see* Sequential compression devices
Sealants, skin, 16-17
Sebaceous glands, 6
Sebum, protection against pathogens
  provided by, 6
Secretions, gastrointestinal, characteristics
  of, 254t
Segmental pressures, 174
Sensation, skin, 7
Sensitivity, screening tools measured by,
  122
Sensory neuropathy, 192
Sepsis, evaluation and treatment of, 253
Sequential Compression Device
  Therapeutic System, 202
Shear
  pressure ulcer formation and, 114-115
  skin injured by, 14-16
Shingles, 22
Silicone mold, fistula pouching using, 269,
  271
Silvadene; *see* Silver sulfadiazine
Silver sulfadiazine, venous ulcers treated
  with, 203
Sinus, fistula and, distinction between, *251*
Sinus tracts, 80-81
Skin, 1-29
  characteristics of, factors altering, 8-10
  cleansing of, fistula pouches and, 278
  damage to; *see* Skin damage
  effect of age on, 8
  functions of, 2, 5-8
  hydration of, 9
  integrity of, 2-10
    fistulas and, 260, 261
  ischemic changes in, in peripheral
    vascular disease, 171
  layers of, 2-4
  manifestation of allergic responses on,
    23-24
  pathology of, 10-25

Skin—cont'd
    perifistular, 261
    peritrauma, assessment of, 83
    photodamaged, 9
    protection of, fistulas and, 262-263
    testing of, for delayed cutaneous
        hypersensitivity, 293
Skin-barriers
    fistula management with, 262-263
    paste used for, 279
Skin damage
    chemicals as cause of, 17-18
    infectious factors in, 20-22
    mechanical, 13-17
    types of, 10-25
    vascular, 19-20
Skin flora, protection against pathogens
        provided by, 6
Skin grafting, 40
    pressure ulcers treated with, 142-143
Skin infections
    herpes simplex as cause of, 21-22
    streptococcal, 21
Skin lesions
    primary, definition of, *11*
    secondary, definition of, *12*
Skin sealants, 16-17
Smoking
    peripheral vascular disease and, 168
    pressure ulcer formation and, 116
Soaps, effect of, on skin, 9-10
Specificity, screening tools measured by,
        122
Spivak gastrostomy, summary of
        procedure for, 219t
Squames, 2
Staging systems, wound classification
        using, 72
Stamm gastrostomy, 215
    summary of procedure for, 216t
Stanozolol, venous ulcers treated by, 202
Staphylococcus aureus, 48
Stasis dermatitis, 198
Stockings, graduated compression, venous
        ulcers treated with, 201
Stratum corneum, 2-3
    protection against pathogens provided
        by, 6
Stratum germinativum, 3
Stratum granulosum, 3
Stratum lucidum, 3
Suction catheters, fistulas managed with,
        271-274
Sulfamylon Cream; *see* Mafenide acetate
Sun, skin characteristics altered by, 9

Sunburn, 9
Support surfaces
    categories of, 128-129
    prevention of pressure ulcers using, 127-
        139
    selection of
        for individual patient, 138-139
        for institution or agency, 136-138
    types of, 333-334
Surgery, peripheral vascular, in diabetic
        patients, 182-183
Surgical incision, assessment of, 96-98
Surgical wounds
    acute, 91-100
        definition of, 92-93
    closure of, 97
    epithelial resurfacing in, 96-97
    factors affecting healing of, 93-96
    local changes at site of, 98
    measurement of, 98-100
    observational and palpation assessments
        of, 99-100
    primary dressing for, 96
Sutures, 97
Sweat glands, 7
Sweating, as thermoregulatory
        mechanism, 6-7
Sympathectomy, lumbar, 184
Synthetic barrier dressings, 52t, 53
    clinical features of, 58

T

Tape, adhesive, application and removal
        of, 16-17
Target cell, 304
TENS; *see* Transcutaneous electrical nerve
        stimulation
Tensor fasciae latae myocutaneous flap,
        greater trochanteric ulcer closed
        with, 147
Tests
    diagnostic, for venous ulcers, 199-200
    invasive, for patients with arterial
        ulcers, 179-180
    noninvasive, for patients with arterial
        ulcers, 174-179
Texas Interface Pressure Evaluator
        System, 127-128
TFEs; *see* Tube feeding enterostomies
TFL flap; *see* Tensor fasciae latae
        myocutaneous flap
TGF-alpha; *see* Transforming growth
        factor-alpha
TGF-beta; *see* Transforming growth factor-
        beta

Thermoregulation, 6-7
TIPE; *see* Texas Interface Pressure Evaluator System
Tissue flaps, pressure ulcers treated with, 143
Tissue interface pressure, 127-128
  measurement of, 112, 127-128
Tissue macrophages, 6
Tissue perfusion, oxgenation and, 42
Tissue plasminogen activity, 197
Tissues
  evaluating damage to, in pressure ulcers, 141-142
  expansion of, for pressure ulcer closure, 144
  extent of damage to, 80
    pressure ulcers and, 119-120
  ischemic, 117
    duration and intensity of pressure and, 113
    redistribution of blood supply in, 119-120
  necrotic, removal of, 48
  tolerance of, to pressure, 113-114
  type of, in wound bed, 81
TLC; *see* Total lymphocyte count
TNF-alpha; *see* Tumor necrosis factor-alpha
Toe pressures, 175-176
Topical antibiotics, 48, 55
Topical antibiotics, venous ulcers treated with, 203
Topical therapy, 46, 48-61
  for arterial ulcers, 186, 187t
  decision making regarding, 60
  for pressure ulcers, 140
  principles of, 48-49
  products for, 330-332
  for stage III pressure ulcers, 142
  for venous ulcers, 202-204
Total lymphocyte count, 293-294
TPA; *see* Tissue plasminogen activity
Tracings, wound, 74-75
Transcutaneous electrical nerve stimulation, 309
Transcutaneous oxygen tension, 177-179
Transforming growth factor-alpha, 303, 305
Transforming growth factor-beta, 303, 304-305
Transparent adhesive dressings, 51, 52t
  clinical features of, 54
Transposition flaps, 143

Trauma
  avoidance of
    in peripheral neuropathy, 193
    in peripheral vascular disease, 191
  venous ulcers and, 198
Trendelenburg test, 199
Trental; *see* Pentoxifylline
Trough procedure, fistula pouching by, 269-270, 273
Tube feeding enterostomies; *see* Gastrostomy; Jejunostomy
Tubes
  empyema, 230-231
    nursing management of, 234
    placement of, 233-234
  gastrostomy and jejunostomy
    advantages and disadvantages of, 225t
    leakage around, 226, 229-230
    nursing management of, 224, 226-230
    site selection for, 224, 226
    stabilization of, 226-229, 230t
    types of, 222-224
  percutaneous; *see* Percutaneous tubes
  percutaneous nephrostomy, 234-235
    nursing management of, 236-240
    obstruction of, 239
    patency of, 239
    placement procedures for, 235-236
    stabilization of, 237-239
Tumor necrosis factor-alpha, 303
Tzanck smear, 22

U

Ulcers
  arterial, 19, 165-191
    assessment of patient with, 171-180
    characteristics of, 172, 173t
    diagnostic tests in patients with, 174-180
    infection in, 186-188
    management of, 180-191
    multidisciplinary team necessary for, 182
    noninvasive for patients with, 174-179
    optimizing wound environment for, 186-189
    perfusion status of, 188-189
    physical examination of patient with, 172-174
    reduce or eliminate cause of, 181-186
    support for patient with, 189-190
    topical dressing algorithm for, 187t
    treatment of, 173t

Ulcers—cont'd
  arterial, venous, and neuropathic,
      comparison of, 173t
  definition of, *12*
  diabetic, 19-20
  greater trochanteric, closure of, 147
  ischemic; *see* Ulcers, arterial
  ischial, closure of, 145-147
  lower extremity, 164-204
    causes of, 165
  neuropathic, 192-193
    assessment of, 173t
    characteristics of, 173t
    multidisciplinary team necessary for,
        182
    treatment of, 173t
  pressure; *see* Pressure ulcers
  radiation, 25
  sacral, closure of, 147
  venous, 19, 195-204
    arterial disease and, 199
    assessment of, 173t
    characteristics of, 173t, 198-199
    cleansing, 202-203
    contributing factors to, 197-198
    control of underlying medical and
        nutritional disorders in, 200
    diagnosis of, 198-200
    elevation of legs and, 199, 200
    fibrin cuff theory for, 196-197
    history and physical examination for,
        198-199
    management of, 200-204
    pathophysiology of, 195-197
    surgical options for, 204
    topical therapy for, 202-204
    treatment of, 173t
Ultrasonic Doppler waveforms, 176-177
Ultrasonography, Doppler, 199
Ultraviolet radiation, exposure of skin to, 9
Undermining, 80-81
Unna boot, venous ulcers treated with,
    201-202

V

Vasodilators, peripheral vascular disease
    treated with, 185
Venography, 179
  contrast, 200
  radionuclide, 199-200
Venous system, anatomy of, 195
Vesicle, definition of, *11*
Visceral proteins, blood levels of,
    nutritional status evaluated by, 293

Vitamin A
  corticosteroids and, 43, 45
  wound healing and, 43
Vitamin C, wound healing and, 43
Vitamin D, synthesis of, in skin, 7
Vitamins, deficiency in, pressure ulcer
    formation and, 115

W

WAI; *see* Wound assessment inventory
Water-filled overlays, 130-131
Waveforms, ultrasonic Doppler, 176-177
WCI; *see* Wound characteristics
    instrument
Wheal, definition of, *11*
Winstrol; *see* Stanozolol
Witzel jejunostomy, summary of
    procedure for, 219t
Wound Assessment Inventory, 78, 99
Wound bed
  arterial ulcer, 172
  type of tissue in, 81
Wound characteristics instrument, wound
    healing evaluated using, 78-79
Wound cleansing, 50
Wound culture, indications for, 44
Wound development, prediction of, 71
Wound dressings, 49, 50-56
  absorption, 52t, 53
    clinical features of, 56
  for autolysis, 59
  biologic, 55
  combination, 53, 55
  epithelial resurfacing and, 97
  foam, 77
  for full-thickness wounds, 59-60
  gauze, 52t, 53
    clinical features of, 57
  gel, 52t, 53
    clinical features of, 58
  hydrocolloid wafer, 52t, 53
    clinical features of, 54
  nonadhesive semipermeable
      polyurethane foam, 52t, 53
    clinical features of, 55
  for partial-thickness wounds, 60
  primary, 96
  synthetic barrier, 52t, 53
    clinical features of, 58
  transparent adhesive, 51, 52t
    clinical features of, 54
Wound gauge, 76-77
Wound healing
  cellular events in, 302

Wound healing—cont'd
  clinical evaluation of, instruments for, 71t
  effect of tissue hypoxia on, 42
  electrical stimulation and, 308-311
  electrical waveforms applied to, 308-309
  factors affecting, 42-46
  full-thickness, 35-42
    defensive phase of, 36-38
    maturation phase of, 40-41
    proliferative phase of, 38-40
  growth factors in, 189, 303-308
  hyperbaric oxygenation for, 311-314
  key events and mediators in, 35t
  macroscopic indices of, 79-83
    documentation of, 84
  moist, 49
  new interventions for, evaluating clinical trials of, 314-316
  nutrients critical to, 43-44
  oxygen-to-volume requirements for, 94-95
  partial-thickness, 34-35
  physiology of, 32-42
  by primary intention, 33
  process of, 33-42
  progress of, assessment of, 78-79
  by secondary intention, 33
  stimulation of, growth factors for, 189
  systemic support for, 47-48
  by tertiary intention, 33
  types of, 33
Wound management
  diet in, 294
  evolving modalities for, 301-316
  molecular regulation in, 302-308
  principles of, 46-61
  topical preparations for, 55, 330-332
Wound molds, 77
Wound surface, moist, 49
Wounds
  access to, fistula pouch and, 266
  acute versus chronic, 41-42
  anatomic location of, 81
  assessment of, 49, 69-79
    accuracy of, 84-85
    frequency of, 84
    grading system for, 99
  causes of
    clues to, 13t
    elimination or reduction of, 46-47
  classification of, 33, 71-73
    according to color, 73

Wounds—cont'd
  classification of—cont'd
    according to tissue layers, 72-73
  clean nonproliferative, 81
  clinical evaluation of, instruments for, 70-71
  closed, assessment of, 78
  contraction of, 40
  dehiscence of, definition of, 250
  depth of, 33
    measuring, 75-76
  draining of, definition of, 250-251
  dressings for; *see* Wound dressings
  duration of, 83
  foreign bodies in, 83
  full-thickness, 33, 35
    topical therapy for, 56-57, 59-60
  full-thickness versus partial-thickness, 73
  infected, cleansing, 50
  in inflammatory phase, 81
  linear measurements of, 73-74, 75-77
  management of; *see* Wound management
  measurement of, 73-78, 98-100
    three-dimensional, 75-78
    two-dimensional, 73-75
  necrotic, cleansing, 50
  noninfected proliferating, cleansing, 50
  open
    assessment of, 78-79
    edge of, 82-83
  partial-thickness, 33, 34
    topical therapy for, 60
  partial-thickness versus full-thickness, 73
  photography of, 75
  pressure as cause of, 13-14
  in proliferative phase, 81
  protection of, from trauma and bacteria, 49
  shear force as cause of, 14-16
  size of, 79-80
  staging systems for, 72
  surgical; *see* Surgical wounds
  thermal insulation of, 49
  tracings of, 74-75
  vascular, grading system for, 80t

Z

Zinc
  deficiency of, venous ulceration and, 198
  wound healing and, 43